ECMO Specialist Training Manual

Third Edition

Editors

Billie Lou Short, M.D.
Lisa Williams, MHA, BSN, RNC-NIC

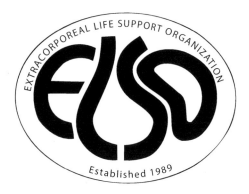

Senior Editor: Billie Lou Short, M.D.
Manuscript Editor: Lisa Williams, MHA, BSN, RNC-NIC
Layout and Production: Peter Rycus, MPH

List of Contributors

Robert H. Bartlett, MD
Professor of Surgery, Emeritus
University of Michigan
Ann Arbor, MI

Stephen Baumgart, MD
Professor of Pediatrics
Division of Neonatology
Children's National Medical Center
Washington, DC

John T. Berger, MD
Medical Director, Cardiac Intensive Care
Divisions of Critical Care Medicine & Cardiology
Children's National Medical Center
Washington, DC

Jeanne Braby, MSN, RN, CCRN
Unit Based Advanced Practice Nurse
Children's Hospital of Wisconsin
Milwaukee, WI

Dominick Carella, RN, MSN
ECMO Coordinator:
St. Christopher's Hospital for Children
Philadelphia, PA

Daniel Conway, MD
ECMO Medical Director:
St. Christopher's Hospital for Children
Philadelphia, PA

Elaine Cooley, RN, RRT
Sr. Clinical Specialist
University of Michigan
Ann Arbor, MI

Heidi J. Dalton MD, FCCM
Chief, Critical Care Medicine
Director, Pediatric/Cardiac ECMO
Phoenix Children's Hospital
Phoenix, AZ

Edward Darling, MS, CCP
Associate Professor/Staff Perfusionist
University Hospital
SUNY Upstate Medical University
Syracuse, NY

Joel Davis, RRT-NPS, AE-C
Advanced Technologies Specialist
Children's Healthcare of Atlanta
Atlanta, Georgia

Patricia English MS, RRT-NPS
ECMO Program Coordinator
Massachusetts General Hospital
Boston, Ma.

Ruth Ferroni, RN
Clinical Instructor, CICU
Children's National Medical Center
Washington, DC

Geoffrey M. Fleming MD
Division of Pediatric Critical Care
Vanderbilt University Medical Center
Nashville, TN

James D. Fortenberry MD
Pediatrician-In-Chief
Children's Healthcare of Atlanta
Associate Professor of Pediatrics
Chief, Critical Care Division and Pediatric ECMO
Emory University School of Medicine
Atlanta, GA

Penny Glass, PhD
Director, Neonatal Neurodevelopmental Clinic
Children's National Medical Center
Washington, DC

Barbara M. Haney, RNC-NIC, MSN, CPNP-AC
Clinical Nurse Specialist and ECMO Coordinator
Children's Mercy Hospitals & Clinics
Kansas City, MO

Daphne Hardison, RN BSN
Manager ECMO Services
Vanderbilt University Medical Center
Nashville, Tennessee

William E. Harris CCP, FPP
Chief Perfusionist, Department of Extracorporeal
Technology
Ochsner Medical Center
New Orleans, Louisiana

Micheal L. Heard, RN
Advanced Technologies Coordinator
Children's Healthcare of Atlanta
Atlanta, Georgia

Darren Klugman, MD, MMS
Departments of Critical Care Medicine & Cardiology
Children's National Medical Center
The George Washington University
Washington, DC

D. Scott Lawson, MPS, CCP
Chief Pediatric Perfusionist, ECMO Liaison
Duke Children's Hospital
Duke University
Durham, NC

Laurance Lequier MD, FRCPC
Director, ECLS Program
Stollery Children's Hospital
Edmonton, Alberta Canada

James E. Lynch, BS, RRT
ECMO Coordinator
Department of Women and Infants
University of Texas Medical Branch – Galveston
Galveston, Texas

William R. Lynch, MD
Director of ECMO Program
Director of Cardiothoracic Intensive Care Unit
University of Iowa Hospitals and Clinics
Iowa City, Iowa

M Patricia Massicotte MD. Msc, FRCPC, MHSc
Director, Vascular Patency and thrombosis Program
Stollery Children's Hospital
Edmonton, Alberta Canada

Sharad P. Menon MD
Cardiac Intensivist
Phoenix Children's Hospital
Phoenix, AZ

Matthew Moront, MD
ECMO Surgical Director:
St. Christopher's Hospital for Children
Philadelphia, PA

Eugenia K. Pallotto, MD
Assistant Professor of Pediatrics, University of
Missouri – Kansas City School of Medicine
Associate Medical Director, Neonatal Intensive
Care Unit, Medical Director, ECMO, Children's
Mercy Hospitals and Clinics
Kansas City, MO

Giles J Peek MD FRCS CTh
Consultant in Cardiothoracic Surgery & ECMO
Head of Service
East Midlands Congenital Heart Centre
Glenfield Hopsital
Leicester, UK

David Powell, MD
Division of Pediatric Surgery
Children's National Medical Center
Washington DC

K. Rais-Bahrami, MD
Division of Neonatology
Children's National Medical Center
Washington, DC

Nancy Rees, RN BSN
ECMO Coordinator
Children's Memorial Hermann Hospital
Houston, Texas

Jennifer Schuette, MD
Division of Critical Care Medicine
Children's National Medical Center
Assistant Professor of Pediatrics
George Washington School of Medicine
Washington, DC

Curt Shelley MEd RRT
ECMO Coordinator
Children's Memorial Hermann Hospital
Houston, Texas

Billie Lou Short, MD
Executive Director, ECMO Program
Chief, Division of Neonatology
Children's National Medical Center
Washington, DC

Christine Small, RN
ECMO Assistant Coordinator:
St. Christopher's Hospital for Children
Philadelphia, PA

Wolfgang Stehr, MD
Senior Fellow, Division of Pediatric Surgery
Children's National Medical Center,
Washington, DC

David C. Stockwell, MD MBA
Executive Director, Improvement Science
Medical Director, Patient Safety and the Pediatric
Intensive Care Unit
Assistant Professor of Pediatrics
Children's National Medical Center
Washington, DC

Jeffrey B. Sussmane MD
Medical Director ECLS
Critical Care Medicine
Miami Children's Hospital
Miami, Florida

John Waldvogel, RRT
Sr. Clinical Specialist
ECMO Program
University of Michigan
Ann Arbor, MI

Lisa Williams, MHA, BSN, RNC-NIC
ECMO Program Manager
Children's National Medical Center
Washington, DC

Edward Wong, MD
Associate Director, Transfusion Medicine
Children's National Medical Center
Washington, DC

Joseph B. Zwischenberger, MD
Johnston-Wright Professor and Chairman
Department of Surgery
University of Kentucky College of Medicine
Lexington, Kentucky

Preface to the 3rd Edition

It is a great pleasure to have participated in the creation of *the 3rd Edition of the ECMO Specialists Training Manual*. This edition is the product of many individuals representing 18 ECMO centers across the country. As Co-Editor of the first edition, it was amazing to see the changes that had occurred between that edition and the second. It's now been 10 years between the 2nd Edition and this 3rd Edition, with enormous changes in the patient populations treated, the equipment used, and clinical management protocols for ECLS support. To that end we have added 8 new chapters outlining physiology of the major categories of patients being treated (neonatal respiratory, pediatric respiratory, adult respiratory and cardiac patients of all ages). We have also added chapters on ECPR, hemofiltration, plasmapheresis, and two exciting chapters on case scenarios and trouble shooting for the ECMO Specialists.

Training of the bedside ECMO specialist remains a priority. This manual was developed to assist ECMO centers in the training and education of the ECMO team in their institution. To further assist in the education of ECMO practitioners, test questions and answers are at the end of each chapter. This manual should be used in conjunction with the existing educational material specific to the individual ECMO center. The material presented in this manual has been written by authors from various ECMO centers, but an attempt has been made to represent general ECMO practice. Techniques specific to a single institution may not be fully covered in this manual, thus requiring each institution to enhance those topics with additional information.

I would like to thank the many individuals who authored and reviewed chapters; it was a pleasure working with all of you. I would like to give a special thanks to my Co-Editors, Lisa Williams and Peter Rycus. If not for their continued support, the 3rd Edition would have been another 10 years in the making.

Billie Lou Short, MD
Chair, Logistics and Education Committee (2007-2009)
ELSO

Table of Contents

1

The History of Extracorporeal Life Support

Robert H Bartlett MD

The first neonatal ECMO survivor is 35 years old this year. In one medical generation the use of prolonged extracorporeal circulation for life support in the intensive care unit has gone from a laboratory curiosity to clinical trials to routine practice. Every major children's hospital has an ECLS program to sustain the life of patients with severe heart or lung failure when other treatments fail. Although the technology was first developed for the care of neonatal respiratory failure, growth and innovation are now primarily in the pediatric and adult intensive care units. In fact, the use of ECLS for neonatal respiratory failure is steadily decreasing as we develop a better understanding of the pathophysiology and better methods of prevention and treatment in the neonatal population. The same will apply to children and adults, as we learn more about pathpphysiology and treatment in those populations.

The heart/lung machine was developed primarily by surgeon John Gibbon, beginning in 1939 and culminating in the first successful heart operation using a heart-lung machine in 1954.[1] For cardiac surgery all the venous return is diverted into the machine and pumped into the systemic circulation, leaving the heart empty long enough to repair intracardiac defects or operate on the coronary circulation. The opportunity to operate directly on the heart was miraculous, but the heart-lung machine itself caused damage to the fluid and solid elements of the blood. In fact, the heart-lung machine caused fatal complications if it was used for more than 2 or 3 hours. The major cause of blood damage was the direct exposure of blood to gas. Interposing a plastic gas exchange membrane between the flowing blood and the gas solved most of the blood-damage problems. By eliminating the gas interface it was possible to use the heart-lung machine for days at

a time, and the physiology and pathophysiology of prolonged extracorporeal circulation was worked out in the laboratory.[2,3,4]

The first successful use of prolonged life support with a heart-lung machine was conducted by J. Donald Hill and his associates in 1971.[5] The patient was a young man suffering from the Adult Respiratory Distress Syndrome. (ARDS was the name applied to a new syndrome of severe respiratory failure complicating pneumonia, shock, trauma, or sepsis. Of course, ARDS had always existed, but was newly recognized and named. The entire discipline we now call Critical Care was evolving at the same time. The concept of chronic intubation and mechanical ventilation was only a decade old, and was itself considered a radical intervention of questionable value.) After Hill's case, several other successful cases were reported in children and adults with severe pulmonary and cardiac failure. At the same time there seemed to be an epidemic of "ARDS" and it looked like extracorporeal support would be the answer. A multi-center clinical trial of prolonged extracorporeal circulation for adults with ARDS was commissioned by the National Institutes of Health in 1975. This was the first prospective randomized trial of a life-support technique in acute fatal illness in which the end point was death. There were many problems with the design and execution of that clinical trial, For example there were 9 study centers, and only 3 of us had any experience with ECMO before entering the first patient. But from the trial we learned that the mortality for all patients with ARDS was 66%, and the mortality for severe ARDS was 90%. We learned that extracorporeal support attempted by inexperienced teams in veno arterial mode for one week, with continuing high ventilator settings did not improve the ultimate survival in severe ARDS. We learned (the hard way) the mistakes to avoid when conducting a prospective trial in acute fatal illness, and we developed a name for the technology: extracorporeal membrane oxygenation (ECMO). The results of that study were published in 1979;[6] laboratory and clinical research on ECLS in adults essentially stopped for a decade. This study is still quoted, but it is irrelevant to modern practice. However, the results in neonatal respiratory failure were very encouraging.

At the planning meeting for the adult NIH-ECMO trial in 1975 we reported the first successful case of ECLS for respiratory failure in a newborn infant.[7] Our laboratory had been studying membrane oxygenator development and prolonged extracorporeal circulation in animals for ten years. We and others had used extracorporeal support for postoperative cardiopulmonary failure in children with the first successful case in 1972.[8] White[9] and Dorson[10] had initiated clinical trials in neonatal respiratory failure without success. Our patient was a full-term neonate with respiratory failure secondary to meconium aspiration. The major cause of hypoxemia was pulmonary hypertension with right to left shunting through the ductus arteriosus and foramen ovale. This was mysterious at the time but we soon recognized that persistence of the fetal circulation physiology (persistent pulmonary hypertension of the newborn, PPHN) is the underlying pathophysiology for most causes of respiratory failure in full-term newborn infants. Using techniques of vascular access, anticoagulation, ventilator management, and extracorporeal circulation which had been developed in the laboratory, we used extracorporeal support for infants with a variety of conditions. Forty newborn patients were treated over the next five years with 50% survival.[11] Neonatologists and surgeons from other institutions joined us to learn the technology. By 1986 eighteen neonatal centers had successful ECMO teams.[12]

As with intubation and mechanical ventilation for newborn infants two decades before, the advent of this new technology met with skepticism and disdain among the relatively new field of neonatology. We conducted the first prospective randomized trial of ECMO in neonatal respiratory failure, using an adaptive design to correct some of the mistakes we had made in the earlier adult trial. After lengthy discussions, the report of this trial was published in *Pediatrics* in 1985,[13] along with invited commentaries criticizing the technology and the trial. This criticism and controversy lead to the second prospective randomized trial carried out by O'Rourke and associates at the Boston Children's Hospital.[14] A similar adaptive trial design was used by the Boston group with similar results (94% survival in the ECMO group). The Michigan trial was criticized for exposing critically ill infants to the high risks of ECMO. Two years later the Boston study was criticized for denying ECMO to the patients in the control group. Academic controversies aside, neonatologists realized that ECMO regularly resulted in high survival rates of happy, healthy children and ECMO became standard treatment for neonatal respiratory failure unresponsive to other measures.

In 1990 the National Institutes of Health held a workshop on the diffusion of high-tech medicine from bench to bedside using neonatal ECMO as an example.[15] Several factors were identified in the neonatal ECMO experience which facilitated the translation from concept to routine application. All aspects of the technology were thoroughly developed in the bench and animal laboratory before clinical trials. Clinical trials progressed through Phases I, II, and III with reporting and discussion at regular intervals but without sensational reports in the lay press. A registry of all cases in all centers was kept from the beginning of clinical application, which proved to be very valuable as the technology grew. The use of ECMO allowed study of patients who would have been dead without it. This unveiled many aspects of neonatal respiratory failure pathophysiology and treatment which in turn resulted in better understanding and the implementation of other simpler techniques. As the technology developed it was standardized, disseminated, studied, and improved in an organized fashion by the actual and potential users. This group of investigators and clinicians was formally organized as the Extracorporeal Life Support Organization in 1989. For the last 20 years that group has developed guidelines and practices, published the standard textbook in the field, and maintained a registry of ECLS cases. ELSO has followed and documented the growth of ECLS in other populations and other diseases. As of January 2010 there were over 40,000 patients in the registry, half of whom are newborn infants. Two other neonatal prospective randomized trials have been reported.[16,17] One of these is the large neonatal trial conducted in the United Kingdom.[17] The design of this trial solved almost all of the problems of prospective randomized trials in acute fatal illness. ECMO is currently used for neonates with respiratory failure unresponsive to other treatment. Overall survival is 85%, ranging from 98% in meconium aspiration to 55% in diaphragmatic hernia.

Based on the success with newborn infants several clinicians returned to children and adults with respiratory failure. Kolobow and colleagues showed that high ventilator inspiratory pressure (lung stretch) and high FiO_2 caused severe lung injury.[18] Gattinoni and Kolobow separated respiration from oxygenation by removing CO_2 by extracorporeal circulation (making ventilation unnecessary) and oxygenating by insufflation. Using extracorporeal CO_2 removal they prevented stretch injury, and reported 56% survival in severe ARDS.[19] These observations led to renewed interest in ECLS for adult respiratory failure. By the 1990s several groups reported similar results.[20,21,22]

Adult Respiratory Failure

The overall mortality for ARDS is 30-40% even with excellent management. ECLS is indicated for those patients who have a high mortality risk within the first week after intubation. These patients have an Aa gradient for oxygen greater than 600 on day 2, 3 or 4 following initial intubation. The mortality risk for those patients is approximately 80% and the recovery rate with ECLS in those patients is approximately 70%.[23,24] Patients on the ventilator more than 5 days pre-ECLS have less chance of recovery, hence the overall survival rate for ECLS treatment of ARDS is approximately 55%. The University of Michigan has reported the largest experience with ECLS for ARDS. In that series the overall survival rate was 52% and 65% since 2002,[25] The series is large enough to characterize the patient population and identify the likelihood of recovery based on age and days on mechanical ventilation. The ELSO registry data on adult respiratotry was reported by Brogan in 2009.[26]

The UK ECMO team in Leicester conducted a prospective randomized trial of ECMO compared to conventional ventilation in ARDS, using the format design used in the definitive neonatal study. The results of this trail (the CESAR trial) were reported in 2009.[27] Survival in patients randomized to conventional treatment was 47% compared to 63% in the patients randomized to Leicester protocol including ECMO.

Pediatric Respiratory Failure

In 1991 the Pediatric Critical Care study group and ELSO conducted a study of 679 pediatric respiratory failure patients in 32 PICUs The overall mortality was 40%. Multivariate regression analysis identified ECMO as the only treatment which had a favorable effect on outcome.[28] Green did a matched pairs study using that database comparing survival in 55 ECMO patients (74%) to survival in110 matched patients managed with conventional ventilation(53%).[29]

Severe respiratory failure in older children is relatively rare, compared to the incidence in newborn infants and adults. The most common cause is viral or bacterial pneumonia. Status asthmaticus is another life-threatening problem in children. ECLS is used when a patient is not responding to other methods of management. The survival rate is approximately 75%, varying to some extent with the primary condition. Most children with respiratory failure can be managed successfully with veno venous access. In children who do not survive, the most common cause of death is progressive lung destruction from the primary infection, or brain damage from the period of hypoxia and ischemia which preceded ECLS. These children are all essentially are normal in followup. Once the lung recovers, pulmonary function and exercise tolerance returns to normal.

Cardiac Failure

ECMO in the venoarterial mode supports function of both the lung and heart. ECMO has been used for cardiac failure since 1972, but that application has grown rapidly in the last decade, primarily in pediatric patients. The reason is that ECMO is the only system (in the US) which can replace cardiac function in children, bridging to recovery, or perhaps transplantation. In adult patients ECMO is routinely used in cardiogenic shock and cardiac arrest, and allows time for evaluation, implantation of a ventricular assist device if indicated, and eventually transplantation.

A new generation of membrane lungs, safe centrifugal pumps, and vasculat access reached the US in 2008. These devices make ECMO safe and simple enough to be managed by the regular ICU staff. This approach (we call ECMOII) has the potential to expand ECMO throughout the hospital for many new applications. ECMO has been possible because of the development of a new specialty: the ECMO technical specialist. Health care professionals from nursing, respiratory therapy, and perfusion have gained the unique knowledge and skills to understand and manage all aspects of prolonged extracorporeal technology. The ECMO specialist has major independent responsibility for the circuit and for care of the patient. A typical protocol order set might be," Adjust the circuit flow and pressure, diuretics, transfusion of blood components, sedation, and ventilator settings to maintain optimal life support". This manual outlines the requirements for an ECMO team, specialist training and qualifications, and details of ECMO management.

References

1. Gibbon JH: Application of a mechanical heart and lung apparatus to cardiac surgery. Minn Med 37:171, 1954.
2. Kolobow T, Zapol W, Pierce J: High survival and minimal blood damage in lambs exposed to long term (1 week) veno-venous pumping with a polyurethane chamber roller pump with and without a membrane blood oxygenator. ASAIO Trans 15:172-177, 1969.
3. Bartlett RH, Fong SW, Burns NE et al: Prolonged partial venoarterial bypass: Physiologic, biochemical and hematologic responses. Ann Surg 180:850-856, 1974.
4. Fong SW, Burns NE, Williams G et al: Changes in coagulation and platelet function during prolonged extracorporeal circulation (ECC) in sheep and man. Trans Am Soc Artif Intern Organs 20:239-246, 1974.
5. Hill JD, O'Brien TG, Murray JJ, et al: Extracorporeal oxygenation for acute post-traumatic respiratory failure (shock-lung syndrome): Use of the Bramson Membrane Lung. N Engl J Med 286:629-634, 1972.
6. Zapol WM, Snider MT, Hill JD et al: Extracorporeal membrane oxygenation in severe acute respiratory failure: A randomized prospective study. JAMA 242:2193-2196, 1979.
7. Bartlett RH, Gazzaniga AB, Jefferies R et al: Extracorporeal membrane oxygenation (ECMO) cardiopulmonary support in infancy. Trans Am Soc Artif Intern Organs 22:80-88, 1976.
8. Bartlett RH, Gazzaniga AB, Fong SW et al: Prolonged extracorporeal cardiopulmonary support in man. J Thorac Cardiovasc Surg 68:918-932, 1974.
9. White JJ, Andrews HG, Risemberg H, et al: Prolonged respiratory support in newborn infants with a membrane oxygenator. Surgery 70:288-296, 1971.
10. Dorson WJ, Baker E, Cohen ML, et al: A perfusion system for infants. ASAIO Trans 15:155, 1969.
11. Bartlett RH, Andrews AF, Toomasian JM et al: Extracorporeal membrane oxygenation (ECMO) for newborn respiratory failure: 45 cases. Surgery 92:425-433, 1982.
12. Toomasian JM, Snedecor SM, Cornell R, et al: National experience with extracorporeal membrane oxygenation (ECMO) for newborn respiratory failure: Data from 715 cases. ASAIO Trans 34:140-147, 1988.
13. Bartlett RH, Roloff DW, Cornell RG et al: Extracorporeal circulation in neonatal respiratory failure: A prospective randomized study. Ped 4:479-487, 1985.
14. O'Rourke PP, Krone R, Vacanti J, et al: Extracorporeal membrane oxygenation and conventional medical therapy in neonates with persistent pulmonary hypertension of the newborn: A prospective randomized study. Pediatrics 84:957-963, 1989.
15. Wright L, ed: Report of the workshop on diffusion of ECMO Technology. NIH Pub. #93-3399, 1993.

16. Schumacher RE, Roloff DW, Chapman R, et al: Extracorporeal membrane oxygenation in term newborns. A prospective cost-benefit analysis. ASAIO J 39:873-879, 1993.

17. UK collaborative randomized trial of neonatal extracorporeal membrane oxygenation. UK Collaborative ECMO Trial Group. Lancet 348(9020):75-82, 1996.

18. Kolobow T: On how to injure healthy lungs (and prevent sick lungs from recovering). ASAIO Trans 34:31-34, 1988.

19. Gattinoni L, Pesenti A, Mascheroni D, et al. Low frequency positive pressure ventilation with extracorporeal CO_2 removal in severe acute respiratory failure. JAMA 1986;256:881-886.

20. Lewandowski K, Rossaint R, Pappert D, Gerlach H, et al: High survival rate in 122 ARDS patients managed according to a clinical algorithm including extracorporeal membrane oxygenation. Intensive Care Med 23:819-835, 1997.

21. Ullrich R, Larber C, Roder G, et al. Controlled airway pressure therapy, nitric oxide inhalation, prime position, and ECMO as components of an integrated approach to ARDS. Anesthesiology 1999; 91:1577-1586.

22. Kolla S, Awad SA, Rich PB, Schreiner RJ, Hirschl RB, Bartlett RH: Extracorporeal life support for 100 adult patients with severe respiratory failure. Ann Surg 226:544-566, 1997.

23. Peek GJ, Moore HM, Sosnowski AW, et al: Extracorporeal membrane oxygenation for adult respiratory failure. Chest 112:759-764, 1997.

24. Linden V, Palmer K, Reinhard J, et al: High survival in adult patients with acute respiratory distress syndrome treated by extracorporeal membrane oxygenation, minimal sedation, and pressure supported ventilation. Intensive Care Med 26:1630-1637, 2000.

25. Hemmila MR, Rowe SA, Boules TN, Miskulin J, McGillicuddy JW, Schuerer DJ, Haft JW, Swaniker FC, Arbabi S, Hirschl RB, Bartlett RH: Extracorporeal Life Support for Severe Acute Respiratory Syndrome in Adults. Annals of Surgery 240(4), 2004.

26. Brogan TV, Thiagarajan RR, Rycus PT, Bartlett RH, Bratton SL. Extracorporeal membrane oxygenation in adults with severe respiratory failure: a multi-center database. Intensive Care Med 2009.

27. Peek GJ, Mugford M, Tiruvoipati R, et al. Efficacy and economic assessment of conventional ventilatory support versus extracorporeal membrane oxygenation for severe adult respiratory failure (CESAR): a multicentre randomised controlled trial. Lancet 2009

28. Timmons OD, Havens PL, Fackler JC. Predicting death in pediatric patients with acute respiratory failure. Pediatric Critical Care Study Group. Extracorporeal Life Support Organization. Chest 1995 September;108(3):789-97.

29. Green TP, Timmons OD, Fackler JC, Moler FW, Thompson AE, Sweeney MF. The impact of extracorporeal membrane oxygenation on survival in pediatric patients with acute respiratory failure. Pediatric Critical Care Study Group. Crit Care Med 1996 February;24(2):323-9.

2

Neonatal Pulmonary Physiology and Pathophysiology

Billie L. Short, MD

Objectives

After completion of this chapter, the participant should be able to:

- Discuss the common pathophysiology of neonatal diseases treated with ECMO
- Discuss the outcome of these patient populations when treated with ECMO
- Outline the risk factors related to ECMO therapy and each disease state

Introduction

Patients who require ECMO therapy in the newborn period may have several disease states and/or pathophysiologic entities.[1] Pulmonary hypertension may be a secondary process in many of the diseases. The near-term infant (34-36 weeks gestation) may present with hyaline membrane disease, but also have underlying pulmonary hypertension or sepsis/pneumonia making their respiratory status very unstable. Meconium aspiration syndrome (MAS), sepsis/pneumonia in larger infants, congenital diaphragmatic hernia (CDH), and idiopathic pulmonary hypertension of the newborn (PPHN) are the most common disorders treated with ECMO.[1] The pathophysiologic states associated with these diseases are the primary focus of this chapter.

Development of Lung Maturity

Surfactant is secreted by type II alveolar cells in the lungs. It is composed of several phospholipids which lower the surface tension forces of alveolar walls.[2] This is important for the initial opening of the alveoli and prevention of subsequent atelectasis.

Diseases Which Accelerate Fetal Lung Maturity:

Maternal
Toxemia
Hypertensive renal disease
Hypertensive cardiovascular disease
Sickle cell anemia
Narcotic addiction
Diabetes group D, E, or F

Fetal
Premature rupture of membranes
Growth retardation

Diseases Which Delay Fetal Lung Maturity:

Maternal
Diabetes group A, B, or C
Chronic glomerulonephritis

Fetal
Hydrops fetalis
Smaller of identical twins

The lack of this substance is the pathophysiologic basis of hyaline membrane disease (HMD), which is characterized by massive atelectasis. The major constituent of surfactant is lecithin. It comprises 50-75% of all the phospholipids. It first appears in significant quantities at 22-24 weeks gestation and continues to increase with gestation. By 35 weeks the ratio of lecithin to sphingomyelin is 2:1 which signifies pulmonary maturity. The presence of another phospholipid, phosphatidyl glycerol (PG), is also an indicator of pulmonary maturity.

Fetal Circulation

The fetal circulation is characterized by the following:
- Presence of anatomical shunts
  - *Foramen Ovale*
  - *Ductus Arteriosus*
  - *Ductus Venosus*
- Presence of the placental circulation (50% of the Cardiac output)
- Minimal blood flow through the lungs (7-10%) secondary to the high pulmonary vascular resistance

In the fetus, blood is oxygenated in the chorionic villi in the placenta, leaves through the umbilical vein, and then crosses between the right and left lobes of the liver. Some blood will perfuse the liver, but most is emptied into the inferior vena cava via the ductus venosus, which empties into the right atrium. The major portion of blood flow from the inferior vena cava empties into the left atrium through the foramen ovale. The remaining volume along with the blood from the superior vena cava is pumped into the right ventricle and then into the pulmonary artery where the majority shunts through the ductus arteriosus into the aorta. The blood which perfuses the pulmonary system (7-10%) returns to the left atrium where mixing of the shunted and the

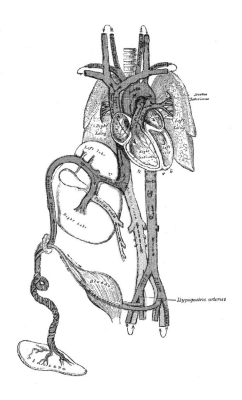

Figure 1: fetal circulation diagram from Wikimedia Commons, originally from 20th U.S. edition of Gray's Anatomy of the Human Body, originally published in 1918 (not copyrightable). Fetal shunts at the foramen ovale and patent ductus arteriosus remain open postnatally in cases where stress occurs at birth resulting in the persistent pulmonary hypertension of the newborn (PPHN), a syndrome that can be idiopathic or associated with other disease states.

Fetal Lung -Vasoactive Mediators	
Vasodilators	**Vasoconstrictors**
– Nitric Oxide	– Endothelin-1
– Prostacyclin	– Platelet-activating factor
– Estrogen	– Leukotrienes
– Adenosine	– Thromboxane

circulated blood occurs. This blood is then pumped into the left ventricle and to the aorta. The descending aorta bifurcates into the right and left iliac arteries. Two arteries branch from these and course upward around the bladder and form the umbilical arteries, which go back to the placenta.

Control of the fetal pulmonary circulation is modulated by several agents. The most important vasodilators are nitric oxide and prostacyclin, while endothelin-1 and platelet activating factor are the predominant vasoconstrictors, with leukotrienes and thromboxane playing a secondary role.[3-10]

Neonatal Diseases Treated with ECMO

Introduction

The most common diseases treated with ECMO as discussed before are depicted in Figure 2 below. With the advent of new therapies such as surfactant, high frequency ventilation, and inhaled nitric oxide, the number of patients requiring ECMO has decreased. A disease such as HMD in the near-term infant is rarely referred for ECMO secondary to the availability of these therapies.[1]

Hyaline Membrane Disease

Hyaline membrane disease is characterized by a lack of surfactant, causing alveolar atelectasis which results in hypoxia.[11] In term infants surfactant production may be turned off by acidosis or hypoxia. The steps leading to hyaline membrane disease are:

- Lack of surfactant or decreased production of surfactant
- Increased work of breathing tires the infant and leads to further atelectasis due to decreased chest wall movement
- Pulmonary hypoperfusion leads to hypoxia and hypercapnia
- Hypoxia leads to anaerobic glycolysis (glucose from glycogen) which produces the by-product, lactic acid, which in turn causes metabolic acidosis (decreased pH and increased BE)
- CO_2 is not blown off due to atelectasis causing hypercapnia and respiratory acidosis (decreased pH and increased pCO_2)
- Hypoxia and acidosis cause vascular spasm resulting in increased pulmonary hypoperfusion. This can cause capillary damage and alveolar necrosis, resulting in subsequent

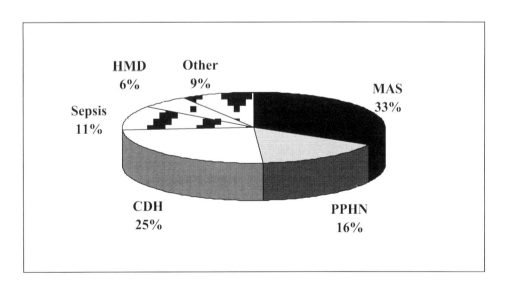

Figure 2. Neonatal respiratory diseases treated with ECMO with percent of ECMO population. Data from Extracorporeal Life Support Organization database, July 2009

decreases in surfactant production and escalation of atelectasis

- Increased vascular resistance (seen more often in term infants) results in right to left shunting through the foramen ovale and/or ductus arteriosus

Primary surfactant deficiency results in this sequence of events and can be linked to the inability to establish alveolar stability.[2] This may occur in utero, secondary to intrauterine asphyxia. The asphyxia would cause pulmonary vasoconstriction, leading to ischemia which damages the alveolar walls and impairs surfactant production. Lung compliance (C_L) is a function of the elasticity of lung tissue and is therefore decreased in HMD. C_L expresses the capacity of the lung to increase in volume in response to a given amount of applied pressure during inspiration ($C_L = V/P$). In HMD far greater pressure is required for expansion of lungs compared to normal lungs. Normal values range from 1 to 4 cc/cmH$_2$O/kg, with levels 1/4 to 1/5 of this seen in HMD and a resultant increased work of breathing. Continuous positive airway pressure (CPAP) therapy helps to open alveoli and decrease atelectasis and thus decreases the work of breathing, increasing lung compliance and oxygenation.

Predisposing factors to HMD:

- Prematurity
- Perinatal asphyxia
- Maternal diabetes (A,B,C)
- History of sibling with HMD
- Second of twins
- Cesarean section without labor
- Male sex

The risks can be decreased by the following:
- Glucocorticoid administration to the mother 24 to 48 hours before birth
- Maternal toxemia
- Premature or prolonged rupture of the membranes
- Lecithin/sphingomyelin ratio of more than 2:1 or presence of phosphatidyl glycerol

Management of HMD:

Artificial and/or calf/pig lung surfactants are now used to treat infants at risk for developing HMD or those exhibiting symptoms of HMD.[11] To date there is no "quick test" to determine if an infant is surfactant deficient, therefore, clinicians must use clinical symptoms and x-ray findings to determine whether surfactant should be given. Infants requiring intubation and an FIO$_2$ greater than 40, should be considered for surfactant therapy.

Infants with HMD who are requiring an FIO$_2$ greater than .50 should be considered for nasal CPAP (continuous positive airway pressure) or high-flow nasal cannula. These therapies help to recruit collapsed alveoli, while keeping other alveoli from collapsing, thus allowing time for natural production of surfactant to occur. If ventilation is a problem, i.e., increasing PaCO$_2$'s, then intubation should be considered. Ventilator strategies should include use of PEEP (positive end expiratory pressure) with IMV (intermittent mandatory ventilation). Peak pressures should be kept as low as possible to decrease the risk of lung injury. Longer inspiratory times ($T_I > .5$ sec) can help recruit alveoli. High frequency oscillatory ventilation (HFOV) is also useful in this population. Patient blood gases and pH should be kept between pH 7.28-7.38, PaCO$_2$ 45-50 mmHg, PaO$_2$ 50-65 mmHg. Oxygen and ventilator therapy both play a role in the development of bronchopulmonary dysplasia (BPD), and therefore infants should be weaned aggressively from these therapies.[12]

Long-term Complications:

BPD is characterized by thickening and eventual necrosis of alveolar walls, basement membranes, and bronchiolar epithelial lining layers.[12] Atelectasis and fibrosis are present and diffusion of oxygen is impaired. 5-30% of patients with BPD will die of infection or cor pulmonale.

Retinopathy of prematurity (ROP) is related to hyperoxemia and/or large swings in oxygenation in the premature. Decreasing gestational age increases the risk for ROP. There are many factors other than hyperoxia which may play a role in its development, i.e., hypotension, acidosis. The disease is characterized by changes in the retinal vasculature that may destroy the normal architecture of the eye, resulting in blindness. In the severe stages retinal detachment can occur.

Meconium Aspiration Syndrome (MAS)

The passage of meconium can occur before birth secondary to acute or chronic hypoxia or stress.[13-17] Infants can aspirate meconium in utero or at the time of delivery when the first breath occurs. The majority of meconium aspiration is mild, but when severe, the patient can exhibit marked respiratory distress resulting from the obstructive nature of the disease. Two forms of lung pathology can occur: (1) emphysema resulting from ball-valving with partial obstruction; and (2) atelectasis resulting from total obstruction (see Figure 2). Both processes are usually present and thus make the management of these infants very difficult.

Meconium can be present in over 10% of deliveries, and should be considered a sign of fetal distress. The infant may do well initially, but then deteriorate as the particles penetrate the peripheral airways. Persistent pulmonary hypertension may be a major component in the pathophysiology of this disease. Air leaks are very common.

Maternal Factors Causing Risk for MAS:

- Toxemia
- Hypertension
- Heavy smoker

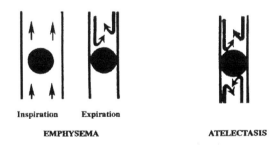

Figure 2. MAS pathophysiology noted with partial or total obstruction of airflow (from CNMC ECMO Training Manual with permission)

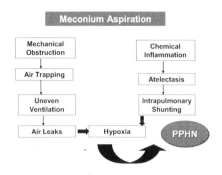

Figure 3. Pathophysiology of severe MAS (from CNMC ECMO manual with permission)

- Chronic respiratory or cardiac disease
- Poor nutrition
- Beyond 42 weeks gestation

Figure 3 shows the mechanisms for lung injury in MAS with mechanical obstruction combined with chemical inflammation resulting in severe hypoxia which in turn can cause the pulmonary vascular resistance to increase and open the fetal shunts resulting in PPHN. This combination is why this population is one of the largest treated with ECMO.

Treatment of MAS:

Although the majority of infants with MAS have mild disease, those who have thick meconium at delivery are at risk for developing the cascade effect noted in the above figure. Attempts at gentle ventilation with lower peak pressures is optimal, and use of iNO for treatment of PPHN is common.[1,14] Their response to high frequency ventilation is variable but should be tried prior to ECMO. Meconium itself and high ventilation appear to turn off surfactant production. Studies have shown that early use of surfactant may improve outcome and reduce the need for ECMO, but it should not be used after they are meeting ECMO criteria.

Persistent Pulmonary Hypertension (PPHN):

Pulmonary hypertension can return or remain high because of perinatal stress such as hypoxia, acidosis, hypotension, and other causes.[1,18,19] If this occurs, as it can with diseases such as MAS, then the infant can continue to shunt right to left through the fetal shunts and remain hypoxic on this basis, creating a vicious cycle. The presence of PPHN with other diseases can make management extremely difficult.

Causes of PPHN:

- Prenatal hypertrophy of muscular layers in the pulmonary arterioles
- Primary failure of the pulmonary artery to relax
- Vasospasm and constriction secondary to hypoxia or acidosis
- Polycythemia, hypocalcemia, and hypoglycemia
- Specific mediators may be through the nitric oxide, prostaglandin, endothelin, and/or leukotriene pathways

PPHN is characterized by:

- Right to left shunts through the patent ductus arteriosus and/or PFO secondary to pulmonary hypertension
- Mixing of oxygenated and unoxygenated blood in the aorta and/or left atrium

  o With a ductal shunt, only blood which is before the entrance of the PDA (preductal) represents oxygenated blood from the lungs, i.e., right radial and temporal artery blood.

  o A difference of 15 torr or greater in the pre- and postductal blood gases agrees with a right to left shunt at the ductal level

  o Shunts only at the PFO, and not the PDA, will not show any difference in pre- and postductal blood gas values because the mixing of oxygenated and unoxygenated blood occurs in the left atrium

Diagnosis of PPHN:

Doppler ultrasound will diagnose directional shunts at both the PDA and PFO. Clinical diagnosis is by the pre- and post ductal blood gas differences for a PDA shunt, and the infant who responds to the hyperventilation-hyperoxia test. Also a presumptive diagnosis can be made in the infant who shows the "flip-flop" phenomenon (acute drop in PaO_2 with small changes in ventilation or stimulation of the infant).

Treatment of PPHN:

- Prevention of hypoxemia; recent data also shows that hyperoxia may cause vasoconstriction so PaO_2 >100mmHg should be avoided
- Rapid correction of acidosis
- Correction of polycythemia by partial exchange transfusion (Hct >65)
- Correction of hypocalcemia, etc.
- Gentle ventilation without hyperventilation is now recommended to reduce lung injury in these infants
- Sedation as needed, try to avoid chemical paralysis
- Inhaled nitric oxide (iNO) - has been shown to keep about 40% of patients off ECMO.[20-22]
- Systemic blood pressure should be maintained, with hypotension treated as per normal protocols
- Milrinone has been used, but studies showing the efficacy have not been done. Hypotension can be a side effect
- Ventilator support including conventional ventilation and HFOV. Ventilator changes should be minimal during the first 1 to 2 days with only one parameter changed at a time, i.e., IMV or FiO_2, but not both

Congenital Diaphragmatic Hernia (CDH)

Congenital herniation of the abdominal contents into the thoracic cavity causes serious respiratory compromise. Herniation occurs most often on the left side and represents a failure of the pleuroperitoneal canal to close completely during fetal development. CDH usually involves thoracic entry of the stomach, a large part of the intestines, and occasionally the spleen and liver. These organs displace the heart and lungs, compromising cardiac output and pulmonary gas exchange. The lung on the affected side is hypoplastic, with varying degrees of hypoplasia on the contralateral side.

Clinically, CDH most often presents as severe respiratory distress in a newborn infant. The physical examination is remarkable for a cyanotic and dyspneic infant with a scaphoid abdomen. If a significant portion of the intestines has herniated, bowel sounds may be audible over the affected side of the thoracic cavity. The diagnosis is usually made on x-ray (Figure 4).

Treatment of CDH

- Proper resuscitation of the newborn in respiratory distress
- Gastric decompression with low continuous suction immediately if diagnosis is considered
- Infant should be positioned with head and thorax higher than the abdomen to facilitate downward displacement of the hernia contents

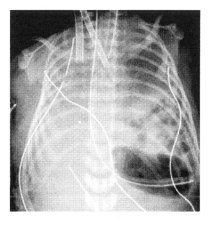

Figure 4. Left CDH noted on x-ray with bowel in left chest. Infant is already on venoarterial ECMO, note ECMO cannula in place

- After stabilization and attempts to correct the acid-base status, the infant should be evaluated for surgery. If the patient is unstable, then ECMO should be considered pre-surgery. Many centers utilize ECMO to stabilize these infants and delay repair until the PPHN has resolved.
- Ventilator management should be as with PPHN although iNO therapy pre-ECMO has not been shown to keep patients off ECMO. It may stabilize them for transport to an ECMO center but the improvement is usually short-term.[24]

PPHN is often associated with infants who are born with CDH.[23] The etiology of PPHN in infants with CDH may be secondary to the hypoxemia caused by the hypoplastic lung, but it has also been noted that the pulmonary artery and branches are structurally abnormal with thickened muscular walls.

Infants with a PaO_2 < 60 mmHg after optimal stabilization, should be considered for ECMO therapy prior to repair. Two approaches to repair exists: one is to repair on ECMO after the infant has shown he/she can be successfully removed from ECMO by idling 8 hours at 10% bypass flows with adequate PaO_2's and $PaCO_2$'s and the second method is to wean the infant off ECMO and repair the patient within 24-48 hours after coming off ECMO. The surgeon and the neonatologist will work together to determine which approach is appropriate.

What to Remember When on ECMO

Infants with HMD are usually premature infants, may be septic and/or have pneumonia. Their risk on ECMO include a higher rate of intraventricular hemorrhage (IVH), 20-40% verses 12% in term infants. Heparinization for these infants should be adjusted for bleeding risk. Any change in neurologic status should raise concern for IVH complication.

Infants with a primary diagnosis of PPHN, or others with PPHN complicating their disease process, may be on iNO when placed on ECMO. It should be remembered that nitric oxide alters platelet function and can be a bleeding risk. In our institution, infants are weaned off iNO quickly after being placed on ECMO. Venoarterial ECMO patients should have no complications from a fast wean while venovenous patients may need to wean slower. No data exist on the type of wean you should attempt.

The infant with CDH is the most challenging of the neonatal cases. If repaired pre-ECMO or on-ECMO you will probably encounter bleeding complications. If 6-12 hours delay can be achieved after repair prior to placing an infant on ECMO, the bleeding risks are less. If surgery is done on ECMO then most centers decrease their heparinization with ACT levels as low as 150-170 seconds depending on the type of ACT monitor you have; increased platelet parameters to >150,000; and may start Amicar to reduce breakdown of fibrin/clot formation. When surgery is done on ECMO, bleeding during the surgery is not usually a problem unless major organs such as the liver or spleen are cut. If the infant can be taken off ECMO within 48 hours of surgery, bleeding complications are less. Many centers are now taking the patient off ECMO and then doing the repair several days after ECMO when the vascular resistance is stable. The CDH patient runs can be long, and therefore the circuit integrity needs to be assessed. We change the circuit when increasing fibrin is seen in the circuit, any clot formation on the arterial side, or when the circuit is 10 days of age (raceway integrity concerns). It is not unusual to have to change a circuit on a CDH patient due to increasing fibrin formation.

References

1. Farrow KN, Fliman P, Steinhorn RH, The Diseases Treated with ECMO: Focus on PPHN, Seminars in Perinatology, 29(1) 2005, 8-14.

2. Jobe AH, Lung development and maturation, In, *Neonatal-Perinatal Medicine: Diseases of the fetus and infant*, 8th Edition, Editors: Martin RJ, Fanaroff AA, Walsh MC, Mosby, 2006.

3. Abman SH, Chatfield BA, Hall SL, McMurtry IF: Role of endothelium-derived relaxing factor during transition of pulmonary circulation at birth. Am J Physiol 259:H1921-H1927, 1990

4. Brannon TS, North AJ, Wells LB, Shaul PW: Prostacyclin synthesis in ovine pulmonary artery is developmentally regulated by changes in cyclooxygenase-1 gene expression. J Clin Invest 93:2230-2235, 1994

8. Leffler CW, Hessler JR, Green RS: The onset of breathing at birth stimulates pulmonary vascular prostacyclin synthesis. Pediatr Res 18:938-942, 1984

9. Teitel D, Iwamoto H, Rudolph A: Changes in the pulmonary circulation during birth-related events. Pediatr Res 27:372-378, 1990

10. Steinhorn RH, Morin FC, 3rd, Van Wylen DG, et al: Endothelium-dependent relaxations to adenosine in juvenile rabbit pulmonary arteries and veins. Am J Physiol 266:H2001-H2006, 1994

11. Rodriguez RJ, Martin RJ, Fanaroff AA, Respiratory distress syndrome and its management, In, *Neonatal-Perinatal Medicine: Diseases of the fetus and infant*, 8th Edition, Editors: Martin RJ, Fanaroff AA, Walsh MC, Mosby, 2006.

12. Bancalari, E, Changes in the pathogenesis and prevention of chronic lung disease of prematurity, Aberican J of Perinatol, 18 (1): 1-9, 2001.

13. Gelfand SL, Fanaroff JM, Walsh MC. Controversies in the treatment of meconium aspiration syndrome. Clin Perinatol 31(3):445-452, 2004

14. Wiswell TE: Advances in the treatment of the meconium aspiration syndrome. Acta Paediatr Suppl 436:28-30, 2001

15. Davey AM, Becker JD, Davis JM: Meconium aspiration syndrome: physiological and inflammatory changes in a newborn piglet model. Pediatr Pulmonol 16(2):101-108, 199324.

16. Soukka H, Viinikka L, Kaapa P: Involvement of thromboxane A2 and prostacyclin in the early pulmonary hypertension after porcine meconium aspiration. Pediatr Res 44(6):838-842, 1998
17. Dargaville PA, South M, McDougall PN: Surfactant and surfactant inhibitors in meconium aspiration syndrome. J Pediatr 138:113-115, 2001
18. Murphy JD, Rabinovitch M, Goldstein JD, Reid LM: The structural basis of persistent pulmonary hypertension of the newborn infant. J Pediatr 1 98(6):962-967, 1981
19. Haworth SG. Pulmonary vascular remodeling in neonatal pulmonary hypertension. Chest 93:133S-138S, 1988.
20. Lotze A, Mitchell BR, Bulas DI, et al: Multi-center study of surfactant (beractant) use in the treatment of term infants with severe respiratory failure. Survanta in Term Infants Study Group. J Pediatr 132:40-137, 1998
21. Clark RH, Kueser TJ, Walker MW, et al: Low dose nitric oxide therapy for persistent pulmonary hypertension of the newborn. N Engl J Med 342:469-74, 2000
22. Neonatal Inhaled Nitric Oxide Study Group: Inhaled nitric oxide in full-term and nearly full-term infants with hypoxic respiratory failure. New Engl J Med 336:597-604, 1997
23. Doyle NM, Lally KP: The CDH Study Group and advances in the clinical care of the patient with congenital diaphragmatic hernia. Semin Perinatol 23:174-84, 2004
24. Neonatal Inhaled Nitric Oxide Study Group: Inhaled nitric oxide and hypoxic respiratory failure in infants with congenital diaphragmatic hernia. Pediatrics 99:838-845, 1997

Chapter 2 Questions

1. The three shunts in the fetal circulation which allow oxygenated blood to flow to the heart and brain are:
   a) placenta, kidney, lung
   b) ductus venosus, foramen ovale, ductus arteriosus
   c) IVC, SVC, ductus venosus
   d) ductus arteriosus, SVC, ductus venosus

2. Infants with persistent pulmonary hypertension (PPHN) have:
   a) elevated pulmonary vascular resistance
   b) shunting right-to-left through the foramen ovale and patent ductus arteriosus (PDA)
   c) hypoxemia
   d) all of the above

3. Which of the following does not decrease pulmonary vascular resistance?
   a) arterial oxygen (PaO2)
   b) nitric oxide (NO)
   c) rise in pH
   d) endothelin

Chapter 2 Answers
1. b
2. d
3. d

3

Pathophysiology of Pediatric Cardiac Disease relevant to ECMO

Darren Klugman, MD and John T. Berger, MD

Objectives

After completion of this chapter, the participant should be able to:

- Understand the common pathophysiology of pediatric cardiac diseases managed with extracorporeal support
- Understand how cardiac physiology dictates extracorporeal support strategies

Introduction

Congenital heart disease affects approximately 1% of all live newborns. The spectrum of disease is wide and heterogeneous in its presentation. While many of these children had limited options only 50 years ago, significant medical and surgical advances have been made since that time. The advent of cardiopulmonary bypass in the late 1950's offered a new set of opportunities to help children who were once without surgical options. Since those early operations, techniques have advanced and many patients undergo primary and complete repair as a neonate, including some patients who are premature.

Along with the advances in surgical technique and cardiopulmonary bypass, perioperative care has also advanced significantly. Advances include prenatal diagnosis by ultrasound, prostaglandin E_1 (PGE_1), nitric oxide (NO), and extracorporeal membrane oxygenation (ECMO). Total mortality for infants with congenital heart disease is currently less than five percent. Extracorporeal support now plays a vital role in the care of many children with congenital and acquired heart disease. Diseases like hypoplastic left heart syndrome were once

considered contraindications to ECMO, but now patients with this diagnosis are routinely placed on ECMO in some centers.[1] The use of ECMO support of the pediatric cardiac patient will be explored in this chapter. The manipulations and various applications in the use of ECMO will be related to the multiple physiologic manifestations of the cardiac lesions discussed. The pathophysiologic states to be discussed in this chapter include:

- Single ventricle physiology
- Total anomalous pulmonary venous drainage (TAPVD)
- Left sided obstructive disease (Pressure loaded LV)
- Left to right shunts (Volume loaded heart)
- Myocarditis
- Cardiomyopathy
- Heart transplant

Single Ventricle Physiology

The group, "single ventricle lesion" includes a diverse variety of congenital cardiac defects where there is only one ventricle capable of pumping blood to the systemic and pulmonary circulation (See Table 1). Additionally, unrepaired patients either have obstructed pulmonary or systemic blood flow, or unobstructed flows to both circulations. This physiology poses complex clinical challenges because these patients often respond differently to supplemental oxygen, mechanical ventilation, medications and ECMO as compared to patients with two normal ventricles. For example, patients with univentricle parallel circulation often require much higher ECMO flow to account for run off into pulmonary circulation. Finally, these patients are palliated in a staged fashion, and the physiology greatly changes after each stage of surgical repair.

Neonate With Univentricle, Parallel Circulation (Unrepaired or Palliated)

The single ventricle patient with obstruction to systemic blood flow usually has unobstructed blood flow to the pulmonary vascular bed. The amount of systemic blood flow is largely dependent on right to left flow at the patent ductus arteriosus and, to a lesser degree, by the amount of systemic outflow obstruction. The degree of right to left shunting at the ductus arteriosus is determined by the relative resistances of the systemic and pulmonary vascular beds. There is mixing of systemic and pulmonary venous return at the atrial level. Single ventricle patients with severe systemic outflow obstruction have "ductal dependent" systemic blood flow. Without prenatal diagnosis or rapid postnatal diagnosis and the initiation of prostaglandin E1 (PGE_1), these patients often present in severe cardiogenic shock as the ductus arteriosus closes.

Conversely, patients with single ventricles and obstruction to pulmonary blood flow usually have unobstructed systemic blood flow. These patients can have very heterogeneous presentations, dependent upon the degree of obstruction to pulmonary blood flow. If pulmonary blood flow is only minimally obstructed, the child may actually have overcirculation of the pulmonary vascular bed at the expense of systemic perfusion. However, as in the case with pulmonary atresia with intact ventricular septum, there is total obstruction to pulmonary blood flow and obligate mixing at the atrial level. Pulmonary blood flow is thus dependent on left to right shunting at the level of the ductus arteriosus. These patients have ductal dependent pulmonary blood flow, and PGE_1 should be started immediately.

All forms of single ventricle physiology have mixing of systemic and pulmonary venous blood at the atrial level. In the immediate postnatal period assessment of atrial communication is crucial. A restrictive atrial septal defect causes severe elevations in pulmonary venous pressure and pulmonary hypertension. Ultimately these patients are profoundly

Physiology	Anatomy
Systemic outflow obstruction	Hypoplastic left heart syndrome Tricuspid atresia with discordant ventriculo-arterial connections. Double inlet left ventricle Double outlet right ventricle (some variations)
Pulmonary outflow obstruction	Tricuspid atresia with concordant ventriculo-arterial connections Pulmonary atresia with intact ventricular septum Critical pulmonary stenosis Severe Ebstein's malformation of the tricuspid valve Double outlet right ventricle (some variations)

Table 1. Anatomic features commonly associated with single ventricle hearts in the newborn

hypoxemic and cyanotic, and emergent balloon atrial septostomy or surgical intervention is required.

Hypoplastic Left Heart Sydrome

Hypoplastic left heart syndrome (HLHS) is the most severe form of single ventricle physiology with obstructed systemic blood flow. The usual underlying anatomy is mitral atresia with aortic atresia or severe aortic stenosis. Preoperatively, these patients require prostaglandin to maintain the ductus arteriousus as a conduit for systemic blood flow. Since distribution of blood flow between the systemic and pulmonary circulation depends on the relative resistances, careful attention to ventilation is crucial. An arterial SpO_2 goal of 75-85% is used to prevent excessive pulmonary blood flow which can lead to pulmonary edema or low systemic perfusion.

Surgical Palliation

Patients with HLHS usually undergo the first stage of their palliation in the first week of life, usually on day of life five to seven. The most recent surgical technique applied is the Norwood operation with Sano modification. The surgery is performed on full cardiopulmonary bypass (CPB), and involves creation of a neoaorta using the native hypoplastic aorta and native pulmonary artery. The neoascending and transverse aorta is created by either a long extended longitudinal augmentation of the native aorta with the pulmonary artery, or an end-to-side anastamosis of the native aorta to the native pulmonary artery. The distal main pulmonary artery is transected, and an atrial septectomy is performed to ensure unrestrictive atrial mixing of systemic and pulmonary venous return. Pulmonary blood flow is established by either a right ventricle to pulmonary artery shunt (Sano modification) or a shunt from the innominate artery to the right pulmonary artery (modified Blalock-Taussig Shunt).

The Sano shunt conveys the hemodynamic advantage of having pulmonary blood flow only during right ventricular systole whereas the MBT shunt has continuous pulmonary blood flow during systole and diastole. As a result of pulmonary blood flow during diastole, coronary perfusion can be compromised

due to the reduction in diastolic blood pressure which decreases coronary perfusion pressure.

Postoperative Management

Care of the postoperative patient with a Norwood must be well coordinated, meticulous, and precise. The challenge of managing the Norwood patient is dictated by the nature of the surgical procedure and the resultant anatomy. Patients have often undergone a prolonged CPB and aortic cross clamp time with deep hypothermic circulatory arrest (DHCA) – the result is significant myocardial dysfunction and end organ ischemia. Thus, the challenge is maintaining adequate cardiac output in the setting of a post-surgical myocardial dysfunction. Often patients require a small amount of inotropy, and hematocrit should be maintained close to 45. Patients should be ventilated to minimize the pulmonary vasodilatory effects of oxygen and respiratory alkalosis in order to maintain adequate systemic perfusion. All patients should get ECGs immediately on arrival to the intensive care unit, and should be further monitored for any signs of coronary ischemia. The single ventricle after the Norwood operation is significantly volume loaded as it is required to pump blood to the pulmonary and systemic circulations. Low cardiac output due to ventricular dysfunction or inadequate central venous volume is poorly tolerated. Systemic perfusion should be followed closely by clinical exam and laboratory markers of perfusion (metabolic acidosis, urine output, mixed venous saturation). Quick response should be made to trends in increasing metabolic acidosis. The postoperative myocardium is exquisitely sensitive to changes in pH and oxygen delivery. Careful attention must be paid to dysrhythmias and filling pressures based on monitored atrial wave forms.

ECMO: When and Why?

Extracorporeal support should be considered in any single ventricle patient with refractory hypotension, circulatory collapse, refractory hypoxemia, dysrhythmia, or inability to wean from CPB. In a study by Allan et al. there was a 48% survival to discharge for patients placed on ECMO after single ventricle staged palliation. Of significance, patients placed on ECMO for refractory hypoxemia had significantly greater survival to discharge compared to those cannulated for hypotension (81% vs 29%).[2] Hoskote et al. studied ECMO survival in functional single ventricle patients and showed that patients with arrhythmias prior to ECLS had significantly lower survival to hospital discharge compared to those without arrhythmias (0% vs 50%).[3] This finding highlights the unforgiving postoperative single ventricle myocardium and the required vigilance of rhythm management. Both of the above studies demonstrate that when used in the correct clinical scenario, ECMO is a valuable support strategy.

Bidirectional Glenn Circulation & Fontan Circulations

The 2nd and 3rd stages of palliation in the patient with a single ventricle moves the source of pulmonary blood flow from the systemic arterial circulation to the superior vena cava (SVC) and inferior vena cava (IVC) respectively. The success of these procedures relies on the patient having low pulmonary vascular resistance since pulmonary blood flow is driven by systemic venous pressure rather than myocardial contraction. The bidirectional Glenn (BDG) circulation is the second stage of a staged palliation for children with a single systemic ventricle. The BDG, usually done between four and six months of age, establishes pulmonary blood flow via connection of the SVC to the pulmonary artery. In the setting of heterotaxy syndromes or other congenital heart disease with bilateral SVC's, a connection is established between both ipsilateral cavae and the pulmonary artery. The establishment of the BDG circulation results in passive pulmonary blood flow. The final stage, the modified Fontan procedure connects the IVC to the pulmonary circulation and completes the separation of the pulmonary and systemic circulations.

Surgical Management

Pre-Glenn cardiac catheterization should be done in all patients to assess PVR, ventricular function, degree of systemic outflow obstruction, and degree of atrioventricular valve regurgitation. The single systemic ventricle is volume unloaded, and the maintenance of its function is essential for the proper functioning of the circulation. Any insult that leads to increased afterload, atrioventricular valve leak, or increased central venous pressures will impede flow through the BDG. Patients are often anticoagulated to limit clots in the passive flow circuit and many are placed on afterload reduction, such as ACE inhibitors, to minimize ventricular work.

Following the BDG, the pulmonary and systemic circulations are completely separated during the Fontan operation or total cavopulmonary connection (TCPC), usually performed at approximately 2 years of age. This procedure introduces the systemic venous return from the IVC to the pulmonary circulation. The connection is created with either an extra-cardiac tube homograft or with an intracardiac baffle using the right atrial free wall. Commonly a fenestration is created between the systemic venous return and the common atria which allows for right to left shunting and maintenance of cardiac output in the setting of elevated central venous pressures. The systemic ventricle now handles only pulmonary venous return, and all pulmonary blood flow is a result of passive flow from the systemic venous return.

Postoperative Management

The postoperative management of the patient with a BDG circuit or Fontan circulation requires particular attention to intrathoracic and central venous pressures. In the setting of passive pulmonary blood flow, the maintenance of low/normal intrathoracic pressure is essential to insure adequate systemic venous return and as a result adequate cardiac output. Typically, postoperative management goals should include early extubation because physiologic breathing patterns are more likely to augment venous return. Positive pressure ventilation on the other hand will increase central venous pressures, PVR, and intrathoracic pressures thus limiting passive pulmonary blood flow. Care should be taken to maintain adequate filling pressures despite attempts at diuresis in the postoperative period. In BDG patients, care should be taken to avoid respiratory alkalosis as it will decrease cerebral blood flow and consequently pulmonary blood flow, as the cerebral circulation represents the majority of SVC flow in the young patient. In the setting of postoperative signs of low cardiac output, particularly in the Fontan patient, clinicians should consider mechanical obstruction to pulmonary blood flow, and prompt investigation with echocardiography should be considered. Patients with a patent Fontan fenestration and low pulmonary blood flow will often be profoundly cyanotic despite maintaining normal pH. Progressive and sustained low postoperative cardiac output requiring massive fluid replacement and inotropy therapy is concerning. Any question of significant mechanical obstruction to pulmonary blood flow should be investigated in the cardiac catheterization laboratory.

ECMO: When and Why?

ECMO should be considered in any postoperative patient with a BDG or Fontan circulation with profound low cardiac output in whom a source of obstruction is not found. In a large single institution experience, Booth et al demonstrated successful support of both BDG and Fontan-type circulations in the immediate post-op setting.[3] However, the support of patients with BDG and Fontan remains a challenge with suboptimal outcome when compared with other cardiac lesions supported with ECMO.[2] Furthermore, patients with Fontan circulation supported with ECMO or ECLS have better outcomes when used for postoperative LCOS rather than for progressive myocardial failure. Patients with Fontan circulation who were at increased risk of death were older patients and those with progressive cardiac failure leading to arrest.[3]

Cannulation of the patient with a BDG or Fontan circulation requires particular attention. When cannulating patients with either BDG or Fontan circulations, initial goal flows should be 100cc/kg/min. This is often challenging, and initial troubleshooting is important. Patients undergoing BDG are usually 4 – 6 months of age, and cannula size is often limited by patient size. Additionally, patients with a BDG circulation have 2 separate systemic venous returns (i.e. the SVC returns to the pulmonary artery and the IVC to the right atrium). As a result, it is often necessary to include an additional venous cannula for further venous drainage. Furthermore, Booth et al demonstrated a number neurologic complications

in BDG/Fontan patients with the use of ECMO.[3] The authors theorize that patients with heart failure and a BDG/Fontan have high central venous pressures and poor cerebral venous drainage. CPR further exacerbates this compromised circulatory state and one should first cannulate the SVC to decompress the cerebral vault and add additional venous cannulas as necessary in order to minimize cerebral venous congestion and bleeding.[3] Despite advances in our understanding and technologic advances long term survival is low.[2,3]

Right Ventricular Outflow Obstruction

The physiology of patients with right ventricular outflow obstruction or inadequate right ventricular size is highly variable depending on the degree of right ventricular outflow obstruction. Some neonates may have only minimal obstruction to pulmonary blood flow, and thus will be virtually asymptomatic or even develop congestive heart failure (mild Tetralogy of Fallot – "pink TET"), while others will have total obstruction to pulmonary blood flow (pulmonary atresia) and be dependent on left to right flow at the level of the ductus arteriosus for pulmonary blood flow. The systemic arterial saturation is dependent on the degree of obstruction to pulmonary blood flow. In the patient with "minimal" obstruction, the newborn may be fully saturated; however, cyanosis can be progressive, and the neonate should be monitored closely.

Neonates with a severely hypoplastic right ventricle or pulmonary atresia should be started on PGE$_1$ and then have an echocardiogram to clearly elucidate sources of pulmonary blood flow. Often in addition to the ductus arteriosus there are multiple aortopulmonary collaterals supplying the pulmonary vascular bed. While on PGE$_1$ close attention should be paid to systemic perfusion as the pulmonary vascular resistance begins to drop in the days after birth. Careful manipulations of FiO$_2$ and volume should be made in order to maximize the balance between Qp and Qs.

Surgical Palliation

Neonates with hypoplastic right ventricle or complete obstruction to pulmonary blood flow usually undergo a right modified Blalock Tausig shunt (RMBTS). As with the Norwood operation, this shunt is conventionally a Gore Tex shunt measuring 3.5mm from the right subclavian artery to the right pulmonary artery. The procedure can be performed without cardiopulmonary bypass.

Postoperative Management

As with all single ventricle patients the postoperative challenge with a MBTS is the delicate balance of Qp:Qs. Although the coronary circulation is significantly more stable than in the postoperative Norwood patient, the MBTS still allows for diastolic run off and potential decreased coronary perfusion due to low diastolic blood pressures. Thus, close attention should be paid to ECG changes. Patients should be maintained on an FiO_2 that maintains arterial SpO_2 between 75% and 85%. The MBTS is a small caliber shunt which is at risk for thrombosis should the postoperative patient become intravascularly depleted. Physical examination as well as laboratory and clinical markers of systemic perfusion should be monitored closely. Immediate attention should be paid to decreasing saturations – a potential early sign of shunt occlusion. Significantly decreased shunt flow usually presents with increasing cyanosis followed by hypotension and metabolic acidosis.

ECMO: When and Why?

Extracorporeal support of the patient with the modified Blalock Tausig shunt can be performed with success and good survival to hospital discharge.[3] ECMO should be considered early in cases of refractory hypotension unresolved with volume and ventilator manipulations, and in refractory/progressive cyanosis. Shunt occlusion or thrombosis is often the precipitating event in postoperative shunt patient. Cannulation should be performed through the chest if the patient has had a sternotomy or through the right neck if the patient had a thoracotomy. Neck cannulation should be performed with venous cannulation of the internal jugular vein and arterial cannulation of the carotid artery.

Once the patient is stable on ECMO, investigation of the shunt should be undertaken with echo-cardiography. If there is concern for shunt occlusion or thrombosis, the patient should undergo cardiac catheterization to further evaluate and potentially treat for shunt occlusion. Once going on ECMO, a number of patients with a MBTS often have paradoxical overcirculation of their pulmonary vascular bed. The chest x-ray may have diffuse opacification, and often a metabolic acidosis persists. In this setting it is sometimes necessary to have the cardiovascular surgeons clip the shunt to limit pulmonary overcirculation. Saturations should be maintained in the 70's and PaO2 should be maintained from 40-50.

Left Ventricular Outflow Tract Obstruction

Clinical presentation of neonates with obstruction to left ventricular (LV) outflow depends on the severity of the obstruction, whether the obstruction occurs rapidly or slowly, and the growth of the left ventricle. On one end of the spectrum is the child with mild coarctation which will likely be progressive as the child grows, at the other end of the spectrum is the child with critical aortic stenosis, critical coarctation, or interrupted aortic arch. The LV is severely pressure loaded. These patients all have ductal dependent systemic blood flow, and without immediate initiation of PGE_1 will present with cardiogenic shock as the ductus arteriosus closes following birth. In many patients the lines are not clearly delineated, and careful evaluation of the degree and levels of obstruction are required. In this setting the infant or neonate should be closely monitored for signs and symptoms of decreased cardiac output. Often the systemic arterial saturation might increase in the face of decreasing pH and PCO_2 – the scenario reflective of decreasing systemic perfusion, lactic acidosis and increasing Qp:Qs.

Surgical Repair

Obstruction to LV outflow at the level of the aortic arch (coarctation of the aorta, interrupted aortic arch) is relieved by surgical repair of the aortic arch. Coarctation of the aorta is repaired through a lateral thoracotomy without cardiopulmonary bypass. Interrupted aortic arch lesions require extensive arch reconstruction and surgery is performed through a sternotomy. The child is placed on cardiopulmonary bypass with cardioplegia and deep hypothermic circulatory arrest. The arch is usually repaired with an extended end-to-end anastamosis, often augmented with Gore Tex or pericardium.

Postoperative Management

Care of the postoperative patient following aortic arch repair is often challenging. The left ventricle has been severely pressure loaded and is often hypertrophied and is now edematous and inflamed following CPB and DHCA. As a result, these patients are at great risk for dysrhythmias and coronary ischemia. Close attention must be paid to the ECG and aggressive arrhythmia management should be standard. Many patients are also paradoxically hypertensive postoperatively due to a prolonged state of hyper-reninemia, and may require nipride and other agents to control blood pressure. Filling pressures, markers of end-organ perfusion, and physical examination should be closely monitored for signs of decreased cardiac output. Low cardiac output should be worked up thoroughly for the underlying cause, and treated aggressively with fluid, packed red blood cells, gentle inotropy, and pacing if necessary.

ECMO: When and Why?

In the postoperative period, neonates with a severely pressure-loaded left ventricle are at high risk for arrhythmias, ventricular dysfunction, and coronary ischemia. If signs and symptoms of low cardiac output state are evident, and correctable causes have been treated and/or ruled out (i.e. intravascular depletion, JET), extracorporeal support should be considered early. The myocardium will not tolerate significant inotropy and beta adrenergic receptor stimulation. Rather than increase cardiac output, excessive inotropy will increase myocardial oxygen demand and consumption and increase the likelihood of arrhythmias. In a study of 35 postcardiotomy patients, Jaggers et al demonstrated no significant difference between those patients placed on ECMO in the OR for failure to wean from CPB versus those patients placed on ECMO in the ICU for low cardiac output. Overall survival to hospital discharge was 60%, and although the data were not statistically significant, those patients placed on ECMO for cardiac arrest had a lower survival to hospital discharge.[4]

During arterial cannulation, care should be taken to avoid fresh suture lines, and minimize the risk of bleeding following cannulation. Ideally the arterial cannula should be placed just proximal to the takeoff of the innominate artery and should not be angled directly at the aortic valve. Position of the arterial cannula toward the aortic valve can cause significant aortic insufficiency and potentially increase LV afterload in an already compromised ventricle. Venous cannula should be in the right atrium just above the tricuspid valve annulus. If radiography does not clearly delineate cannula position, echocardiography should be performed to confirm cannula positioning. Arrhythmias should be treated in order to minimize further myocardial stress and oxygen consumption. In addition close attention should be paid to the quantity and quality of chest tube output and bulging of the sternotomy patch, which can be further signs of excessive bleeding. Frankly bloody and increasing chest tube output with a bulging sternotomy patch are ominous signs for ongoing post-ECMO bleeding.

Left to Right Shunts (Volume Loaded LV)

Left to right shunts which place the LV under volume loaded conditions include ventricular septal defect (VSD), large patent ductus arteriosus (PDA), and aorto-pulmonary (AP) window. The degree of shunting, and thus volume load on the left ventricle, is dependent upon the size of the defect and most importantly the down-stream resistance in the pulmonary and systemic vascular beds. In the first few days of life, there is often little hemodynamic consequence of a large VSD or PDA due to high pulmonary vascular resistance (PVR) in utero and in the days following birth. As PVR drops in the first days and weeks of life, the degree of left to right shunting increases significantly. Long-standing large left to right shunts cause significant LV dilatation, left atrial hypertension, and ultimately pulmonary artery hypertension.

Surgical Repair

Surgical repair of left to right shunts is straight-forward. A large PDA in a premature infant which is causing hemodynamic and respiratory compromise should be surgically ligated if medical therapy such as indomethacin has failed, or is contraindicated. A large PDA noted on exam of an older child can be closed in the cardiac catheterization laboratory with an intravascular device. When diagnosed, AP windows should be closed. Once pulmonary vascular resistance falls after birth, an AP window exposes the pulmonary vascular bed to high systemic level pressures and very high flow. Untreated, these patients are at high risk for irreversible, fixed pulmonary hypertension.

Large ventricular septal defects should be closed in the newborn period if they cause significant heart failure, cause an inability to wean from mechanical ventilation, or there are signs of early pulmonary hypertension. Smaller ventricular septal defects should be closed in patients who develop aortic insufficiency or recurrent endocarditis.

ECMO: When and Why

It is uncommon for a postoperative VSD repair to need extracorporeal support. ECMO support of the postoperative VSD patient is required most often for refractory arrhythmias or severe ventricular dysfunction. When severe arrhythmias or ventricular dysfunction occur following VSD repair, coronary injury or ischemia should always be considered if all treatable causes have been ruled out.

Total Anomalous Pulmonary Venous Drainage (TAPVD)

Total anomalous pulmonary venous drainage is a group of congenital heart defects where the pulmonary veins connect to a residual embryologic vein rather than to the left atrium. Anomalous pulmonary venous drainage can involve some or all of the pulmonary veins. The physiology of partial anamolous pulmonary venous drainage (PAPVD) with one or two veins joining to a systemic vein, such as the superior vena cava, is akin to the physiology of an atrial septal defect. Patients with PAPVD are unlike

to require ECMO. In patients with total anomalous pulmonary venous drainage (TAPVD), the anatomy and physiology varies widely including where the anomalous vein connects, the presence of other intracardiac defects, and the degree of pulmonary venous obstruction. Approximately one third of patients with TAPVD have associated cardiac defects such as single ventricle physiology, atrioventricular canal defects, or transposition of the great vessels.

A brief review of normal fetal development is helpful in order to understand the anatomy of TAPVD. During early development the lungs do not drain directly to the heart but instead pulmonary venous blood flows through the common cardinal and umbilicovitelline veins. These fetal veins form many parts of the systemic venous system such as the SVC and IVC. As development proceeds an outgrowth from the left atrium forms and connects to the pulmonary veins, after which the pulmonary veins gradually lose connections with the cardinal and umbilicovitelline veins. Any interruption in this process leads to variable abnormalities in the pulmonary venous connections. There are four major types of TAPVD depending on the location of the anomalous connection:

- Supracardiac: The pulmonary veins join in a confluence which is drained by an ascending vertical vein to join the innominate vein.
- Cardiac: The pulmonary veins connect either to the coronary sinus or the right atrium.
- Infracardiac: The pulmonary veins drain via a descending vein to a variety of infradiaphragmatic veins. Frequently, there is pulmonary venous obstruction.
- Mixed: Any combination of the 3 previous types.

Cardiac output in all patients with TAPVD is dependent upon an atrial right to left shunt. The combination of left to right shunt and a variable degree of pulmonary venous obstruction (PVO) results in a wide clinical spectrum. The pathophysiology of TAPVD depends most importantly on the degree of pulmonary venous obstruction. The site of pulmonary venous obstruction can occur by several mechanisms. In supracardiac TAPVD, the vertical vein can be compressed between the pulmonary artery and the bronchus. In the infracardiac type, pulmonary venous obstruction can occur at multiple sites including the diaphragm or where the anomalous vein joins the portal system. The degree of pulmonary venous obstruction can vary between patients and is the primary determinant of the urgency of surgical repair. Pulmonary venous obstruction results in pulmonary venous hypertension, secondary pulmonary arterial hypertension, and severe pulmonary edema. In addition to the severe hypoxemia and respiratory failure produced, cardiac output may also be limited by the anatomic obstruction or a restrictive atrial communication. The clinical presentation of extreme obstruction often mimics persistent pulmonary hypertension of the newborn with meconium aspiration syndrome or severe neonatal sepsis. Severe pulmonary venous obstruction is refractory to medical management and either requires emergent cardiac surgery or preoperative ECMO to maintain hemodynamic stability and organ perfusion.

A small percentage of neonates with TAPVD have no venous obstruction. The anomalous pulmonary venous connection is often to the coronary sinus, and patients are largely asymptomatic in the newborn period. There is a mild degree of arterial desaturation and a large volume load on the right ventricle. Children present later in childhood with signs and symptoms of congestive heart failure from the chronic RV volume overload.

The preoperative management of the critically ill neonate with obstructed TAPVD is directed at careful delineation of the anatomy and maintaining adequate systemic oxygen delivery. Echocardiography is the diagnostic modality of choice, and is helpful in identifying the neonate with TAPVD rather than neonatal sepsis or PPHN. Initial echocardiogram must not only delineate all four pulmonary veins, but must also clearly show the pathway for return of pulmonary blood to the heart. Intracardiac anatomy is also important to delineate, given the variability in the underlying anatomy. Preoperative treatment includes mechanical ventilation, ionotropic agents, and PGE_1 to manage the pulmonary artery hypertension and cardiogenic shock. An important factor to remember is the recognition of the failure of medical management and when the

patient should undergo urgent cardiac surgery or be placed on ECMO.

Surgical Correction

Despite widespread advances in neonatal cardiac surgery, correction of TAPVD remains challenging with most mortality within the first year of repair.[5] Neonates with TAPVD most commonly require repair in the newborn period. The degree of pulmonary venous obstruction (PVO) usually dictates the urgency with which repair is undertaken. Patients with severe PVO require emergent surgery or preoperative ECMO if medical therapy can not stabilize the patient. Surgical repair involves ligation of the vertical vein connecting the pulmonary venous confluence to the systemic venous drainage. The pulmonary venous confluence is then sutured to the posterior wall of the left atrium with closure of the atrial septal defect.

Postoperative Pathophysiology

During the postoperative period, the major concerns are low cardiac output syndrome and pulmonary hypertensive crises. Pulmonary hypertensive (PH) crises (episodes of acutely elevated PA pressure resulting in low cardiac output or severe cyanosis) are common after repair of TAPVD, particularly in patients with significant preoperative pulmonary venous obstruction. Cardiopulmonary bypass further injures the pulmonary endothelium and is a potent stimulus for pulmonary hypertension. Low cardiac output syndrome can occur from pulmonary artery hypertension and RV failure and more rarely from LV dysfunction. LV dysfunction occurs from the acutely increased volume load and increased afterload. Pulmonary artery hypertension can also compromise LV function when the intraventricular septum shifts leftward and interferes with LV filling. One major goal of postoperative management is to prevent PH crises by minimizing noxious stimuli and hypoxia, providing adequate sedation, and optimizing mechanical ventilation. Often judicious use of catecholamines is also necessary to maintain and augment cardiac output. Inhaled nitric oxide is a useful therapeutic adjunct for severe, refractory, or recurrent pulmonary hypertensive crises after

TAPVD repair.[6] Patients with refractory pulmonary hypertension despite use of inhaled NO may require postoperative ECMO support. In a single institution series of one hundred and twenty-three patients, single ventricle physiology was the only independent risk factor for postoperative death.[7]

A late complication of TAPVD is pulmonary vein stenosis. Pulmonary vein stenosis can occur at the site of surgical anastomosis or as progressive fibrosis of the pulmonary veins. unrelated to the surgical procedure. Stenosis at the surgical site results from tension on the suture line or an underestimation of the degree of stenosis when creating the baffle. Postoperative restenosis occurs over time, usually days to weeks. The etiology of progressive pulmonary vein stenosis has not been clearly elucidated; however, it is believed that many of patients with TAPVD have intrinsically abnormal pulmonary vasculature which is often diffusely hypoplastic.

ECMO: When and Why?

Extracorporeal support for the neonate with TAPVD should be considered in any patient with preoperative or postoperative refractory hypoxemia. Patients with severely obstructed TAPVD are often severely hypoxemic and cyanotic preoperatively due to decreased pulmonary venous return and resultant elevated PA pressures. As previously described, these patients may develop low cardiac output and symptoms of cardiogenic shock with poor end-organ perfusion and metabolic acidosis. While inhaled NO is useful in the postoperative patient with pulmonary hypertension, in the preoperative patient with severe PVO, inhaled NO will worsen an already challenging situation. Ideal management is urgent surgical repair; however, in critically ill infants, ECMO is a means by which cardiac output and end-organ perfusion can be maintained. The morbidity and mortality for neonatal cardiac surgery is even greater when patients are in extremis with severe metabolic acidosis, low cardiac output, and severe hypoxemia. Thus, ECMO allows for stabilization prior to surgical repair

The use of ECMO in the postoperative patient following TAPVD repair is usually due to severe refractory pulmonary hypertension Patients with severely obstructed TAPVD and premature infants have the greatest risk postoperatively. One should have a low clinical threshold for the use of ECMO with these patient populations. It is, however, important to use all of the clinical data in the context of the patient's underlying preoperative and postoperative anatomy. Neonates with severely obstructed TAPVD preoperatively often have suprasystemic PA pressure, and in the postoperative period often have a PA line in place. Care must be taken to accurately interpret the available postoperative data. The postoperative patient may have brief, transient self-limited elevation in PA pressure without significant hemodynamic consequence while others may have PA pressures that are persistently ¾ systemic without hemodynamic effects. These patients do not require ECMO support. Those patients that do require extracorporeal support will benefit from the early institution of ECMO and avoidance of cardiopulmonary resuscitation

Myocarditis

Myocarditis is classically defined as an acute inflammatory disease of the myocardium, usually caused by a viral infection. In clinical practice myocarditis and dilated cardiomyopathy are opposite ends of a spectrum of myocardial disease. The diagnosis of myocarditis is challenging and often missed due to the nonspecific symptoms. Children can present at any age, and there is no predisposition for males or females. Myocarditis should be considered in any patient who presents with congestive heart failure or cardiogenic shock and a structurally normal heart. The presentation can vary from mild myocardial dysfunction and indolent illness to acute fulminant myocarditis presenting with severe arrhythmias and cardiogenic shock.

Patients with fulminant myocarditis usually present with one or more of the following: a short viral prodrome, cardiogenic shock, ventricular arrhythmias, heart block, or sudden death. The arrhythmias are due to diffuse myocardial inflammation and infiltrative processes. Children at the other end of the spectrum present with a longer viral prodrome and congestive heart failure instead of shock. The treatment for myocarditis should be aggressive, and is largely supportive with the goals of reducing myocardial oxygen demand and maintaining end organ perfusion.. Medical management often requires the use of anti-arrhythmics, mechanical ventilation, and inotropic support. Despite significant morbidity and mortality early in the course of illness, patients with acute fulminant myocarditis have good prognosis for recovery of myocardial function.[8]

ECMO: When and Why?

When treating patients with myocarditis, extracorporeal support should be considered when routine medical therapies are failing and it can be life saving in patients with cardiogenic shock or cardiac arrest. Initially, ECMO was viewed as a bridge to heart transplantation but now is often a bridge to recovery especially in patients with fulminant myocarditis. The main objective of ECMO in myocarditis is myocardial rest and recovery. Left ventricular distention resulting from either inadequate unloading of the LV with ECMO or inability of the LV to eject will impair myocardial recovery and worsen pulmonary edema. LV distension can be diagnosed by echocardiogram and LA pressure monitoring. If LV distension occurs, decompression by placement of left atrial cannula or catheter-based atrial septostomy should be considered. Adequate coronary oxygen supply should be provided by maintaining adequate although not excessive mechanical ventilation. If myocardial recovery is not evident by day 7-10 of ECLS support, then evaluation for heart transplant should be considered. Survival with ECLS and ECMO for myocarditis is generally good, and multiple studies have reported success.[9, 10] Tsai et al report success specifically with arrhythmia management, and suggest early consideration and prompt initiation when ECMO is considered.[11]

References

1. Ungerleider, R.M., et al., Use of routine ventricular assist following the first stage Norwood procedure. Cardiology in the Young, 2004. 14 Suppl 1: p. 61-4.
2. Allan, C.K., et al., Indication for initiation of mechanical circulatory support impacts survival of infants with shunted single-ventricle circulation supported with extracorporeal membrane oxygenation. Journal of Thoracic & Cardiovascular Surgery, 2007. 133(3): p. 660-7.
3. Hoskote, A., et al., Extracorporeal life support after staged palliation of a functional single ventricle: subsequent morbidity and survival. Journal of Thoracic & Cardiovascular Surgery, 2006. 131(5): p. 1114-21.
4. Jaggers, J.J., et al., Extracorporeal membrane oxygenation for infant postcardiotomy support: significance of shunt management. Ann Thorac Surg, 2000. 69(5): p. 1476-83.
5. Karamlou, T., et al., Factors associated with mortality and reoperation in 377 children with total anomalous pulmonary venous connection. Circulation, 2007. 115(12): p. 1591-8.
6. Atz, A.M. and D.L. Wessel, Inhaled nitric oxide in the neonate with cardiac disease. Semin Perinatol, 1997. 21(5): p. 441-55.
7. Hancock Friesen, C.L., et al., Total anomalous pulmonary venous connection: an analysis of current management strategies in a single institution. Ann Thorac Surg, 2005. 79(2): p. 596-606; discussion 596-606.
8. English, R.F., et al., Outcomes for children with acute myocarditis. Cardiol Young, 2004. 14(5): p. 488-93.
9. Duncan, B.W., et al., Mechanical circulatory support for the treatment of children with acute fulminant myocarditis. J Thorac Cardiovasc Surg, 2001. 122(3): p. 440-8.
10. Wu, E.T., et al., Children with fulminant myocarditis rescued with extracorporeal membrane oxygenation. Heart, 2006. 92(9): p. 1325-6.
11. Tsai, F-C., et al. Extracorporeal life support to terminate refractory ventricular tachycardia, Critical Care Medicine, 2007. 35(7): p1673-5.

Chapter 3 Questions

1. What is the most common immediate postoperative complication following repair of TAPVD which necessitates the use of ECMO?
    a) Arrhythmias
    b) Incomplete repair
    c) Pulmonary venous obstruction
    d) Refractory pulmonary hypertension and hypoxemia

2. When placing a single ventricle patient with a modified Blalock-Taussig shunt on ECMO, signs of pulmonary overcirculation include:
    a) Hypoxia
    b) Metabolic acidosis
    c) Diffuse opacification on chest x-ray
    c) Persistently elevated oxygen saturations
    e) All of the above
    f) B,C, and D only

3. Which of the following are anticipated postoperative complications of patients with repaired left ventricular outflow tract obstruction?
    a) Arrhythmia
    b) Coronary ischemia
    c) Severe myocardial depression
    d) All of the above

Chapter 3 Answers

1. d
2. f
3. d

4

Pediatric Pulmonary Physiology and Pathophysiology

Curt L. Shelley, BS RRT-NPS AE-C and Nancy J. Rees, RN BSN

Objectives

After completion of this chapter, the participant will be able to:

- List the common diagnoses that necessitate ECMO.
- Explain the mechanism which viral pneumonias causes gas exchange mismatch.
- List the most common bacterial pneumonias.
- List common bacteria that may cause aspiration pneumonia.
- List objective observations that define ARDS.

Introduction

Pediatric ECMO is defined as an age group >30 days of life to <18 years. This patient population is characterized by conditions which were acquired after birth. Discounting "other," viral pneumonia, bacterial pneumonia and aspiration pneumonia are the three most common reasons that require ECLS.

The clinical experience of pediatric patients on ECMO is less than that of neonatal patients. According to the July 2009 ECLS Registry Report, there have been 9660 pediatric patients, with 27432 neonatal patients. These numbers represent respiratory, cardiac and ECPR patients. As it has been for years past, the most common diagnoses for the pediatric pulmonary group remains viral pneumonia, followed by acute respiratory failure, non-ARDS. The

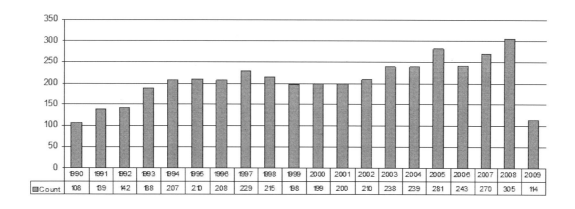

	1990	1991	1992	1993	1994	1995	1996	1997	1998	1999	2000	2001	2002	2003	2004	2005	2006	2007	2008	2009
Count	108	139	142	188	207	210	208	229	215	198	199	200	210	238	239	281	243	270	305	114

Figure 1: Annual respiratory pediatric runs as reported by ELSO, July 2009[1]

	Total Runs	Percent of Total	Percent Survived
Viral Pneumonia	926	22%	63%
Bacterial Pneumonia	478	11%	57%
Pneumocystis Pneumonia	30	1%	50%
Aspiration Pneumonia	200	5%	66%
ARDS, post-op/trauma	102	2%	61%
ARDS, not post-op/trauma	373	9%	53%
Acute respiratory failure, non-ARDS	741	17%	50%
Other	1413	33%	51%

Figure 2: Pediatric Respiratory Runs by Diagnosis[1]

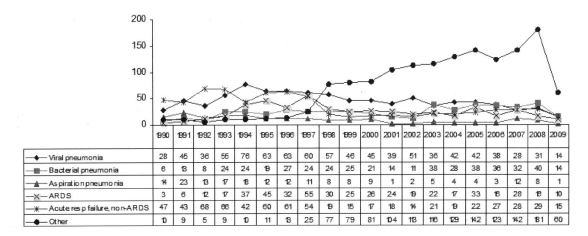

Figure 3: Pediatric Respiratory Diagnoses by Year as reported by ELSO[2]

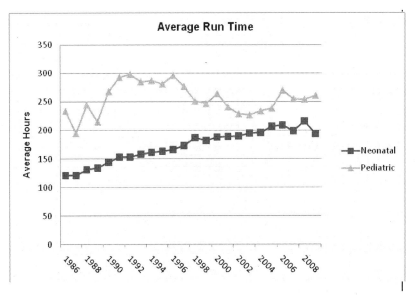

Figure 4: Average Run Times for neonatal and pediatric cases[1]

cumulative survival rate for all pediatric pulmonary diagnoses is 55%.[1]

Inclusion and Exclusion Guidelines

Due to advances in experience with pediatric ECMO, most cases are evaluated on a case-by-case basis as no universally agreed upon criteria have been identified.

Inclusion criteria for pediatric ECMO are:
- Potentially reversible respiratory failure associated with high risk of mortality without ECMO
- Acute hypoxemia unresponsive to maximal medical management
- Oxygenation index >40 for greater than 2 hours
- Hypercarbic respiratory failure with pH <7.2
- Persistent air leak on maximal ventilator support

Exclusion Criteria
- Non-pulmonary disease associated with high risk of mortality
- Pulmonary and/or cardiac failure unlikely to be reversible in fourteen days
- Ongoing multisystem failure defined as pulmonary or cardiac failure associated with two additional major organ systems
- Fixed elevated pulmonary vascular resistance
- Evidence of severe or irreversible brain damage
- Hemorrhagic condition that would be uncontrollable with heparin therapy necessary to prevent clotting in the ECMO circuit

Relative Contraindications
- High morbidity disease condition
- Recent CNS hemorrhage
- Recent invasive procedure or trauma
- Creatinine >3.0
- Profound shock refractory to medical management
- Overwhelming sepsis with capillary leak
- Prolonged ventilatory therapy >14 days
- Prolonged pre-ECMO CPR
- Immunosuppression?

All patients who are considered for ECLS are, by definition, in critical condition. The probability of profound morbidity and mortality is high. "Con-ventional" medical management, at this point is usually considered non-productive. At this point in the patient's management, the airways have been subjected to high airway pressures and oxygen concentrations. Most are fluid overloaded with a concurrent low urinary output. Multi-organ failure can be present along with coagulopathy due to deficient clotting factors and liver insufficiency.

In light of this cascading organ failure and undesirable patient trajectory, it is important to remember that VV ECMO will only provide gas exchange. While VA ECMO will augment the cardiac output. Complete cardiac support will be limited by the upper limit of pump flow, which is limited by the venous return and the venous cannula(s) inner diameter as well as arterial resistance by the arterial cannula size. The ultimate goal, once ECLS has been initiated, is to preserve remaining lung function by limiting barotrauma and hyperoxic/reperfusion insult, while meeting oxygen demand.[3]

Pathophysiology

Viral Pneumonia

Viral pneumonia is the most common listed reason for pediatric ECMO on the ELSO International Summary.[1] Viruses invade the cells lining the airways and the alveoli. This infection often results in cell destruction either through direct killing by the virus or by self-destruction through apoptosis. Further damage to the lungs occurs when the immune system responds to the infection. White blood cells, in particular lymphocytes, are responsible for activating a variety of cytokines, which cause leaking of fluid into the alveoli. The combination of cellular destruction and fluid-filled alveoli interrupts the gas exchange capability of the lungs.

Viral pneumonia is an acute infectious disease of the lungs that causes the parenchymal tissue to become inflamed and fill with fluid. Most viral pneumonia cases result from exposure to infectious aerosolized secretions. Although half of all pneumonias are believed to have a viral etiology, mixed viral and bacterial infections are common. Viral pneumonias may be caused by influenza types A, B or C (most common in adults); respiratory syncytial virus (RSV) (most common in infants and young children); parainfluenza 1, 2, 3, or 4; adenovirus; cytomegalovirus (CMV) (particularly in the immunocompromised); varicella zoster virus (chicken pox); herpes simplex virus (HSV); rubella (measles); enterovirus; coronavirus; Epstein-Barr virus; and hantavirus.[4] Complications of viral pneumonia include superimposed bacterial infections, respiratory failure, pulmonary fibrosis, acute respiratory distress syndrome, noncardiogenic pulmonary edema and Reye's syndrome. Viral pneumonia is usually self-limiting (lasting several days to a week) and usually has a good prognosis, but death can occur, particularly with adenovirus and influenza infections in pediatric or elderly populations.[4]

Risk factors include newborns, infants, elderly, smokers, immunocompromised, pregnant, history of recent upper viral infections, asthma, COPD, cardiac disease and those living in crowded conditions.

While viral pneumonia accounts for approximately 4 to 39% of pneumonia cases in adults, viral pneumonia is the most common pneumonia in children, accounting for approximately 90% of cases.[4]

While most episodes of viral pneumonia improve without treatment within a few days to three weeks, some episodes may last longer and, if lung impairment becomes so severe that the ability to support the patient's oxygen demand is severely compromised, ECMO may be needed.

Bacterial Pneumonia

Bacterial pneumonia is an acute infection within the lung parenchyma that causes a severe inflammatory response that fills alveoli and prevents them from exchanging gas normally.[5] It is the third most common diagnosis for pediatric ECMO.[1] Acute respiratory distress syndrome and bacterial pneumonia are the most common conditions in sepsis that may require ECMO.[6] Two of the most common bacteria that could necessitate ECMO are staphylococcus aureus and beta-hemolytic streptococci (GBS). Fortunately, venovenous ECMO can effectively provide adequate oxygenation for the majority of this patient population.[7,8] In addition to maintaining the normal flow of blood through the body, another benefit of venovenous ECMO is that particulate

matter or emboli returning from the ECMO circuit to the patient will be trapped in the vascular system of the lungs.

The use of VV ECMO, while preferable for multiple reasons, may not be able to support the profoundly compromised patient who has severe lung injury and cardiac dysfunction as well. Although the prognosis for patients with previously normal lungs and adequate host defenses is generally good, the mortality rate is higher in the setting of advanced age, multilobar disease, severe hypoxemia, extrapulmonary complications and bacteremia. Severe pneumonia with destruction of lung tissue may result in severe hemorrhage. Some centers have reported use of activated factor VII to control severe bleeding without having thrombosis within the ECMO circuit.[9] Other anecdotal and case reports have noted clotting with administration of factor VII and this therapy should be used with caution and always with a back-up circuit available.

Streptococcus pneumonia is the most common bacterial pneumonia. Other causes of bacterial pneumonia are haemophilus influenza, chlamydia, moraxella catarrhalis, legionella, pseudomonas and klebsiella.[11] Similar to viral pneumonia, infection is via infectious aerosolized secretions. Alternatively, it may be distributed through hematogenous (blood borne) or lymphatic dissemination. Complications may include septic shock, hypoxemia, respiratory failure, empyema, bacteremia, endocarditis, pericarditis, meningitis, lung abscess and pleural effusion.[11]

Streptococcus pneumonia generally resides in the nasopharynx and is carried asymptomatically in approximately 50% of healthy individuals. A strong association exists with viral illnesses, such as influenza. Viral infections increase pneumococcal attachment to the receptors on activated respiratory epithelium. Once aerosolized from the nasopharynx to the alveolus, pneumococci infect type II alveolar cells. The pneumonic lesion progresses as pneumococci multiply in the alveolus and invade alveolar epithelium. Pneumococci spread from alveolus to alveolus through the pores of Kohn, thereby producing inflammation and consolidation along lobar compartments.[10]

Aspiration plays a central role in the pathogenesis of nosocomial pneumonia. Approximately 45% of healthy subjects aspirate during sleep, and an even higher proportion of severely ill patients aspirate routinely. Depending on the number and virulence of the pathogenic organisms reaching the lower respiratory tract and on the host defense factors, pneumonia may develop. The oropharynx of hospitalized patients may become colonized with aerobic gram-negative bacteria within a few days of admission. Therefore, nosocomial pneumonia is often caused by gram-negative bacilli. In the current era, the incidence of staphylococcus aureus lower respiratory tract infection is increasingly common in the hospitalized and institutionalized patients and must now be considered a possible pathogen for nosocomial pneumonia.[11] Fungal pneumonia can also occur as a nosocomial pathogen.

Aspiration Pneumonia

Aspiration pneumonia, also known as anaerobic or necrotizing pneumonia, is an inflammation or infection of the lungs and bronchial tubes caused by inhaling foreign material, usually food, drink, vomit, or secretions, into the lungs. Aspiration of these substances usually causes impaired airway protections, particularly in those patients with an altered level of consciousness and/or abnormal swallowing reflexes. Because of aspiration, the injured lungs may become infected with such anaerobic bacteria as prevotella melaninogenica, fusobacterium necleutum, porphyromonas gingivalis, norcardia asteroids, klebsiella pneumonia, and bacteroids fragilis or with such mixed oropharyngeal flora organisms as peptostreptococcus magnus or microaerophilic streptococci (S. pneumoniae or S. pyogenes). The infection can cause pus to collect in the lungs (empyema) or if surrounded by a protective membrane, form a lung abscess.[11, 12]

Aspiration of gastric liquid may also result in a chemical pneumonitis, which the patient may either recover rapidly, progress to acute respiratory distress syndrome (ARDS) or develop a bacterial infection. The patient's response depends upon the characteristics and amount of the aspirated substance, and/or the level of acidity of the aspirate, the severity of the resulting pneumonia, the type of organism and the extent of the lung involvement.[12]

Aspiration pneumonia represents less than 15% of all community-acquired pneumonia, and

5% of respiratory diagnoses by year as reported by ELSO.[13, 1]

Treatment should include maintenance of airways and clearance of secretions with tracheal suctioning, oxygen supplementation, mechanical ventilation if the patient is unable to maintain adequate oxygenation, early use of positive end-expiratory pressure (PEEP), and administration of intravenous fluids. Routine use of corticosteroids is not indicated.[14] Early prophylactic use of antibiotics is controversial because no evidence indicates that bacterial infection plays a role in the initial events. Bacterial pneumonia that may occur later (eg, days after the aspiration event) as a complication of chemical pneumonia and should be treated with appropriate antibiotics.[13]

Acute Respiratory Distress Syndrome

Acute Respiratory Distress Syndrome (ARDS) is defined as an acute condition characterized by bilateral pulmonary infiltrates and severe hypoxemia in the absence of evidence for cardiogenic pulmonary edema. By these criteria, the severity of hypoxemia necessary to make the diagnosis of ARDS is defined by the PaO_2/FiO_2 ratio less than 200, and in acute lung injury (ALI), this ratio is less than 300. In addition, cardiogenic pulmonary edema must be excluded either by clinical criteria or pulmonary capillary wedge pressure of less than 18 mm Hg.[14]

Early ARDS is characterized by an increase in the permeability of the alveolar-capillary barrier leading to an influx of fluid into the alveoli. The alveolar-capillary barrier is formed by the microvascular endothelium and the epithelial lining of the alveoli. Hence, a variety of insults resulting in damage either to the vascular endothelium or to the alveolar epithelium could result in ARDS. The main site of injury may be focused on either the vascular endothelium (eg, sepsis) or the alveolar epithelium (eg, aspiration of gastric contents).

Injury to the endothelium results in increased capillary permeability and the influx of protein-rich fluid into the alveolar space. Injury to the alveolar lining cells also promotes pulmonary edema formation. Two types of alveolar epithelial cells exist. Type I cells, comprising 90% of the alveolar epithelium, are injured easily. Damage to type I cells allows both increased entry of fluid into the alveoli and decreased clearance of fluid from the alveolar space. Type II cells are relatively more resistant to injury. However, type II cells have several important functions, including the production of surfactant, ion transport, and proliferation and differentiation into type I cells after cellular injury. Damage to type II cells results in decreased production of surfactant with resultant decreased compliance and alveolar collapse. Interference with the normal repair processes in the lung may lead to the development of fibrosis.[15]

ARDS is an inhomogeneous process. Relatively normal alveoli, more compliant than affected alveoli, may become overdistended by the delivered tidal volume, resulting in barotrauma (pneumothorax and interstitial air). Alveoli already damaged by ARDS may experience further injury via volutrauma. In addition to the mechanical effects on alveoli, these forces promote the secretion of proinflammatory cytokines with resultant worsening inflammation and pulmonary edema. The use of positive end-expiratory pressure (PEEP) to diminish alveolar collapse and the use of low tidal volumes (4 to 6 ml/kg)[15] and limited levels of inspiratory filling pressures appear to be beneficial in diminishing the observed ventilator-associated lung injury.

ARDS often occurs along with failure of other organ systems, such as the kidneys or liver. This resultant end-organ damage appears to be ultimately responsible for the mortality rate of 30 to 40%. If associated with sepsis, the mortality rate may reach 90%. The most common causes of ARDS include pneumonia, septic shock, trauma, aspiration of gastric contents, near drowning, pancreatitis, massive blood transfusion, pulmonary emboli, drug overdose, and toxic chemical inhalation.[16]

ARDS is often associated with pulmonary hypertension resulting from elevated pulmonary vascular resistance. Pulmonary artery vasoconstriction likely contributes to ventilation-perfusion mismatch and is one of the mechanisms of hypoxemia in ARDS. Normalization of pulmonary vascular resistance and elevated pulmonary artery pressures occurs as the syndrome resolves. The development of progressive and sustained pulmonary hypertension is associated with a poor prognosis.

Editorial

Heidi J. Dalton, MD, FCCM

Many processes can combine to cause lung injury of such severity that gas exchange is limited. Viral and bacterial pneumonias are often the precipitating events which lead to hypoxemia and respiratory failure. Secondary lung injury by ARDS can occur from sepsis, trauma or many other factors. ECMO can help optimize oxygen delivery and allow reduction of toxic ventilator and oxygen levels to limit barotrauma to the already injured lung. Support of the patient can often be adequate with venovenous ECMO, although patients with concomitant hemodynamic compromise may require venoarterial support.

References

1   ECMO Registry of the Extracorporeal Life Support Organization (ELSO), International Summary, Ann Arbor, Michigan, July 2009.

2   ECMO Registry of the Extracorporeal Life Support Organization (ELSO), International Trend Summary, Ann Arbor, Michigan, July 2009.

3   Van Meurs K, Lally K, Peek G, Zwischenberger J, eds. *ECMO Extracorporeal Cardiopulmonary support in Critical Care.* 3rd ed. Ann Arbor, Mi: Extracorporeal Life Support Organization; 2005.

4   Sharma S. Pneumonia, Viral. *eMedicine.* Retrieved February 15, 2005 from http://www.emedicine.com/med/topic1854.htm.

5   Pneumonia, bacterial. Buckley L *Cinahl Information Systems*, Retrieved February 18, 2008 from http://web.ebscohost.com.ezproxy.lib.uh.edu/ehost/pdf?vid=15&hid=8&sid=e3762c15-c9bf-4e71-a099-898ce07f2df0%40sessionmgr106.

6   Maclaren G, Butt W. Extracorporeal membrane oxygenation and sepsis. Crit Care Resusc. 2007 Mar;9(1):76-80.

7   Pettignano R, Fortenberry JD, Heard ML, Labuz MD, Kesser KC, Tanner AJ, Wagoner SF, Heggen J. Primary use of the venovenous approach for extracorporeal membrane oxygenation in pediatric acute respiratory failure. Pediatr Crit Care Med. 2003 Jul;4(3):385-6.

8   Zahraa JN, Moler FW, Annich GM, Maxvold NJ, Bartlett RH, Custer JR. Venovenous versus venoarterial extracorporeal life support for pediatric respiratory failure: are there differences in survival and acute complications? Crit Care Med. 2000 Feb;28(2):521-5.

9   Stroud MH, Okhuysen-Cawley R, Jaquiss R, Berlinski A, Fiser RT. Successful use of extracorporeal membrane oxygenation in severe necrotizing pneumonia caused by Staphylococcus aureus. Pediatr Crit Care Med. 2007 May;8(3):294-6.

10 Sharma S. Pneumonia, Bacterial. *eMedicine.* Retrieved February 18, 2008 from http://www.emedicine.com/med/topic1852.htm.

11 Swaminathan A. Pneumonia, Aspiration. *eMedicine.* Retrieved February 18, 2008 from http://www.emedicine.com/emerg/topic464.htm.

12 Buckley L. Pneumonia, Aspiration (Anaerobic). *Cinahl Information Systems*, Retrieved February 18, 2008 from http://web.ebscohost.com.ezproxy.lib.uh.edu/ehost/pdf?vid=19&hid=8&sid=e3762c15-c9bf-4e71-a099-898ce07f2df0%40sessionmgr106.

13 Varkey A. Pneumonia, Aspiration. *eMedicine.* Retrieved February 18, 2008 from http://www.emedicine.com/med/TOPIC175.HTM

14 Harman E. Acute Respiratory Distress Syndrome. *eMedicine.* Retrieved February 18, 2008 from http://www.emedicine.com/med/topic70.HTM.

15 The Acute Respiratory Distress Syndrome Network. Ventilation with lower tidal volumes as compared with traditional tidal volumes for acute lung injury and the acute respiratory distress syndrome. N Engl J Med. 2000;342:1301-1308.

16 Buckley L. Acute Respiratory Distress Syndrome. *Cinahl Information Systems.* Retrieved February 18, 2008 from http://web.ebscohost.com.ezproxy.lib.uh.edu/ehost/pdf?vid=29&hid=105&sid=e3762c15-c9bf-4e71-a099-898ce07f2df0%40sessionmgr106.

Chapter 4 Questions

1. The combination of cellular destruction and fluid-filled alveoli is what interrupts gas exchange during viral pneumonia.
   a) True
   b) False

2. The ultimate goal of ECLS is?
   a) To maximize oxygen delivery.
   b) To hyperoxygenate the brain.
   c) To preserve remaining lung function by limiting barotrauma.
   d) To minimize oxygen consumption.

3. The most common bacterial pneumonia is caused by:
   a) Streptococcus
   b) Staphylococcus aureus
   c) Klebsiella
   d) Pseudomonas aeruginosa

Chapter 4 Answers

1. A
2. C
3 . B

5

Extracorporeal Life Support (ECLS) Physiology

Nancy J. Rees, RN BSN and John Waldvogel, RRT

Objectives

After completion of this chapter, the participant should be able to:

- Present the physiology of oxygen exchange and how it relates to ECMO
- Present the function of the membrane lung used in ECMO and the mechanisms for improving oxygenation on ECMO
- Review the blood gas management on VA and VV ECMO

Introduction

Though conventional patient management continues to improve with new technology and research, there remains a need for ECLS. The use of ECLS has broadened to support a wide range of pathophysiology in the critically ill neonatal, pediatric and adult populations. The physiologic goal of ECLS is to sufficiently supply oxygenated blood to meet metabolic requirements and facilitate the removal of metabolic waste. Understanding the physiology of ECLS is paramount to the comprehensive and safe management of the patient on extracorporeal life support.

Native Gas Exchange

In the native state, oxygen and carbon dioxide are exchanged at two levels, the alveolar level in the lungs, and at the tissue level. Pulmonary respiration is the exchange of oxygen and carbon dioxide between blood and inspired gas in the lungs. Tissue respiration is the exchange of gas at the cellular level. The exchange of oxygen and carbon dioxide on both levels is driven by diffusion gradients, caused by the difference in partial pressures of gases between environments. The net movement of gas is from a

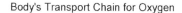

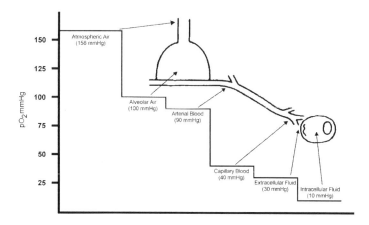

Body's Transport Chain for Oxygen

Figure 1

higher to a lower partial pressure. The partial pressure of gas is measured in Torr or mmHg.

Figure 1 demonstrates the pathway of oxygen transport from atmospheric air to the cellular level. The PO_2 of ambient air is roughly 158 mmHg. Once it has reached the cellular level the PO_2 is 6-10 mmHg.

Carbon dioxide is driven by the partial pressure from plasma to be excreted by the lungs. As with oxygen, this is achieved with its diffusion gradients, similar to those of oxygen. Carbon dioxide builds up in the peripheral tissues and diffuses out, across the capillary wall into the blood. The blood carries the CO_2 back to the lungs for elimination. Carbon dioxide is carried in the blood in 3 ways. A small amount, only about 5%, is dissolved in the blood plasma. A small amount (~10%) is carried chemically combined with hemoglobin (carbaminohemoglobin). Most of the CO_2 is carried in the form of HCO_3.

Membrane Lung Gas Exchange

The Avecor membrane is described in depth in chapter 8. This oxygenator was used widely in the United States until recent years when hollow fiber technology became commercially available. Briefly, a thin silicon rubber sheet with a plastic screen spacer inside is wound around a polycarbonate core and encased in a silicon rubber sheath. This design allows blood to flow on one side of the sheet and gas to flow on the other. The partial pressures of oxygen and carbon dioxide are the driving forces of diffusion across the screen spacer.

An important factor of this membrane is the concentrations of CO_2 on either side of the membrane. Carbon dioxide transfers at a rate six times that of oxygen. This can necessitate the use of a carbon dioxide enriched gas to be blended in. A flow meter and blender are used to regulate gas flow to the membrane. The characteristics of this membrane limit the gas flow so if the gas phase pressure exceeds the blood phase, air emboli can occur. Another important factor is that the transfer of carbon dioxide is independent of blood flow but dependent on the membrane's surface area. Loss of surface area will affect carbon dioxide transfer. The third important factor of CO_2 exchange is the gas flow rate. Increasing the total gas flow rate by increasing the oxygen gas flow will result in a decrease of the concentration of CO_2 gas in the sweep gas across the membrane, and thus decreasing the CO_2 content in the blood. The opposite will increase the CO_2 content in the blood.

The partial pressure of oxygen is high in the sweep gas causing a larger driving force for oxygen to cross the silicone membrane quickly. The red blood cells entering the oxygenator in proximity to the membrane become saturated with oxygen. The oxygen diffuses further into the blood flow, increasing the pO_2. The blood path thickness is an important factor to consider in oxygen exchange. The pattern of blood flow through the silicon membrane is laminar, which decreases the exposure of blood to the membrane. The blood flow in the center of the blood phase is less saturated. Increasing the flow rate will drive more blood across the surface of the membrane and improve oxygenation, to a certain point, then it will become too short of a time period

CO2 Exchange (air flow variable)	O2 Exchange (blood flow variable)
Independent of blood flow	Independent of sweep gas flow rate
Dependent on gas diffusion gradient	Dependent on blood flow rate
Dependent on sweep gas flow rate	Dependent on blood path thickness
Dependent on membrane surface area	Dependent on membrane diffusion thickness
	Dependent on O2 concentrations
	Dependent on membrane surface area

for the oxygen to reach the flow center. The larger the surface area of an oxygenator means more blood is exposed to oxygen. The flow rate of the sweep gas will not affect the oxygen content of the blood since the oxygen content of the sweep gas is greater than that of the blood.

Oxygenators are flow rated. This is the highest blood flow rate recommended for maximal oxygen delivery by each specific device. (See Figure 2)

Now that it is commercially available, use of the polymethylpentene hollow fiber non-microporous membrane is increasing. Even though the surface area is decreased, the design of this oxygenator optimizes the blood flow path. The principles of oxygen and carbon dioxide transfer are the same. As with the silastic membrane, the hollow fiber membranes are given rated gas and blood flow limits by the manufacturers. The low resistance of this membrane makes it easy to prime and blood flow through it is efficiently distributed.

Pathophysiology of Membrane Lungs

Understanding the gas exchange characteristics of the membrane oxygenator are an important factor in diagnosing its potential malfunctions. Membrane oxygenators can develop pulmonary edema, ventilation/perfusion mismatch, pulmonary emboli, and other functioning abnormalities.

Perfusion of the membrane can be affected by thrombosis of the inlets, distribution ports, membrane cells, or blood leakage into the gas phase. This not only decreases the diffusion of oxygen and carbon dioxide, but increases the blood flow resistance. Measurement of the pre-oxygenator pressure can give some indication of changes in resistance to blood flow which may correlate with thrombus or improper functioning of the membrane. Elevations in the patients arterial resistance or increases in post-oxygenator pressure can also be reflected in changes in the pre-oxygenator pressures as well. Pre-oxygenator (and often post-oxygenator) pressures are transduced to help follow the resistance to blood flow. Water vapor buildup within the oxygenator from warm blood interacting with the cooler sweep gas can result in a decrease in performance of the oxygenator in both ventilation and oxygenation. The sweep gas flow rate can be increased to help clear the fluid and blow off more carbon dioxide, similar to native increases in minute ventilation which increases carbon dioxide clearance. Membranes are gas flow rated to reduce the risk of air emboli from the gas phase into the blood phase. If gas is diverted to areas of the membrane that are not well perfused or blood flow is through areas that are not well ventilated, ventilation/perfusion mismatch occurs.

The Concept of Rated Flow

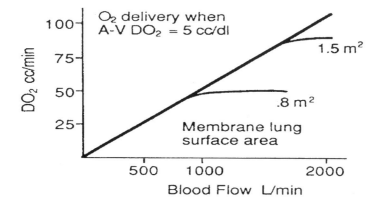

Figure 2

Figure 3 illustrates potential problems of the membrane lung. Pre and post membrane gases and membrane pressure transducing can indicate and diagnose abnormalities in function. The design of the hollow-fiber nonmicroporous membrane allows for blood to flow in a low-resistance manner and this may decrease the potential for thrombus formation within the oxygenator as compared to the silicone lung. Thrombus at stagnant areas of blood flow within microporous oxygenators can occur, however, especially at very low blood flow rates.

Oxygen Kinetics and Tissue Respiration

In normal cardiopulmonary physiology, distribution of cardiac output varies among organ systems. Metabolic rate drives oxygen consumption and as such determines blood flow to organs such as the brain, heart, skeletal muscle, kidneys, and splanchnic area; blood flow to the skin is thermally mediated. Venous blood flows from the vascular beds of these organ systems through central venous conduits (inferior and superior vena cavae)

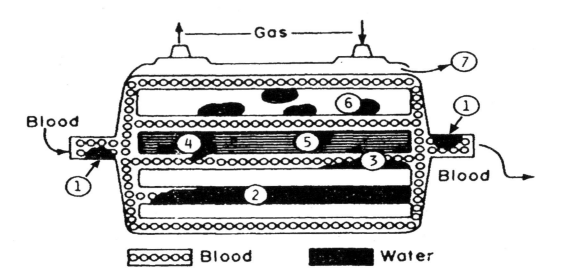

Blood Flow Obstruction	ΔO_2	ΔP	ΔCO_2
1) Inlet or Outlet Thrombosis	↓↓↓	↑↑↑	↓↓↓
2) Complete Thrombosis of cells	↓	↑	↓↓
3) Partial Thrombosis of cells	–	–	–
4) Blood Leak (may cause 5 or 6)			
Gas Flow Obstruction			
5) Complete Obstruction of Cell (Water or Blood)	↓	–	↓↓↓
6) Partial Ventilation/Obstruction of Cell (Water)	↓	–	↓↓
7) Gas Leak (may cause 6)			
Ventilation Perfusion Mismatch			
8) Poor Ventilation (6 7) in area of High Flow due to (1 2 3 4) or Design	↓	–	↓

Figure 3

to the right heart. In the pulmonary artery, oxygen saturation of mixed venous hemoglobin represents a balance of oxygen after total systemic perfusion. The variable relationships of blood flow (oxygen delivery) and oxygen extraction (consumption) in each organ are microcosms of the relationships that are measurable at the bedside (i.e., cardiac output and SVO_2). Although it is currently beyond our control to regulate individual organ perfusion in the intensive care setting, an awareness of this diversity lends itself to a better understanding of some of the intricacies of extracorporeal support and management. That said, we are driven to monitor and react to those things that reflect global support of oxygen delivery and consumption.

Within the limits of normal physiology, the cardiopulmonary system maintains an oxygen delivery to consumption ratio of 4:1. This equates to a mixed venous saturation of 75%. Since oxygen content in arterial blood is generally "fixed" cardiac output becomes the "first responder" to increase when systemic oxygen demand increases.

Oxygen Consumption

Oxygen consumption (VO_2) is the amount of oxygen utilized by tissue in aerobic metabolism. Normal resting rates for newborn infants – 5-8 ml/kg/min, children – 4-6 ml/kg/min, and adults – 3-5 ml/kg/min. These are increased by muscular activity, infection, hyperthermia, and high levels of catecholamine and thyroid hormones.

Regardless of pulmonary function, in steady state conditions, the amount of oxygen absorbed across the lung in gas exchange is equal to the amount consumed by peripheral tissue during metabolism (The Fick Principle). Oxygen consumption (VO_2) can be calculated as the product of Stroke Volume x Heart Rate x A-V O_2 difference.

Oxygen Delivery

Whereas oxyhemoglobin is the primary determinant of oxygen content in whole blood, blood flow is of equal importance in delivering oxygen to the tissues. Recall that oxygen delivery is determined by multiplying cardiac output times oxygen content. In terms of oxygen demand, cardiac output is variable so that the oxygen delivery to consumption ratio is maintained at 4:1. Thus the physiology of oxygen delivery to the tissues is such that at "fixed" oxygen content (stable Hgb, O_2 saturation) blood flow increases or decreases based on metabolic demand. SVO_2 serves as a marker of this supply demand relationship. See figure 4.

Monitoring venous saturation (SVO_2) in the management of ECMO patients is very important. The arterial blood may be fully saturated, but if the SVO_2 is low, it is obvious that consumption is disproportionate to delivery.

Oxygen Delivery / Consumption Relationship

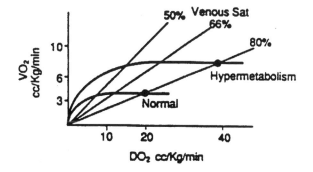

Figure 4

Oxygen Content

Oxygen content is not usually measured in the clinical applications, but is a vital consideration in the ECMO setting. In bedside assessment and management of oxygenation, focus is generally directed at PO$_2$ since it is a universally accepted parameter that reflects lung ventilation/perfusion matching. In addition, it serves as a "lab report" that enables the clinician to make adjustments in supplemental oxygen therapy and correlate patient response to the severity of lung dysfunction. Aside from this, PO$_2$ is of limited value when assessing oxygen content, since it represents oxygen dissolved in plasma, or approximately 2% of all oxygen in whole blood. The content of oxygen dissolved in plasma is calculated by multiplying PO$_2$ times the solubility coefficient of oxygen in plasma (.003).

The advent of commercially available pulse oximeters in the 1980s provided instantaneous, non-invasive assessment of oxygenation in the form of saturation of hemoglobin in arterial blood. Thus, SPO$_2$ and "sat" became common language and pulse oximetry became another vital sign. Yet, arterial oxygen saturation represents saturation of available hemoglobin only, and as such yields limited information related to oxygen content if hemoglobin concentration is unknown.

Hemoglobin is the pack mule in whole blood, accounting for 98% of transported oxygen. Each gram of hemoglobin is capable of binding 1.34cc of oxygen when all four heme sites are loaded. See Figure 5. When this state of oxygen binding occurs,

saturation of hemoglobin is 100%. Consider the following oxygen content equation:

O$_2$ content = [(Hgb x 1.34) x O$_2$ saturation] + (PaO$_2$ x .003), where Hgb = 15 gm/dl, O$_2$ saturation = 1.0 and PaO$_2$ = 90 mmhg. The equation sets up as:

Arterial O$_2$ content = [(15 x 1.34) x 1.0] + (90 x .003)

= 20.1 + 0.27

= 20.37 cc of oxygen/dl arterial blood, also expressed as 20.37 cc volume %. In this example, 98.6 % of oxygen is transported bound to hemoglobin.

Substituting different values for the variables (Hgb, O$_2$ saturation, and PO$_2$) in this equation allows for comparison of oxygen content in whole blood over a wide range of possibilities. For example, calculate the oxygen content in whole blood using the following 2 sets of variables:

Hgb 10, O$_2$ saturation 98%, PO$_2$ 100
Hgb 15, O$_2$ saturation 70%, PO$_2$ 40

Variable set "a" with an impressive PO$_2$ and O$_2$ saturation yields an O$_2$ content of 13.43 cc of oxygen per deciliter of whole blood.

Variable set "b" with a much lower PO$_2$ and O$_2$ saturation yields an O$_2$ content of 14.19 cc of oxygen per deciliter of whole blood.

By comparison, variable set "b", because of a higher hemoglobin concentration, has higher oxygen content than variable set "a". There are some take home messages. When it comes to oxygen content, blood gas reports can be misleading, but hemoglobin matters!

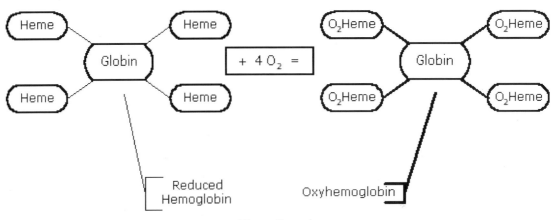

Figure 5

Oxygen - Hemoglobin Dissociation Curve

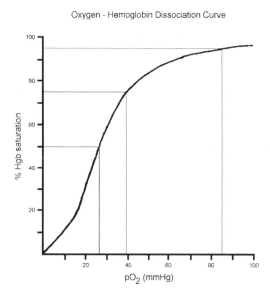

Figure 6. The oxyhemoglobin dissociation curve demonstrates oxygen saturation (SO2) and partial pressure of oxygen in the blood (PO2), and is determined by how readily hemoglobin acquires and releases oxygen molecules from its surrounding tissue. See Figure 6.

Left Shift of Oxygen - Hemoglobin Dissociation Curve

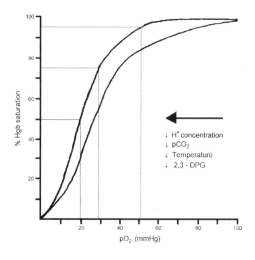

Figure 7. The curve shifting to the left results in decreased oxygen delivery to the tissue, regardless of the PO2. See Figure 7

Right Shift of Oxygen - Hemoglobin Dissociation Curve

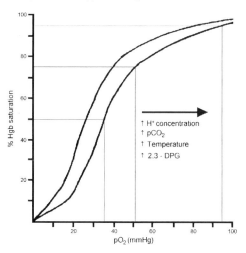

Figure 8. The curve shifting to the right results in increased oxygen to the tissues regardless of the PO2. Driving the PO2 to extreme highs has little effect on oxygen delivery if the available hemoglobin is fully saturated.

Hemodynamics

ECLS

Extracorporeal life support is indicated when cardiac and/or pulmonary failure is not amendable to conventional support. The mode of extracorporeal support is in large part driven by specific organ failure (lungs or heart). Respiratory failure with hemodynamic stability can be supported with venovenous (VV) ECLS. Hemodynamic collapse secondary to cardiac failure is an indication for the circulatory support found in the venoarterial (VA) mode of ECLS.

The concept of ECLS, whether venovenous or venoarterial, is relatively simple. Blood is drained from central venous circulation into the ECLS circuit, pumped through an extracorporeal lung, and returned to the patient. However, a thorough understanding of extracorporeal physiology including flow, circuit pressures, and gas transfer is essential to safe, effective management in addition to troubleshooting endeavors.

With extracorporeal support, flow goeth as flow cometh. Said another way, you can't make flow, you get flow. To understand this is to appreciate the importance of right heart filling pressure, venous cannula size, pump preload, and pump speed, since these are the primary determinants of flow. As Mick Jagger and the Rolling Stones once chorused, "You can't always get what you want…" In ECLS, the challenge is to find out why.

In human physiology, arterial blood pressure is a product of heart preload, rate, contractile force of the left ventricle, and resistance to flow (SVR). By comparison, central venous blood pressure is much lower, and is determined by venous blood volume and venous vascular tone. This arterial/venous pressure relationship is mimicked by extracorporeal circuit physiology. Pressure in the arterial limb of the circuit is determined by pump pre-load, pump flow, and resistance to flow (tubing, circuit components, cannula, pt. blood pressure). As flow increases, arterial limb pressure increases. Pressures as high as 300 mmhg are considered safe, although the risk of blood leaks and circuit rupture increases as pressure rises. Pressure in the venous limb is low,

since flow is generated via passive siphon or pump generated negative pressure. When pressure in the venous limb becomes sub-atmospheric, the risk for air entrainment (e.g., through a stop cock) increases. With excessive negative pressure, blood cavitation and red blood cell damage can occur.

Blood draining from central venous circulation determines pump pre-load and as such, limits pump flow, regardless of the type of perfusion system used.

Placement of the return cannula determines the mode of ECLS. The cannula should be large enough to accommodate the flow expected to support the patient so that excessively high circuit pressures are avoided. Extracorporeal blood returning to a cannula in a vein denotes venovenous support. Conversely, blood returning to a cannula in an artery denotes venoarterial bypass. Depending on the mode of ECLS, the extracorporeal physiology is said to be "in series" (VV) or "in parallel" (VA) with native cardiopulmonary physiology. Each will be covered separately.

Venovenous ECLS

VV ECLS provides respiratory gas exchange (oxygen loading, CO_2 removal) in venous blood before it reaches the right ventricle, and is indicated in the management of severe respiratory failure when conventional support methods are unsuccessful. Since blood is drained from and returned to central venous circulation, no hemodynamic support is derived from this mode of ECLS. Critical to the delivery of venovenous extracorporeal support is the ability to pump a sufficient amount of blood through the ECLS circuit so that "total" gas exchange support is provided. This is accomplished by placing a venous drainage cannula that allows for blood flow rates of 120 ml/kg/min. for neonates, 90 ml/kg/min. for pediatrics, and 60 ml/kg/min. for adults. To this end, it is common practice to select a venous drainage cannula with the shortest length and largest internal diameter so that resistance to blood flow is minimized.

The circuit components should be configured with these flow rates in mind. For instance, the extracorporeal lung should be capable of gas transfer (oxygen and carbon dioxide) well beyond the maximum anticipated metabolic requirements of the patient. This is best determined by comparing the "rated flow" capacity of the lung to the flow rates intended for the patient. The arterial cannula should be large enough to accommodate anticipated ECLS flow so that complications seen with high circuit pressures and blood shear are minimized.

Although the term "bypass" is used interchangeably with ECLS, it is in fact a misnomer when used in the context of VV ECLS, since the system functions in series with the native cardiopulmonary system. Said another way, blood is drained, oxygenated, ventilated, and returned to central venous circulation before leaving the right side of the heart. This is accomplished in one of several ways. In neonates and small pediatric patients, VV ECLS support is provided via a double lumen cannula. With placement in the right internal jugular vein (RIJ) advanced to the right atrium, blood drains through the venous lumen into the ECLS circuit and returns through the venous lumen into the ECLS circuit and returns through the arterial lumen side hole ports directed at the tricuspid valve. Having passed through the extracorporeal lung, the returning blood is oxygen enriched and ventilated to desired $PaCO_2$. As this blood exits the arterial side ports of the cannula, it mixes with native venous return in the right heart. Mixing is complete as blood exits the right ventricle. The net effect of this is improvement in oxygen content per deciliter of blood and restoration of $PaCO_2$ and pH. A newer design of venovenous cannula (Avalon, Inc), consists of 2 drainage lumens, one placed in the inferior vena cava and one in the superior vena cava, and a single return lumen which is directed at the tricuspid valve. While excellent flow and minimal recirculation can be obtained with this catheter, optimal placement requires echocardiography or fluoroscopy at the bedside. Cannulas are available in sizes from neonate to adult,

In the late stages of respiratory failure, the blood gas values in the pulmonary artery approximate systemic arterial blood gas values since native pulmonary function is severely compromised. Although VV ECLS offers no direct hemodynamic support, arterial admixture of mixed venous blood in this mode of extracorporeal support increases availability of oxygen to the coronary circulation as it ejects from the left ventricle.

In larger patients, traditional VV ECLS may involve 2-site cannulation. Cannulae are placed into the RIJ and either the right or left femoral vein. Direction of flow (venous outflow and arterial return) is at the discretion of the ECMO physiciani, being influenced by anatomical factors (e.g., vessel size, obesity) that would impact on the ability to siphon sufficient blood to provide full support to the patient.

"Recirculation" is an aspect that is common only to venovenous ECLS and is seen with either method of cannulation (1 or 2 cannulae), as some oxygenated blood is inadvertently siphoned into venous drainage. This occurs because blood is drained from and returned to the same blood path. The end result of this is arterial "contamination" of venous blood which invalidates circuit SVO_2 as a true marker of oxygenation support. More importantly, recirculation limits the efficacy of VV support since that portion of blood never reaches native circulation. To compensate for this, higher ECLS blood flow is required, but flows >400-500 mL/min will result in higher recirculation and my in fact reduce oxygenation." As a result, arterial oxygen saturations of 80-95% are seen at maximum flow. To the ECLS specialist, increasing recirculation is recognized as falling arterial oxygen saturation (SPO_2) simultaneous with an increasing circuit mixed venous oxygen saturation (SVO_2). This is amendable with head/neck repositioning in the patient cannulated with a dual lumen neck cannula. Recirculation with 2-site cannulation is seen when the tips of the drainage and reinfusion cannulae are in close proximity, and may be amendable with cannula repositioning Direction of 2-site VV blood flow may influence the extent of recirculation, with a decrease in recirculation often obtained by drainage from the femoral cannula and return into the IJ site.

Venoarterial ECLS

Unlike VV ECLS, venoarterial (VA) ECLS offers hemodynamic support (in addition to respiratory gas exchange). As with VV support, central venous circulation serves as the source for ECLS pump pre-load. The return cannula however, is placed into an artery, thus creating a cardio-pulmonary bypass system that parallels native cardio-pulmonary physiology. By design, VA ECLS does not capture all venous return to the right heart as is seen with CPB in the OR. Thus, only a portion of the blood, determined by pump speed, is drained into the ECLS circuit, routed through an extracorporeal lung, and returned to arterial circulation. The remainder of venous return to the right heart follows the physiologic pathway across native lungs to the left heart where it is pumped into the aorta. Gas exchange across the native lungs is a function of ventilation to perfusion relationship and the extent of any pulmonary impairment. The net change in arterial oxygen content and $PaCO_2$ depends on native cardiac output, native pulmonary function, ECLS sweep, ECLS flow, oxyhemoglobin, and site of convergence of ECLS perfusate and native circulation. Site placement of the arterial cannula affects how, and to what extent, the 2 circulations mix. Cannulation of the right common carotid artery (RCCA) or transthoracic cannulation of the aorta ensures adequate mixing of both circulations, resulting in improved systemic oxygen delivery and pH balance. Selective perfusion of the right arm from streaming of arterialized blood down the RCCA and subclavian vessel invalidates arterial blood gas sampling from the right radial artery as a marker of total body gas exchange support.

In large pediatric and adult patients, cannulation of the femoral artery provides hemodynamic support, but delivery of oxygenated perfusate to the aortic arch and coronary arteries can be compromised in the presence of respiratory failure with significant native cardiac output. In this configuration, cardiac output "competes" with retrograde flow of ECLS perfusate in the descending aorta and may prevent perfusion of the arch vessels and aortic root with oxygenated blood. In this situation, pulmonary capillary blood, with poor ventilation/perfusion matching in the lungs, returns essentially as mixed venous blood to the left heart where it is ejected into the aorta. As a result, the coronary and cerebral circulations are perfused with hypoxemic blood. This relationship should be suspected when hypoxemia exists, as evidenced by right radial arterial blood gas analysis (site of choice with femoral arterial cannulation), or by disparity in SPO_2 obtained from different sites (left hand SPO_2 > right hand SPO_2). This may be amendable to increased extracorporeal flow, or may require placement of a cannula into a large vein (RIJ), thus changing the

mode of support to venoarterial venous (V-AV). In this configuration, a split in the arterial limb of the circuit is created so that a portion of this oxygenated perfusate is delivered to the right heart, mimicking VV ECLS. This allows for oxygen enrichment of mixed venous blood with improvement in oxygen delivery to the coronary and cerebral circulations. The hemodynamic support of this configuration remains intact, since the balance of ECLS flow is delivered to arterial circulation. Distribution of V-AV flow is determined by assessment of oxygenation and hemodynamic support. Left unchecked, extracorporeal perfusate would take the path of least resistance, flowing to central venous circulation, and robbing arterial circulation of blood flow intended for hemodynamic support. Taken to the extreme, the potential for left-to-right shunting through the ECLS circuit would occur if aortic antegrade flow exceeded extracorporeal flow, thus creating an "A-V" loop, resulting in severe hypotension. For this reason, distribution of flow is controlled by application of an external clamp to the venous "return" line to the patient. Adjusting tension on the clamp controls blood flow to this limb of the circuit, enabling the specialist to affect the desired oxygen saturation and hemodynamic support. Inotropes or pressors may be required to maintain desired mean arterial blood pressure (MAP) if this strategy compromises hemodynamic support.

Extracorporeal blood flow is non-pulsatile. In the VA mode of support, this characteristic affects arterial pulse pressure contour. Increasing pump speed obligates more venous blood to drain into the circuit, thus decreasing right and left heart preload. As a consequence, left ventricular stroke volume decreases, as evidenced by a dampened contour of the arterial blood pressure tracing. With increasing extracorporeal flow, the arterial pressure tracing dampens further, and pulse pressure narrows, although MAP remains fairly constant. For this reason, MAP, rather than systemic blood pressure, is assessed as a marker of hemodynamic support. A flat pressure tracing with no pulse pressure is indicative of total bypass, although lower ECLS flow with residual pulsatility is desirable in most instances. Typically, extracorporeal flow is managed between 60%-80% of predicted resting cardiac output.

Absence of pulsatility as seen with cardiomyopathy or cardiac stun may be a harbinger of pulmonary hemorrhage despite right heart preload reduction with VA ECLS, since any filling of the left atrium (thebesian and bronchial venous drainage) elevates left heart filling pressure in the absence of left ventricular contractility. In this setting, an atrial septostomy allows high left atrial pressures to vent to the right atrium, which has been cannulated for venous drainage to the ECLS circuit. Alternatively, cannulation of the left atrium with connection to the venous limb of the ECLS circuit effectively reduces left heart pressures. Either method introduces left heart blood to the venous circulation of the ECLS circuit, and circuit SVO_2 may be skewed if native pulmonary function oxygenates any blood that traverses the pulmonary capillary circuit. This is more likely to occur with atrial septostomies since mixing occurs in the right atrium. With left atrial cannulation, placement of an external SVO_2 probe proximal to the convergence of right and left heart circuit drainage ensures that SVO_2 is not contaminated by left heart blood.

Summary

A thorough understanding of cardio-pulmonary physiology is essential to management of cardio-pulmonary failure. Advancements in medicine and medical technology enable care providers to successfully treat heart and lung failure that would otherwise carry high mortality rates. Extracorporeal Life Support is among those technologies, although not necessarily on the front line. The management arsenal for treatment of pulmonary failure includes low stretch mechanical ventilation with permissive hypercapnea, high frequency oscillatory ventilation (HFOV), synthetic surfactants, and inhaled nitric oxide. Each (or any combination) of these treatment options are likely to be selected before considering extracorporeal life support. Those patients who have refractory failure thus present a serious challenge to management with ECLS, since time, disease progression, and organ damage begin closing a window of opportunity for healing and meaningful recovery. Management of cardiac failure takes on a different look, typically relying on inotropes, vasoactive agents, and fluids to affect end organ perfusion. Treatment options for cardiac failure not amendable to these strategies include several extracorporeal support options such as tandem hearts, ventricular

assist devices, and ECLS. As with pulmonary failure, successful management of cardiac failure with extracorporeal support is predicated on timeliness and appropriateness of intervention.

Editorial

Heidi J. Dalton, MD, FCCM

Understanding the physiology of the ECMO circuit is paramount to proper assessment of the adequacy of ECLS support and to identify problems. The goal of support is to improve oxygen delivery, provide ventilation by carbon dioxide removal and allow reduction of toxic ventilator settings to promote lung healing. Provision of enhanced oxygen delivery by the ECLS system can help "rest" the heart, the lungs and give needed oxygen nourishment to secondary organs. Understanding of the role of hemoglobin, oxygen tension and factors that affect oxygen delivery will help the specialist provide better care at the bedside to the patient. Identifying changes between venovenous and venoarterial cannulation setups is also important to accurate interpretation of parameters assessed during ECMO such as blood gas information, venous saturation data and blood pressure.

References

ECMO Specialist Training Manual. 2nd Edition. Krisa Van Muers, MD, [et al]. ELSO; 1999.

Bartlett RH. ECMO Extracorporeal Cardiopulmonary Support in Critical Care 3rd Edition. *Physiology of Extracorporeal Life Support. ELSO; 2002.* p.2-25

Meyer, Dan M, Jessen, Michael E, *Extracorporeal Life Support. Landes Bioscience, 2001.*

Maquet. Quadrox D Overview page. Available at: http://www.maquet.com. Accessed January 19, 2008.

Chapter 5 Questions

1. Oxygenation exchange in a membrane lung is effected by all except the following:
    a. Blood flow rate
    b. Blood path thickness
    c. Sweep gas flow
    d. Oxygen concentration

2. Membrane failure can be characterized by a raising pump CO_2 level because of the following
    a. changes in blood flow patterns caused by clot formation
    b. changes in sweep gas flow patterns caused by clot formation
    c. alteration in membrane surface area caused by fibrin formation
    c. changes in oxygen concentrations due to fibrin formation

3. ECMO improves oxygen delivery by which mechanism:
    a. improving oxygen content through stabilization of hemoglobin saturations
    b. improving oxygen content by taking over at least 60% of the blood flow through a functioning membrane lung, away from the sick native lung
    c. stabilizing oxygen delivery by taking over at least 60% of the cardiac output through the ECMO pump
    d. all of the above

Chapter 5 Answers

1. c
2. c
3. d

6

Extracorporeal Membrane Oxygenation Cannulation and Decannulation

K. Rais-Bahrami, MD. and David M. Powell, MD.

Objectives

After completion of this chapter, the participant should be able to:

- Outline the equipment, personnel, medications needed for an ECMO cannulation and decannulation
- Discuss risks associated with cannulation and decannulation
- Discuss Pro/Con of VA vs VV ECMO

Venoarterial Extracorporeal Membrane Oxygenation—Cannulation

Indications:

Placement of carotid arterial and internal jugular venous catheters for use in venoarterial ECMO. Venoarterial ECMO should be used in patients with significant cardiovascular instability.

Precautions:

1. Ensure that the patient is paralyzed and sedated before placement of the venous catheter, to prevent air embolus.
2. Recognize that:
   a. Internal jugular lines placed for intravenous access prior to ECMO may cause clot formation, resulting in the need for thrombectomy before the placement of the venous ECMO catheter.
   b. Excessive manipulation of the internal jugular vein may cause spasm and in-

ability to place a catheter of appropriate size.
   c. A ruptured vessel may result in the need for a sternotomy for vessel retrieval. Appropriate instruments should be on the bedside tray. A backup unit of blood should be available in the blood bank.
   d. Blood loss sufficient to produce hypotension can occur during a difficult ECMO cannulation. Emergency blood should be available at the bedside (10 to 20 mL/kg).
   e. The vagus nerve is located next to the neck vessels and may be injured or manipulated during isolation of the vessels. Manipulation can cause bradycardia or other cardiac arrhythmias.
   f. Vital signs and pulse oximetry values must be monitored at all times because clinical observation of the patient is prevented by the use of surgical drapes.
   g. If the patient has been hand bag ventilated for stabilization, do not place the Ambu bag on the bedside when surgical drapes are placed. The bag may entrap oxygen, which can result in a fire when electrocautery is used.

Personnel, Equipment, and Medications[1]

Personnel
1. Surgical team
   a. An experienced pediatric, cardiovascular, or thoracic surgeon with assistant
   b. A surgical scrub nurse and circulating nurse

2. Medical team
   a. A physician trained in management of ECMO patients and cannulation techniques, who will administer anesthetic agents and medically manage the patient during the cannulation procedure
   b. A bedside intensive care nurse who will monitor vital signs, record events, and draw up medications as needed by the ECMO physicians
   c. A respiratory therapist who will manage the ventilator settings as necessary
3. Circuit specialists
   a. Cardiovascular perfusionist, nurse, or respiratory therapist specially trained in this procedure who will prime the ECMO pump
   b. A bedside ECMO specialist with special training in ECMO who will manage the ECMO system after the patient is on ECMO

Equipment:

Sterile

1. Arterial and venous catheters[2]
   a. Arterial
      (1) The size of the arterial catheter determines the resistance of the ECMO circuit, because it is the part of the ECMO circuit with the smallest internal diameter and thus the highest resistance.
      (2) This catheter should be as short as possible, with a thin wall and a large internal diameter (resistance is directly related to the length of the catheter and inversely related to the diameter). An example of a suitable catheter is the Bio-Medicus Extracorporeal Circulation Cannula 8 to 10 French (Fr) (Bio-Medicus, Minneapolis, MN, U.S.A.).
   b. Venous
      (1) Venous catheter should have as large an internal diameter as possible to allow maximal blood flow (patient's oxygenation is directly related to the rate of blood flow)
      (2) Should be thin walled with a large internal diameter. An example of a suitable catheter is the Bio-Medicus Extracorporeal Circulation Cannula 8 to 14 Fr. (Bio-Medicus, Minneapolis, MN, U.S.A.).
2. Surgical instruments required include:

Sterile

- Gowns and gloves
- Saline for injection
- Syringes (1 to 20 mL) and needles (19 to 26 gauge)
- Povidone–iodine solution
- Povidone–iodine ointment
- Semi-permeable transparent membrane-type dressing
- Absorbable gelatin sponge, for example Gelfoam® (Upjohn, Kalamazoo, MI, U.S.A.)
- Surgical lubricant, bacteriostatic

Nonsterile

- Surgical head covers and mask
- Pulse oximeter
- Surgical head light
- Electrocautery
- Wall suction
- Shoulder roll, for example a small blanket, to place under patient's shoulders
- Tubing clamps

Medications

1. A long-acting paralyzing agent, for example pancuronium bromide (0.1 mg/kg)
2. Fentanyl citrate (10 to 20 Microgram/kg)
3. Sodium heparin (75 to 150 Units/kg)
4. Topical thrombin / Gelfoam®
5. Xylocaine, 0.25% with epinephrine
6. Xylocaine, 1% plain (without epinephrine)
7. Cryoprecipitate, thawed or commercially available fibrin sealant (optional)

Technique–Preparation for Cannulation

1. Place patient with head to "foot" of the bed..
2. Anesthetize the patient with fentanyl (10 to 20 Microgram/kg).
3. Paralyze the patient with pancuronium (0.1 mg/Kg).
4. Hyperextend the patient's neck with a shoulder roll, and turn the head to the left (Figure 1). Make sure that the Bovie ground pad is placed.
5. Monitor vital signs and give additional fentanyl and/or pancuronium as needed.
6. Clean a wide area of the right neck, chest, and ear with Betadine solution.
7. Drape the infant and entire bed with sterile towels.
8. Use Steri-Drapes®(3M Health Care, St. Paul, MN, U.S.A.) to secure the towels to the skin.
9. At the point of incision, infiltrate the skin with Xylocaine (AstraZeneca, Wayne, PA, U.S.A.) (0.25% with epinephrine) (Figure 1).
10. Wait at least 3 minutes for anesthesia to be effective.
11. Make a 1- to 2-cm vertical incision over the right sternocleidomastoid muscle, starting approximately 1 cm above the right clavicular head, using the electrocautery set on cutting current (Figure 2).

12. Continue to use the electrocautery to cut through the subcutaneous tissue.
13. Coagulate all visible bleeding sites.
14. Spread the fibers of the sternocleidomastoid muscle apart with a hemostat and retract using hemostats clamped onto the muscle (Figure 3).
15. Open the carotid sheath, taking care to avoid the vagus nerve.
16. Irrigate both common carotid artery and internal jugular vein with 1% plain Xylocaine to vasodilate the vessels.

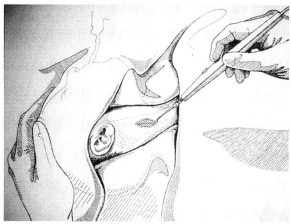

Figure. 2. Landmarks over the sternocleidomastoid muscle for making the incision with electrocautery. (From Short BL. CNMC ECMO training manual. 2005, with permission)

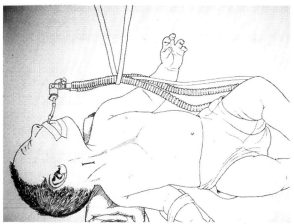

Figure 1. Infant positioned for cannulation with shoulder roll present and head extended to the left. Position of neck incision is indicated. (From Short BL. CNMC ECMO training manual. 2005, with permission)

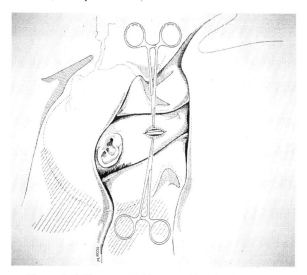

Figure 3 Split sternocleidomastoid and open carotid sheath. (From Short BL. CNMC ECMO training manual. 2005, with permission)

17. Encircle the artery with silicone loop, and proximal and distal 2-0 silk ties held with clamps but not tied. Avoid "sawing" the ties on the artery.
18. Avoid excessive handling of the internal jugular vein. Some isolate the vein after cannulation of the carotid artery to avoid spasm.
19. Estimate the length of the cannula to be inserted.
    a. Identify the sternal notch and the xiphoid process.
    b. The arterial catheter is inserted approximately one-third of the distance between the sternal notch and the xiphoid process. This is typically between 3-4 cm.
    c. The venous catheter is inserted approximately one-half the distance between the sternal notch and the xiphoid process. This is typically between 7-7.5 cm.
    d. Mark these distances on the catheters with a 2-0 tie, or note the distance if the cannula is marked.
20. Heparinize the patient with a bolus of 75 to 150 U/kg of sodium heparin, depending on the estimated risk of bleeding, and wait 60 to 90 seconds before proceeding with cannulation.

Arterial Cannulation

1. Tie the distal ligature on the carotid artery, and place a bulldog clamp on the proximal portion of the artery. Allow blood to dilate the artery before placing the bulldog clamp.
2. Make an arteriotomy using a no. 11 scalpel blade, and place two traction sutures of 6-0 Prolene (Ethicon, Somerville, NJ, U.S.A) on the proximal side of the arteriotomy (Figure 4). Always use traction sutures to prevent intimal tears.
3. If desired, lubricate Garrett dilators with sterile surgical lubricant and dilate the artery to the approximate size of the catheter.
4. Place a sterile tubing clamp on the catheter. Lubricate the catheter and insert the catheter into the vessel as the bulldog clamp is removed.
5. Secure the catheter with a 2-0 silk ligature tied over a 0.5- to 1-cm vessel loop (Figure 5A).
6. Place a second 2-0 silk ligature. Tie the distal tie around the catheter, and then tie the distal and proximal ties together. Some

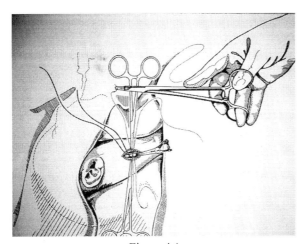

Figure 4 A

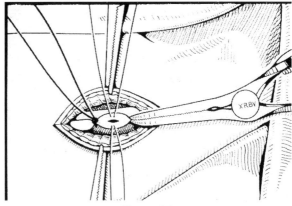

Figure 4 B

Figure 4 A & B
4A: Carotid artery isolated with vessel clamp in place and with arteriotomy site showing the placement of the 6-0 Prolene traction sutures. 4B (inset): Magnified view of A.
(From Short BL. CNMC ECMO training manual. 2005, with permission)

surgeons place two ties proximally and one distal for added security.

7. Allow blood to back up into the catheter to remove air.

Venous Cannulation

1. Dissect the vein free and isolate with two 2-0 silk ties. Do not apply traction to the vein with the ties, to avoid spasm.

2. Place a bulldog clamp on the proximal end of the vein, allowing blood to distend the vein. Then tie the distal end of the vein with the 2-0 silk tie.

3. Make a venotomy with a no. 11 scalpel blade, and place two stay sutures of 6-0 Prolene as traction sutures, as for arterial cannulation.

4. Lubricate the venous catheter, place a sterile tubing clamp on the catheter, and dilate the venotomy.

5. Insert the catheter as an assistant places traction on the proximal tie, and apply pressure over the liver to increase the backflow of blood out of the catheter (to decrease the risk of an air embolus). There will be a slight impedance to catheter advancement at the thoracic inlet—pushing against resistance will tear the vein. Use gentle downward and posterior pressure.

6. Secure, as for the artery, and return blood into the catheter by pressing gently on the liver.

7. If desired, pack the wound with absorbable gelatin sponge soaked in topical thrombin or commercially available topical fibrin sealant, Tisseel-HV® Fibrin Sealant (Baxter

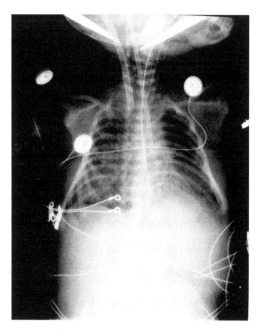

Figure 6. X-ray at cannulation, showing proper placement of the arterial and venous catheters. Note the radiopaque dot indicating the end of the Bio-Medicus venous extracorporeal membrane oxygenation catheter (arrow). (From Short BL. CNMC ECMO training manual. 2005, with permission)

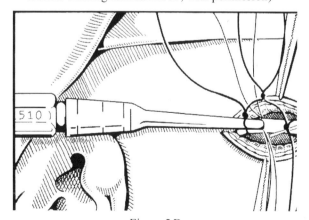

Figure 5 A   Figure 5 B

Figure 5 A & B. A: Securing the catheter with proximal and distal ties onto a "bootie." B (inset): Magnified view of A. (From Short BL. CNMC ECMO training manual. 2005, with permission)

Hyland Division, Glendale, CA, U.S.A.) to assist in hemostasis.

8. Confirm catheter placement by chest x-ray and/or cardiac echocardiography, if the patient is stable (Figure 6).[3] If unstable, the patient can be placed on ECMO and the x-ray taken when adequate oxygenation is achieved but prior to closing the surgical wound.

Venovenous Extracorporeal Membrane Oxygenation—Cannulation

More than 60% of neonatal ECMO patients reported in the ELSO registry have received treatment with venoarterial bypass.[4] In neonates with respiratory failure, venoarterial ECMO is gradually being replaced by a venovenous technique, which uses a single double-lumen catheter (Figure 7). The catheter is placed in the right atrium, where blood is drained and reinfused into the same chamber, thus requiring cannulation of only the right jugular vein, sparing the carotid artery. Other advantages of VV ECMO include maintenance of normal pulsatile blood flow, and the theoretical advantage that particles entering the ECMO circuit enter by way of the pulmonary rather than the systemic circulation. The design of the original VV catheter resulted in significant recirculation, limiting its use when ECMO flows >350 ml/min were required. Research by Rais-Bahrami et al. resulted in development of a new catheter design which significantly lowers the degree of recirculation.[5] The double-lumen catheter should be placed within the right atrium, directing the oxygenated blood from the return lumen through the tricuspid valve to minimize recirculation. Availability of this catheter design in 12, 15, and 18 Fr. sizes allows the use of VV ECMO in a greater number of patients.[6]

Advantages of Venovenous Bypass
1. Provides excellent pulmonary support
2. Avoids carotid artery ligation
3. Oxygenated blood enters pulmonary circulation.
4. Particles coming from the ECMO circuit enter the venous circulation instead of the arterial circulation.

Disadvantages of Venovenous Bypass
1. Lack of cardiac support
2. ECMO support is dependent on the patient's cardiac function.
3. Catheter position and rotation are extremely critical.
4. Amount of recirculation

Cannulation Technique

The cannulation technique for venovenous ECMO is essentially the same procedure as venous cannulation for venoarterial ECMO, with the following exceptions:
1. Both internal jugular vein and carotid arteries are identified and dissected, although the internal jugular vein is the only vessel cannulated with the double-lumen venovenous catheter. A silastic loop may be tied loosely around the artery to facilitate potential conversion to venoarterial flow. Both vessels are isolated in case a rapid conversion to venoarterial bypass becomes necessary.

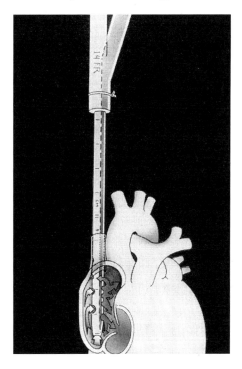

Figure 7. Schematic of the venovenous extracorporeal membrane oxygenation catheter placed in the midright atrium. (From Short BL. CNMC ECMO training manual. 2005, with permission)

2. The catheter is advanced in a direction with the arterial side upward and anterior to the venous limb of the double-lumen cannula. The correct position of the catheter helps direct the oxygenated blood return toward the tricuspid valve, thus minimizing the recirculation of the oxygenated blood back to the ECMO circuit.

3. The proximal end of the internal jugular vein is also cannulated for cephalad drainage, which is, a jugular bulb catheter. This catheter is connected to the venous tubing of the ECMO circuit via a 3-way luer connector. For this, we use a custom-made Carmeda® heparin-coated Bio-Medicus venous catheter, made specifically for use as a cephalad catheter. This allows additional venous drainage to the ECMO circuit, preventing venous congestion, and also allows for cephalic venous saturation measurement.

4. If using a jugular bulb catheter to measure cerebral saturations, care should be used when entering the circuit; air will draw into the venous side of the circuit rapidly if a stopcock is loose or left open.

Placing Patient on the Extracorporeal Membrane Oxygenation Circuit

The circuit has been previously primed with packed cells/albumin. The priming procedure and the surgical placement of the ECMO catheters should be timed so that the two are completed at the same time. Priming of the circuit is beyond the scope of this chapter.

1. Fill catheters with sterile saline. Connect them to the ECMO circuit by inserting the 1/4 x 1/4 inch connectors into the tubing as the assistant drips sterile saline into the ends of the circuit tubing and the catheter, to ensure that all residual air is eliminated prior to connection.
   a. Do not squeeze the tubing while attaching; air will enter when the tubing is released.
   b. If air is seen in the tubing, the catheters must be disconnected from the circuit. Prior to reconnection, air is removed, and the catheters are reconnected as described.

2. Remove all sterile tubing clamps from the catheters, and have an assistant hold the catheters.

3. Place the patient on ECMO by removing the arterial clamp, and removing the venous clamp. This will remove all clamps from the circuit.

4. Increase ECMO flow in 50-mL increments over 20-30 minutes, until adequate oxygenation is achieved (usually at 120 mL/kg/min).

5. Decrease the ventilator settings and oxygen concentration gradually as the ECMO circuit flows are increased.

Closure of the Neck Wound

1. Ensure x-ray confirmation of appropriate catheter position and the achievement of an adequate flow rate through the ECMO circuit, prior to closure of the neck wound.

2. Cut and remove traction sutures.

3. Approximate the skin with a running 4-0 Vicryl (Ethicon) suture on an atraumatic needle.

4. Tie the Vicryl suture, and use the tails of the suture to secure each catheter.

5. Tie catheters together with another silk tie.

6. Anesthetize the area behind the ear with 0.25% Xylocaine with epinephrine.

7. Use 2-0 silk suture on a non-cutting needle to place a stitch behind the ear and tie around the catheter to secure in place. Place a separate stitch for each catheter.

8. Tie catheters together, dress the incision with povidone–iodine ointment, and cover the area with semi-permeable membrane dressing.

9. Tape the circuit tubing securely to the bedside to reduce traction on the catheters.

Complications

1. Torn vessels, more commonly the vein
   a. This risk is decreased if the 6-0 Prolene stay sutures are always used.

b. Do not attempt to use too large a catheter.
2. Aortic dissection associated with arterial cannulation (7)
3. Blood loss, particularly during the venous cannulation, when side holes in the catheter are outside the vein
4. Venous spasm, resulting in inability to place a large enough venous catheter to meet the required ECMO flow to adequately support the patient
5. Arrhythmias and/or bradycardia can occur, owing to stimulation of the vagus nerve

Extracorporeal Membrane Oxygenation— Decannulation

Precautions

1. The patient must be paralyzed during the removal of the venous catheter to avoid an air embolus.
2. The vessels are fragile and may tear. A backup unit of blood should be available at the bedside.

Personnel, Equipment, and Medications

Personnel

Same as for cannulation, with the exception of the perfusionist

Equipment

Sterile
- Surgical tray with towels and suture as for cannulation
- Semi-permeable transparent dressing
- Povidone–iodine ointment
- Syringes (1 to 20 mL) and needles (18 to 26 gauge)
- Unit of blood
- Absorbable gelatin sponge

Nonsterile
- Same as for cannulation

Medications

1. Fentanyl (10 to 20 Microgram/kg)
2. Vecuronium bromide (0.2 mg/kg). A short-acting paralyzing agent is preferred because of the relatively short duration of the procedure.
3. Xylocaine 0.25% with epinephrine
4. Topical thrombin
5. Protamine sulfate (1 mg)

Technique

Post-decannulation vessel reconstruction is beyond the scope of this chapter.

1. Place the neck in an extended position, using the shoulder roll.
2. Give fentanyl for relaxation, prior to giving vecuronium.. Because of the risk of air embolism during the removal of the venous catheter, the patient must NOT be allowed to breathe during decannulation.
3. Increase ventilator setting to a rate of 40-50 breaths/min, a peak inspiratory pressure of 20-25 cm H_2O (depending on chest movement), and FiO_2 of 0.30-0.40 after paralytic agent is given.
4. Clean the neck, and drape as for cannulation.
5. Anesthetize with 0.25% Xylocaine with epinephrine.
6. Cut and remove the Vicryl suture.
7. Remove absorbable gelatin sponge packing, exposing the catheters and vessels.
8. Jugular bulb catheter should be clamped off before its' removal, after the patient is taken off bypass. Be aware that removing the catheter while on bypass without a clamp in place will result in the introduction of air into the circuit.
9. Separate the catheter from surrounding tissue by blunt dissection.
10. Encircle the vein with a 2-0 silk tie, which is used for traction and hemostatic control.
11. Place a Satinsky clamp around the vein to stabilize the catheter (Figure 8).
12. Place a 2-0 silk tie proximal to the clamp.
13. Cut the silk ties securing the catheter in the vein with a no. 11 scalpel blade. The two proximal ties should be cut where they cross the vessel loop.

14. The ECMO specialist to remove the patient from the ECMO circuit.
15. Monitor vital signs and oxygen saturation as an indication that ventilator settings are appropriate. Settings may have to be increased when the patient is removed from the ECMO support.
16. Provide an inspiratory "hold" on the ventilator while the surgeon places pressure on the liver and removes the venous catheter. Failure to do this can result in air embolus.
17. Replace any significant blood loss.
18. Cut the 2-0 silk traction suture and tie the suture proximal to the Satinsky clamp. Remove the Satinsky clamp.
19. Isolate the arterial catheter, dissect free, and remove. The decannulation procedure is the same as for the venous catheter, with the exception that an inspiratory hold is not required.
20. Give protamine (1 mg IV.) after removal of both catheters. Administration of protamine is not mandatory if there is no significant bleeding.
21. Irrigate the wound with sterile saline and cauterize any bleeding sites.

22. Close the neck incision using subcuticular horizontal sutures of 4-0 Vicryl.
23. Remove the sutures holding the cannula behind the right ear.
24. Place povidone–iodine ointment over the incision and cover with semi-permeable transparent dressing.

Complications

1. Vessel laceration.
2. Excessive blood loss
3. Venous air embolus

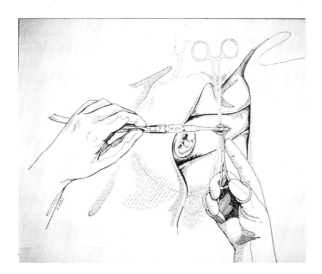

Figure 8. Placement of Satinsky vessel clamp prior to removal of extracorporeal membrane oxygenation catheter. (From Short BL. CNMC ECMO training manual. 2005, with permission)

References

1. Allison P, Kurusz M, Graves D, et al. Devices and monitoring during neonatal ECMO: survey results. *Perfusion* 1990;5:193.
2. Van Meurs K, Mikesell G, Seale W, et al. Maximum blood flow rates for arterial cannulae used in neonatal ECMO. *ASAIO Trans* 1990;36:M679.
3. Irish M, O'Toole S, Kapur P, et al. Cervical ECMO cannula placement in infants and children: recommendations for assessment of adequate positioning and function. *J Pediatr Surg* 1998;33:929.
4. Neonatal ECMO Registry of The Extracorporeal Life Support Organization (ELSO). Ann Arbor, MI, July 2007.
5. Rais-Bahrami K, Rivera O, Mikesell G, et al. Improved Oxygenation with Reduced Recirculation During Venovenous Extracorporeal Membrane Oxygenation: Evaluation of a Test Catheter. *Crit Care Med* 1995;23:1722.
6. Rais-Bahrami K, Walton D, Sell J, et al. Improved Oxygenation with Reduced Recirculation During Venovenous ECMO: Comparison of Two Catheters. *Perfusion* 2002;17:415.
7. Paul J, Desai H, Baumgart S, et al. Aortic dissection in a neonate associated with arterial cannulation for extracorporeal life support. *ASAIO* 1997;43:92.

Chapter 6 Questions

1. The following are advantages of VV- ECMO support in neonates, Except:
a) Major advantage of VV-ECMO is that it avoids ligation of carotid artery
b) VV-ECMO Provides excellent pulmonary support
c) Oxygenated blood enters pulmonary circulation
d) Particles coming from the ECMO circuit directly enter the patient's cerebral circulation.
e) None of the above

2. What are the major disadvantages of VV-ECMO support in neonates?
a) ECMO support is dependent on the patient's cardiac function.
b) Catheter position and rotation are extremely critical.
c) In VV-ECMO the circuit venous saturation is mixed with arterial recirculation loosing its monitoring value
d) In VV-ECMO the flow required to support the patient may be limited by its recirculation
e) All of the above

3. For which of the following patients would you prefer VA vs. VV-ECMO support?
a) An infant with severe respiratory failure
b) A newborn with echo-cardiographic evidence of cardiomyopathy
c) A Pre-ECMO, ultrasound evidence of grade 1 IVH.
d) A 3 day old, 2.8 Kg infant, born at 36 weeks gestational age with MAS
e) None of the above

4. What are the potential complications during ECMO cannulation?
a) Torn vessels, more commonly during the vein than arterial cannulation
b) Aortic dissection associated with arterial cannulation
c) Blood loss, particularly during the venous cannulation, when side holes in the catheter are outside the vein
d) Cardiac arrhythmias and/or bradycardia
e) All of the above

Chapter 6 Answers

1. d
2. e
3. b
4. e

7

Principles and Practice of Venovenous and Venoarterial Extracorporeal Membrane Oxygenation

Micheal L. Heard, RN, Joel Davis, RRT-NPS, AE-C, James D. Fortenberry, MD

Objectives

After completion of this chapter, the participant should be able to:

- Describe the advantages and disadvantages of VA and VV ECMO
- Discuss the selection process in choosing VA or VV ECMO
- Discuss the management of patients on VA or VV ECMO
- Discuss the weaning and trial off procedures for either VA or VV ECMO

Introduction

Delivery of extracorporeal life support (ECLS) can be accomplished with a variety of cannulation approaches to meet specific needs for ECMO support. The two most common approaches employed are venoarterial (VA) and venovenous (VV) support. Various permutations of these two approaches can be used to provide support in unique situations, or for conversion approaches, but this discussion will focus on the basic VA and VV physiology and configurations. This chapter will define these two approaches, compare advantages/disadvantages and indications, and describe specific details of cannulation and management.

VA support is defined as a technique in which cannulas are placed to allow drainage of deoxygenated blood from a large vein or veins. The blood is then circulated through extracorporeal circuitry, which includes an artificial lung that oxygenates the blood, which is then returned to a major artery, usually the aorta. VV ECMO, in contrast, utilizes both venous drainage of deoxygenated blood and return of oxygenated blood to the right-sided venous system (Figure 1). The most widely used strategy for ECMO perfusion support has traditionally been

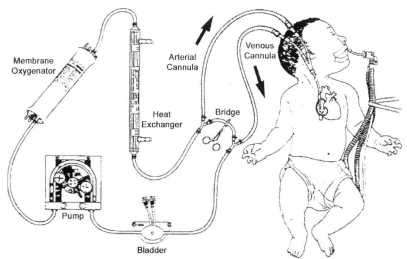

Figure 1: One Site Double Lumen Cannula VV ECMO
(from CNMC ECMO Manual with permission)

VA ECMO. Established as a recognized therapy for respiratory failure in neonates in 1982, VA support has been used in over 19,000 ECMO cases for all respiratory failure patient populations through 2008, according to the ELSO Registry Database. However, VV ECMO has slowly been gaining ground as a technique used in neonates. VV ECMO was first described in 1969 by Kolobow[1], who established that adequate oxygen delivery could be provided during acute respiratory failure when blood was drained to the pump from the internal jugular vein and returned to the circulation at the level of the right atrium via a catheter placed in another major vein.

The original VV cannula consisted of two thin-walled, steel tubes located inside each other. It was inflexible and had the potential to lacerate vascular or cardiac structures. The double lumen catheter (DLC) has been improved over the years to achieve ideal wall thickness, stiffness, and inflow/outflow characteristics and now constitutes one of the greatest advantages to using VV ECMO[2]. Studies have shown that a large number of patients who qualify for VA ECMO can be successfully supported with adequate oxygen delivery using VV ECMO.[3-6]

VA and VV ECMO: Advantages and Disadvantages

VV and VA ECMO differ significantly in ways that offer both advantages and disadvantages for use of each approach. Most major risks inherent to VA bypass apply similarly to VV ECMO since instrumentation, systemic anticoagulation, and long-term perfusion are required. However, VV ECMO provides several potential safety advantages over VA cannulation. Primarily, VV ECMO avoids instrumentation and ligation of the carotid artery. The advent of VV cannulas and the use of percutaneous VV cannulation techniques may allow for shorter cannulation times with decreased long-term morbidity, such as ligation of the jugular vein. Additionally, use of a double lumen VV cannula could provide significant time savings from cannulating one vessel rather than multiple sites.

The potential for direct ischemic lung injury from decreased pulmonary blood flow during VA ECMO is also eliminated with the use of VV ECMO, as VV support provides well oxygenated blood to the lungs. This could contribute to decreased pulmonary inflammation; recent animal studies suggest diminution of bronchoalveolar cytokine response with VV cannulation compared to VA.[7]

VV cannulation has potential advantages for the brain. VA cannulation requires ligation of the carotid artery that potentially is permanent. VV cannulation routes possible thromboemboli arising from the ECMO circuit to the pulmonary rather than the systemic and cerebral circulation as seen with VA support. During VV ECMO, blood entering the cerebral circulation is not as highly oxygenated nor is it under as much pressure as during VA ECMO. This could decrease the risk of cerebral reperfusion injury, particularly in infants with cerebral auto regulation altered by prior insult. Studies have shown varying effects of VA and VV ECMO on cerebral blood flow.[8-11] However, both a recent human infant study[9] and a neonatal lamb study[10] using continuous laser Doppler flow found persistent decreased cerebral blood flow velocities in VA compared to VV cannulation. The decline in cerebral blood flow with VA support could be related to observed decreases in cardiac output, increases in cerebral vascular resistance, and diminished vascular pulsatility.

The primary disadvantage of VV ECMO is that it does not provide direct circulatory support. Maximum achievable oxygen delivery with VV ECMO in some cases may be inadequate to meet demand. Oxygenation with VV support also may be lower than on VA ECMO because of the mixing of ECMO return blood with desaturated systemic venous blood. The problem of blood oxygen desaturation can also be exacerbated by recirculation, a disadvantage unique to VV ECMO and reviewed later in this chapter. Refractory hypotension or increased metabolic rate, as with sepsis, accentuates these problems on VV ECMO.

While it does not provide direct cardiac support, VV ECMO does offer a variety of advantageous circulatory effects relative to VA ECMO. VV support does not decrease right ventricular preload, pulmonary blood flow, left atrial return, or left ventricular output, since the volume of blood drained from and returned to the central venous system must be equal. In contrast, VA ECMO decreases right ventricular preload and pulmonary blood flow, and it increases left ventricular afterload.[12-15] The absence of a change in left ventricular afterload with VV support may eliminate the isolated left ventricular "stun" syndrome seen in a subset of VA-supported patients.[8] Occasionally, however, some patients placed on VV ECMO manifest symptoms consistent with right ventricular stun. These patients develop severe pulmonary hypertension with right ventricular dilation. The dilated right ventricle can cause bowing of the ventricular septum into the left ventricle, reducing filling, and compromising cardiac output. Careful management of preload, myocardial contractility and afterload can reverse this problem without the need for conversion to VA support.

Echocardiographic studies demonstrate that patients managed on VV ECMO have normal cardiac function.[12] VV ECMO may indirectly improve cardiac performance by increasing mixed venous oxygen content returning to the pulmonary circulation. Compared to VA ECMO, the oxygen saturation of the blood delivered to the pulmonary artery is higher because oxygenated blood is delivered to the RA, not the aorta. The higher mixed venous oxygen saturation in the pulmonary arteries may decrease pulmonary vascular resistance and right ventricular afterload. In addition, avoidance of increased left ventricular afterload with improved oxygen delivery to the coronary arteries may improve myocardial performance.

VV perfusion also provides potential cardiovascular benefit by preservation of physiologic pulsatility. When compared to non-pulsatile flow, pulsatile flow decreases vascular resistance, decreases afterload, and improves organ perfusion. Differences in pulsatile and non-pulsatile flow could also produce differing effects on renal function. However, experimental animal studies show comparable effects of VV and VA support on blood pressure, renal blood flow, and plasma renin activity.[22]

VV ECMO is also more dependent on optimal venous drainage (i.e., maximum venous cannula size and appropriate position) than VA support because of the inefficiency imposed by recirculation between venous cannulas. VV ECMO may also require separate surgical sites if two-site VV support is being provided, as opposed to the placement of both catheters in the neck for VA ECMO. This disadvantage is obviously minimized with use of a DL cannula.

Finally, interpretation of blood gas data is conceptually different with VV ECMO compared to VA support, requiring some re-education for teams whose experience is limited to VA ECMO. Recirculation is a concept that must be taught and understood completely by the ECMO practitioners to enable successful use of VV ECMO.

Circulatory Effects of ECMO

VA and V ECMO produce circulatory characteristics which will affect the patient differently. VV and VA ECMO are referred to as "bypass" however, VA ECMO is best described as partial bypass, meaning the arterial, or return blood, mixes in the aorta with left ventricular blood which has traversed the lungs. During VA ECMO, the effect of pump flow is very different than during VV ECMO. It can have dramatic effects on blood pressure; cardiac output, and even heart function in general.

Venoarterial ECMO and its Effects

Pulsatile vs. Non-Pulsatile Flow

The effect of VA bypass on systemic perfusion is reflected in the pulse contour and pulse pressure. The ECMO pump creates a flow that is essentially non-pulsatile. Consequently, as more blood is routed through the ECMO circuit, the systemic arterial pulse contour becomes flatter, then intermittent, then is stopped altogether when total bypass is reached. At total bypass the left ventricle gradually distends with thebesian venous return and ejects when it is full, leading to an occasional pulsatile beat. (Figure 2)

Reaching total bypass is unusual on VA ECMO as long as there is cardiac function. Typically, VA ECMO achieves approximately 60-80 percent of normal resting cardiac output, allowing 20 percent or more of the blood to pass through the lungs and left heart, resulting in a diminished yet discernible pulse contour. As long as total blood flow is adequate, the presence of a pulse contour is not important physiologically. Pulsatile and nonpulsatile perfusion do not differ if adequate blood flow (>100 mL/kg/min) and adequate mean pressure exist.

Low levels of blood flow (<40 mL/kg/min) may result in inadequate oxygen delivery, shock, anaerobic metabolism, and acidosis. During ECMO, all of the management effort is placed on maintaining normal oxygen delivery; therefore non-pulsatile flow has minimal negative effects. The kidney is most sensitive to non-pulsatile flow, usually requiring some amount of diuretics to overcome the effects.[16-18]

ECMO Blood Flow Effect on Physiology

In VA support, forward flow results from the sum of ECMO pump contribution via arterial return plus the native left ventricular (LV) cardiac output. A reduction in preload leads to inadequate forward flow and hypotension. The left atrial (LA) pressure or pulmonary capillary wedge pressure (PCWP) is used to reflect LV preload. Similarly, central venous pressure (CVP) is used to reflect right ventricular preload. CVP, while used as an indicator of intravascular volume status, is not an accurate monitor on ECMO. Due to the continuous draining of blood from the RA, the resultant low CVP could be inaccurately construed as decreased intravascular volume (or decreased RV preload).

The unloading of the left atrium results in decreased filling of the LV, or decreased LV preload, and decreased preload decreases native cardiac output. It must also be considered that the arterial

return blood from the ECMO pump is delivered to the aortic arch, and is directed towards the aortic valve. This may increase afterload on the LV. With increased afterload, the LV has difficulty ejecting effectively, which actually results in over distention of the ventricle and compromises native cardiac output.

In the presence of adequate preload and adequate forward flow (cardiac output plus pump output), hypotension is related to a drop in systemic vascular resistance (SVR). Increasing forward flow can restore adequate pressure. This can be accomplished by increasing preload in the system (intravascular volume) or by increasing the flow rate of the ECMO pump. If the flow rate of the pump is maximized, intravascular volume is increased, and mean arterial pressure (MAPs) remains low, additional intervention is required. Increasing LV afterload, or systemic vascular resistance, (SVR), may result in higher MAPs. MAP is a direct measurement of afterload. Drugs that increase afterload include inotropes such as dopamine and vasoconstrictors such as epinephrine and norepinephrine.

RV afterload is usually elevated on VA ECMO due to lung collapse and pulmonary arterial constriction. This increases pulmonary vascular resistance and pulmonary arterial pressure. This increase in afterload against which the RV ejects can decrease RV output. This will actually result in decreased cardiac output, which may produce decreased MAPs. The intervention in this scenario would be to decrease afterload by vasodilation, thus improving cardiac output and MAPs. Drugs that decrease afterload include dobutamine, nitroprusside, milrinone and priscoline.

Pressure is defined as the force exerted per unit area of surface. As with any closed circuit, pressure is directly proportional to flow and resistance (Poiseuilles's Law), described as: Pressure = Flow * Resistance. As flow or cardiac output increases, the pressure increases. As the resistance (systemic vascular resistance) increases, the pressure increases. Given a fixed resistance, pressure can be maintained with adequate forward flow.

Systemic blood pressure is determined by cardiac output and systemic vascular resistance. Cardiac output is the product of heart rate and stroke volume. The inotropic state of the heart, preload, and afterload all combine to determine stroke vol-

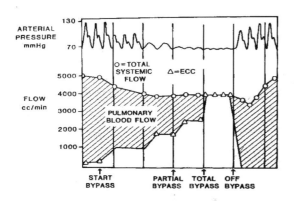

Figure 2: Arterial Pulse Contour on VA ECMO

ume. In infants and young children, cardiac output is generally increased by increasing heart rate, due to developmental constraints on increases in stroke volume. However, during ECMO, the first objective is to optimize oxygen delivery, which is done primarily by adjusting the ECMO flow and minimizing the negative effects on native cardiac output. Maintaining a normal mean blood pressure by balancing afterload and preload with adequate contractility is the key to management on VA ECMO and must be individualized.

Left Ventricular Stun

Left ventricular ejection is a major component of VA ECMO. If the LV is not ejecting adequately, overdistention may become a problem. Ejection fraction may be impeded by myocardial injury such as hypoxemia or by a phenomenon known as myocardial stun. If the left side of the circulation becomes over-distended, cardiac damage and pulmonary edema may occur. It is most important to prevent this from occurring. This is usually not a significant problem in neonatal VA ECMO, due to the presence of the PDA. Periods of non-pulsatile flow may exist in the neonate for 12 to 24 hours without obvious severe left sided myocardial injury. However, even a few minutes of left sided overdistention can cause myocardial damage in the older patient.

The diagnosis of LV stun should be expected when there is a loss in pulse pressure that is not secondary to hypovolemia, pneumothorax, pneumopericardium, hemothorax, or hemopericardium. This diagnosis should be confirmed by an echocardiogram that shows very little LV wall motion. In patients with LV stun, it is tempting to increase ECMO pump flow to improve oxygen delivery. In some cases, this is the wrong thing to do.

During VA ECMO, increasing ECMO flow decreases ventricular preload, increases LV afterload, and can increase myocardial oxygen consumption. In patients with cardiac stun, these effects can cause the LV to dilate, the mitral valve to become insufficient and increase the risk for pulmonary hemorrhage. In patients with LV stun, decreasing ECMO flow can reduce afterload and improve intrinsic cardiac function.

Unfortunately, decreasing pump flow so as to optimize the pre-load/afterload balance may not be possible since the patient's injured heart may not compensate by proportionately increasing cardiac output. The result may be inadequate perfusion. Additional volume to improve right heart filling, the use of cardiotonic agents to improve left heart emptying, maximizing post-membrane oxygen content and thus total oxygen delivery, and reducing afterload with vasodilators may all be helpful measures.

LV stun often resolves over a 48-hour period. Failure to see improvement after 4-5 days of ECMO is an ominous sign and suggests myocarditis or myocardial infarction. Surgical decompression of the overdistended LV may be crucial to preventing irreversible damage to the LV and the lungs. Decompression is generally performed in the cardiac catheterization laboratory by balloon septostomy with or without stent placement. Additionally, a catheter may be placed in the LA or LV to assist in decompressing. These catheters may be connected easily to the venous drain line of the ECMO circuit.

Venovenous ECMO and its Effects

VV ECMO does not really 'bypass' anything. Since the volume of blood drained from and returned to the central venous system is equal, VV ECMO does not decrease RV preload, pulmonary blood flow, LA return, or LV output. The absence of a change in LV afterload may eliminate the isolated LV "stun" syndrome seen in a subset of VA-supported patients.

However, RV stun is a complication that has been associated with VV ECMO. The consequences of right and left ventricular stun are similar. Neonates who develop RV stun often have severe pulmonary hypertension before initiation of ECMO. Once on ECMO, the RV becomes dilated and works poorly. The dilated RV causes the ventricular septum to bow into the LV. LV filling is compromised and cardiac output can be decreased. Careful echocardiographic assessment and subsequent use of pharmacologic agents directed at reducing RV afterload can be helpful at reversing these problems.

Oxygenation During ECMO

VA ECMO

The most important principle to understand about VA ECMO is that oxygen delivery is controlled through the ECMO pump by simply increasing or decreasing flow. For example, assuming no lung function at maximal flow, 80 percent of blood is circulating through the ECMO pump. This blood is 100 percent saturated and delivered to the patient at 120 mL/kg/min. The resultant arterial content is approximately 19 volumes percent. By increasing or decreasing the flow, the content delivered is also increased or decreased. Reviewing calculation of oxygen content and delivery in another chapter of this manual is worthwhile.

Patient arterial PaO_2 or oxygen saturation may not be reliable indicators of tissue oxygen sufficiency during VA ECMO. Oxygen sufficiency is evaluated in VA ECMO by evaluating mixed venous oxygen saturation and content returning to the right heart as an indication of whether borderline levels of oxygen supply are leading to increased extraction of oxygen from hemoglobin with each pass. If a patient needs more oxygen, his tissues will take more of what is offered until that is inadequate. True end organ perfusion (or "what is left over") is measured with a "mixed venous" specimen taken from the pulmonary artery. Normal pulmonary artery saturations are 65 to 75 percent. Pulmonary artery saturations in this range indicate the tissues and organs are receiving and utilizing enough oxygen to maintain normal state of health. If pulmonary artery saturations are below this range, the worry is that oxygen demands may not be satisfied. In ECMO we rarely have access to the pulmonary arterial circulation for direct evaluation of mixed venous saturations. While pre-membrane saturations do not represent true mixed venous saturations, it is the closest and most consistent indicator of oxygen delivery in VA ECMO. Therefore, in VA ECMO we monitor pre-membrane saturations, not patient arterial saturations or PaO_2's, to evaluate adequate oxygen delivery.

It should be noted that in clinical practice, oxygenation can be significantly affected by the patient's lungs, even on low ventilator settings and with severe disease. The magnitude of the pulmonary contribution to oxygenation will depend on the settings used on the ventilator (usually with pressures of 26/10-14 cm H_2O, a rate of 10 breaths per minute, an inspiratory time of 0.6 seconds, and 21-30% inspired oxygen) and on the severity of the pulmonary dysfunction. As the patient's lungs contribute progressively more to oxygenation, the ECMO specialist is able to maintain the venous saturation within the desired range (usually 65-75%) while decreasing pump flow.

As the patient recovers, lung function improves and the transfer of oxygen through the pulmonary bed increases. The mixture of ECMO blood flow and pulmonary blood flow produces higher oxygen content, signaling that ECMO blood flow may be reduced.

VV ECMO

The success of VV ECMO is dependent upon the manipulation and management of various factors unique to this therapy. Since VV ECMO provides no direct circulatory support, it can be difficult to achieve the same level of oxygen delivery as during VA ECMO. However, when recirculation fraction is minimal and cardiac output is supported, oxygen provided to the patient from the ECMO circuit can be similar to that seen with VA ECMO. Oxygenation is optimized when the hemoglobin concentration is around 15 grams/dL, when the recirculation fraction is low, and when the venous drainage catheter is large enough to achieve approximately 120-140 mL/kg/min pump blood flow.

In practical terms, four variables can be used to monitor oxygenation during VV ECMO: arterial oxygen saturation, pre-oxygenator pO_2 or saturation, cerebral venous oxygen saturation, and calculated oxygen consumption "across the oxygenator." The arterial oxygen saturation, sampled by blood gas or pulse oximetry, is a good reflection of oxygen sufficiency in a patient on VV ECMO. Since it is readily available, this measurement is most often used to monitor VV patients. However, there is more to monitoring oxygenation than merely this value.

During VA ECMO, the pre-oxygenator saturation is used as a mixed venous saturation, and therefore the determining factor of adequacy of oxygenation. There is no straightforward measurement of oxygenation during VV ECMO. Mixed venous saturation readings from the pulmonary artery are not interpretable due to the highly oxygenated blood returned from the ECMO circuit to this side of the circulation. Pre-oxygenator venous saturation readings do not reflect changes in the patient's mixed-venous saturation alone, because this number is strongly influenced by the recirculation fraction. An increase in the pre-oxygenator saturation can occur both in the settings of patient improvement or deterioration. When recirculation is high, blood sampled from the pre-oxygenator site will have a high saturation, even if the patient's mixed-venous saturation is dropping and oxygen delivery is inadequate. In order to understand this, the practitioner must understand the concept of recirculation, which will be discussed in depth in the next section.

The third approach to measuring oxygenation is to measure a venous saturation not affected by recirculation as an approximation of mixed-venous saturation. For example, oxygen saturations can be measured from a catheter in the jugular venous bulb to provide an estimation of oxygen sufficiency. Unfortunately, measurements of jugular venous bulb saturations are not very sensitive to changes in the patient's cardiopulmonary status since cerebral blood flow is preserved even in patients with life-threatening cardiopulmonary failure. Even so, the use of a cephalad catheter can provide another site to measure oxygenation in addition to augmenting the amount of oxygen provided to the patient by decreasing recirculation. It has been shown that the ECMO flow required to support adequate gas exchange during DLVV ECMO with a cephalad drain in place is similar to the flow required during VA ECMO.[10] In contrast, the flow required to support adequate gas exchange in DLVV ECMO without a cephalad drain in place is higher. While cephalad saturations do not readily reflect the changes in cardiopulmonary status, they have been found to be very sensitive to changes in ventilatory status. As one would expect with intact auto-regulation, changes in $PaCO_2$ directly affect the rate of blood flow measured in the cephalad cannula. As $PaCO_2$ levels increase, the rate of blood flow measured in the cephalad cannula also increases. As $PaCO_2$ levels decrease, the rate of blood flow measured in the cephalad cannula also decreases. Similarly, cephalad saturations also rise and fall with changes in levels of $PaCO_2$.[10]

The fourth method to monitor oxygenation during VV ECMO is to actually calculate oxygen uptake across the oxygenator. This does have one major limitation, in that it does not reflect any oxygen added to the blood by the native lungs. Therefore, unless there is no gas exchange in the lungs, this measurement will underestimate total oxygen consumption.

Recirculation During VV ECMO

An understanding of the concept of recirculation is critical to the successful application of VV ECMO as well as appropriate interpretation of blood gas results obtained from patients on VV ECMO. Recirculation is defined as the portion of blood returning to the ECMO circuit immediately after being infused to the patient from the ECMO circuit. Figure 3 graphically demonstrates this concept for a DLC.

All patients on VV ECMO have some element of recirculation. Clinically, recirculation may present as decreasing patient arterial saturations, increasing pre-membrane saturations, and decreasing $AVDO_2$. Additionally, it can be noted that the blood draining from the right atrium is the same color as the blood

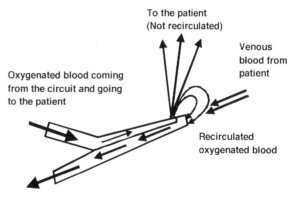

Figure 3: Schematic diagram of the principles of recirculation within a Double Lumen Cannula for VV ECMO

returning from the pump. Mathematically, recirculation fraction (R) can be estimated as:

$$\text{Recirculation} = \text{S preOx} - \text{SvO}_2 / \text{S postOx} - \text{SvO}_2$$

S preOx is the oxygen saturation of the blood entering the oxygenator, S postOx is the oxygen saturation of the blood exiting the oxygenator, and SvO_2 is the true mixed venous oxygen saturation in the patient. For example, if the pre-oxygenator saturation is 90% and the mixed venous saturation is 55% (post-oxygenator saturation is always 100%) then the recirculation fraction is 77 percent--this is very BAD!! However, if the pre-oxygenator saturation is 78% and the mixed venous saturation is 65% the recirculation fraction is 37%--this is better. 30% recirculation is considered typical in VV ECMO.

Unfortunately, it is impossible to measure mixed venous saturation during VV ECMO since oxygenated blood from the ECMO circuit has been added to the blood in the pulmonary artery. Approximations of the mixed venous saturation during VV ECMO may be obtained by sampling blood from another major vein not affected by recirculation.

It is less important to calculate recirculation fraction than it is to understand the factors that affect it. Four factors can affect recirculation: pump flow, catheter position, cardiac output, and right atrial size (or intravascular volume).

Pump Flow

The impact of pump flow on recirculation is straightforward. If pump flow is high, the negative pressure drawing blood from the right atrium back into the ECMO circuit is higher. The increased suction pressure causes streaming of oxygenated blood from the oxygen delivery catheter into the venous drainage catheter. Recirculation fraction increases almost linearly with increasing pump flow. The amount of oxygen provided to the patient first increases and then decreases as pump flow increases beyond optimal flow and minimal recirculation.

Note that in this idealized diagram (Figure 4) the point at which "effective oxygen delivery" begins to decrease is at 500 mL/min flow. The reason for the decreased effective oxygen delivery is that the

recirculation proportion has limited the amount of oxygen provided to the patient. In numerical terms, effective flow may be described by the equation:

Effective Flow = Total Flow - (Total Flow * Recirculation Fraction)

When total flow is zero, the effective flow is zero. At maximal flow the recirculation fraction is 100%, and effective flow again becomes zero. Ideal pump flow provides the highest effective flow at the lowest revolutions per minute of the pump, yielding the best oxygen delivery. As pump flow increases, the effective flow first increases, stabilizes, and then decreases.

Pump flow is the factor affecting recirculation over which the ECMO specialist has the most control. If recirculation is high (i.e., patient sats are 85%, pre-membrane sats are 86%, venous sats are 53%), WEAN the pump flow by 10 – 30 mL/min, dependent on patient size. If patient saturations improve or stay the same, wean again. If saturations decrease, go back up on flow and seek other causes for recirculation. This is referred to as 'Defining the Curve'. The ECMO Specialist should keep a visual picture of figure 4 in their minds as they begin this process. If defining the curve does not significantly improve oxygenation, there are at least three other factors that affect the recirculation fraction. Remember that the recirculation curve should be re-defined frequently. As the patient status changes, so does the effective flow.

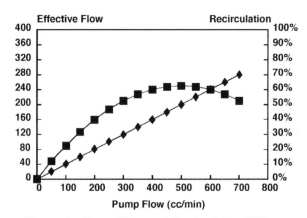

Figure 4: Pump Flow and Recirculation Effects on VV ECMO. The change in effective pump flow (■) and recirculation (♦) compared with set pump flow in VV support.

Catheter Position

Catheter position is another major factor of recirculation. Surgical positioning during cannulation is critical for optimal support during VV ECMO. For example, if the double lumen cannula (DLC) is positioned high in the SVC, blood flow from the catheter will tend to remain within the confines of the vessel and be drained back into the ECMO pump before it reaches the RA. When using the DLC, the patient's head should be almost midline, and the arterial reinfusion port should be flat against the patient's neck behind the ear. In larger patients, if the tips of the drainage and infusion catheters (e.g., catheters inserted in the femoral vein and the internal jugular vein) are directed at each other from close range, the recirculation fraction will be high.

If recirculation appears to be high, inadvertent changes in catheter position should be ruled out. Catheter position can change when degree of lung inflation changes, neck edema increases, or the patient moves. Catheter position problems may be diagnosed with a chest x-ray. If catheter position is the problem, try repositioning the patient's head, add or remove neck rolls (depending on whether high or low), or add slight tension on the cannula. If the non-invasive techniques are unsuccessful, then surgical repositioning must be considered.

The use of a cephalad venous catheter has been shown to decrease recirculation and increase the amount of oxygen that can be added to the blood as it passes through the membrane lung.[10] Blood draining from this catheter is more desaturated than the blood in the right atrium because it is not mixed with blood returning from the ECMO circuit. Initially this catheter was employed to decompress the cerebral venous circulation in order to decrease the incidence of intracranial pathology. Extra-axial fluid was a common finding on cranial ultrasound, and many centers believed that use of this catheter would reduce the incidence of its occurrence.

An additional benefit is that the flow from the cephalad catheter augments the amount of venous drainage, thereby increasing the amount of maximum obtainable pump flow. Typically, 1/3 to 1/2 of the total ECMO flow is obtained from a well placed cephalad cannula. This flow can be measured continuously using a flowprobe. If flow changes are observed, the Specialist can intervene as required. Also, a venous saturation measurement from the cephalad cannula can be applied to the recirculation fraction equation. Of note, this saturation will be the last to be compromised due to autoregulation and physiologic attempts to maintain cerebral oxygenation.

From a practical standpoint, compare the color of the blood draining from the cephalad to the color of the blood draining from the right atrium . . . if the colors are similar then recirculation is low, if the colors are very different (cephalad dark or "blue" and the RA is bright or red) then the recirculation is high. Using this simple assessment as a guide, the specialist can manipulate the cannula or patient position to try and improve the color differential (and therefore decrease recirculation).

Cardiac Output

Cardiac output also affects recirculation. If the oxygenated blood delivered to the right atrium is rapidly moved into the right ventricle, it is less accessible to the drainage catheter. In contrast, during cardiac standstill, all of the oxygenated blood flowing into the right atrium would drain back into the ECMO circuit, since it has nowhere else to go.

Cardiac output (CO) is the product of heart rate and stroke volume. Tachycardia should be managed with adequate sedation and a minimum stimulation environment, and if necessary adenosine or cardioversion for supraventricular or ventricular tachycardia. Stroke volume should be optimized by increasing intravascular volume and use of cardiotonic drugs as indicated.

Right Atrial Size

Intravascular volume or more precisely, right atrial volume, also influences recirculation. When oxygenated blood is delivered to a very small right atrium, it is more likely to be aspirated directly back into the ECMO circuit than if the oxygenated blood is diluted in a larger volume of desaturated blood in a normal right atrium. A visual example: if a DLC is placed in a thimble or in a bathtub, one could see how the chance for recirculating the same blood that was just re-infused into a thimble would be much higher than if it was re-infused into a bathtub. Assess the need for volume expanders and blood products, if hypovolemia is the issue and give as indicated.

Patient Selection

Each ECMO center has protocols in place that define selection criteria based on the degree of illness and potential for morbidity and mortality. These criteria do not determine which technique to use, only that the patient would benefit from extracorporeal support. Determining which mode of ECMO to use will depend on patient diagnosis, severity of illness, vessel size, and/or physician preference.

In the past, VV ECMO has been reserved for patients with only moderate respiratory failure. Many centers do not consider VV support for patients with severe cardiorespiratory failure. If a patient was categorized as "too sick", then VA ECMO would have been chosen. However, it has been demonstrated that no specific diagnosis (except for primary cardiac disease), PaO_2 range, hemodynamic status, or level of support precludes the use of VV ECMO.[6, 19-24]

Decisions about the use of VV ECMO for patients with circulatory compromise are not straightforward. VV ECMO does not provide direct circulatory support and may not provide sufficient support in patients with inadequate cardiac performance. However, numerous patients with right, left, or biventricular compromise have been reported to recover with VV support.[6, 12] Many hypotensive patients with biventricular failure have oxygenated well, improved mean arterial pressures, and have weaned from cardiovascular drugs within a few hours of instituting VV ECMO.[25, 26] The use of VV ECMO for patients with myocardial failure following recent cardiac surgery, a history of recent and severe cardiac arrest, or with refractory rhythm disturbances associated with systemic hypotension is not advocated. These patients require direct circulatory support that only VA ECMO can provide.

For children with cardiac depression associated with respiratory failure and its treatment, VV ECMO can be effectively employed. After venous cannulation, ECMO is initiated. If the patient's oxygenation and mean arterial pressure improve progressively over the subsequent 15-30 minutes, VV support is continued. If the patient does not improve, or if he/she worsens at any time, a catheter is placed in the carotid artery and the patient is converted to VA support. All venous lines are connected together using "Y" connectors to access venous drainage. If a double lumen cannula (DLC) is in place, both lumens are connected together for venous drainage.

Patient size was previously a limiting factor for use of VV ECMO. The 14 Fr DLC initially was the only cannula available for neonates and patients smaller than 3 kg required VA ECMO. Because of the concern for venous congestion, patients between 4.5 and 10 kg could not be cannulated femorally and also required VA ECMO. However, the addition of 12, 15 and 18 Fr DLC have virtually eliminated requirement for VA ECMO based on patient size alone. Limiting factors for VV ECMO do still include inadequate size of the jugular vein, an excessively prominent first rib, or mediastinal shift due to congenital diaphragmatic hernia. The recent availability of newer double lumen cannulas ranging from 13 Fr to 31 Fr allows for an entirely new patient population to have the benefits of single site VV ECMO.

Cannulation Techniques

When determining the type of ECMO to use, the discussion of how many cannulation sites are available will come into play. The diversity of catheter sizes that are available allows a wide range of choices. In neonatal ECMO, it is assumed that it will be one site, meaning only the neck will be accessed. Once the practitioner moves into the pediatric or adult realms, the availability of the femoral vessels allows for multiple-site ECMO. The practitioners will discuss the various sites and technique to be used in a particular patient and then proceed with obtaining surgical access.

In VA ECMO, the most common vessels used in neonates are the internal jugular vein and the common carotid artery. In larger patients, femoral veins and arteries may be used, requiring multiple cannulation sites.

In VV ECMO, the internal jugular vein is used to accommodate the double lumen catheter in neonates. The use of the ascending internal jugular, or cephalad vein, may also be used as a secondary venous drain. Simultaneous venous drainage from a 10 Fr or 12 Fr cephalad-directed internal jugular catheter may extend the useful weight range of the 15 Fr DLC up to 4.5 kg. Cephalad-directed venous catheters can access one-third to one-half of total drainage, providing better venous return to the circuit and augmenting oxygen delivery. [25]

Ideally, the tip of the double lumen catheter should be in the lower third of the RA. This directs the arterialized blood preferentially to the tricuspid valve, as well as assures that all side drainage holes are in the atrium. Placement of the catheter too high in the right atrium will result in arterialization (increased redness) of the venous drainage from recirculation effect. It may also lead to possible perforation of the SVC if a side hole remains in the vessel. In infants, the junction of the IVC and the RA is approximately 0.5 centimeters above the diaphragm; thus the catheter may be considered to be in optimal position if its tip is visible on chest radiograph ~ 1 centimeter above the diaphragm.

Unfortunately, this relationship changes regularly with alterations in ventilator settings on ECMO even if the catheter is properly secured in the vessel by suture to the skin of the neck and behind the ear. Prior to cannulation, the patient's lungs are often maximally inflated. With lung rest on ECMO support and lower mean airway pressure, mean lung volume falls, and the diaphragm rises. If the catheter position in the chest does not change secondary to the rise in the diaphragm, then the heart will rise on the catheter, moving the catheter toward or into the IVC. This may result in increased recirculation fraction and falling saturation. Traction on the circuit tubing connected to the catheter will move it in the cephalad direction enough for correction. It is rarely necessary to re-open the incision and reposition the catheter. The reverse situation with cannula position can occur as lung healing brings improved compliance and higher mean lung volumes. Releasing traction on the circuit tubing can restore optimal cannula position. A chest radiograph is recommended if there is any question regarding the catheter's position. In general, it is best not to try to reposition a catheter that is functioning well.

Radial orientation or rotation of the DL cannula is also important. These catheters are designed with venous and arterial side holes positioned opposite each other. The arterial or return side holes will be directed toward the tricuspid valve if the catheter is secured to the neck (usually just behind the ear) with the red-labeled arm of the "Y" (arterial return) directed upward or anterior to the venous arm. This orientation will further help to minimize recirculation.

For large children and adults, the surgical approaches that have been most widely used require cannulation of both the internal jugular vein and of one or two of the femoral, saphenous, or iliac vessels. Drainage of blood from the femoral vessels and return of oxygenated blood to the patient through the internal jugular vein has a marked advantage of minimizing recirculation, and is increasingly being used. Smaller pediatric patients may have decreased recirculation and improved access to venous drained blood volumes by draining the right atrium and returning to a femoral vessel.

Surgical vascular access for ECMO cannulation is best described in Chapter 7 of the ECMO Red Book, 3rd Edition, 2005.

Initiation Of Bypass

Preparing to cannulate a patient is discussed in a separate chapter in this manual. Assembling and priming extracorporeal circuitry is determined by each ECMO center and can be unique to the individuals who designed the program. The blood prime and its components is one of the most important aspects of a successful initiation. VA ECMO is the most forgiving of an imperfect blood prime. Even if a patient is initiated with a crystalloid prime mix, a low hematocrit or unbalanced electrolytes, most patients will overcome the prime and maintain appropriate vital signs. VV ECMO however, requires a perfectly balanced circuit prime with initiation of bypass.

Blood Prime

The characteristics of the blood used to prime the circuit are the basis for a successful prime. Fresh blood, no more than 5 days old, will assure that potassium levels and red cell viability are optimized. The use of packed red blood cells will allow achievement of a higher hemoglobin concentration, optimally 15 gm/dl. Leukoreduced cells add the additional benefit of removing of potentially harmful cells.

Once blood has arrived, the addition of other components will assure a physiologic prime for initiating ECMO.[6]

To each unit of fresh (< 5 day old), leukoreduced, packed red blood cells, add

1. 40 mL 25% Albumin
2. 25 mL THAM
3. 10 mEq NaHCO$_3$
4. 100 units (1/1000) heparin
5. After gentle agitation add, 300 mg Calcium Gluconate

Once blood prime is circulating, add an additional 300 mg Calcium Gluconate for neonatal circuits, or, 100 mg per unit of pRBCs used for other sized circuits.

This recipe generally results in a serum sodium concentration of 136 mEq/L, potassium of about 3.5 – 6 mEq/L, (dependent on age of blood), a total protein level of 4 gm/dL, an albumin concentration around 3 gm/dL, an osmolarity of about 280 mOsm/L, and a hematocrit of 45 – 55%. The importance of normalizing the ionized calcium has been shown to prevent changes in cardiac function with the initiation of VV bypass.[23] A normalized ionized calcium may be the most important ingredient to the successful application of VV ECMO, and may ease VA ECMO initiation as well.

Gas Prime

Once the blood prime is circulating, a "gas prime" is performed. The most common way of achieving gas exchange across the oxygenator is to turn on the sweep gas flow with a FiO$_2$ of 100% at 2 LPM for 2-3 minutes. After time is complete, the gas is removed from the oxygenator and a circuit gas is drawn to measure the resulting pO$_2$ and pCO$_2$. Another method is to use carbogen, a 95% O$_2$ / 5% CO$_2$ mixture, at 2–4 LPM for 20 minutes. This hyperoxygenates the prime to a pO$_2$ of approximately 500 mmHg, and equalizes the pCO$_2$ to 35–40 mmHg. One benefit to using carbogen instead of oxygen as sweep gas is that the primer does not have to remove the gas after achieving gas

exchange. After 20 minutes of stabilization, circuit blood gases, electrolytes, hematocrit, and activated clotting time should be drawn. The carbogen may be left on the oxygenator, without compromising the levels of pH, pO$_2$, and pCO$_2$, whereas if the oxygen sweep gas was left running, the result would be an extremely low pCO$_2$. Once laboratory results are received, ionized calcium levels should be treated, if required, and levels checked again if time permits, before going on ECMO.

Circuit Capacity

Circuit capacity is another component of the prime that may contribute to a successful initiation of ECMO. When an extracorporeal circuit is primed with crystalloid fluid, then blood primed, there is a certain distensibility of the tubing that remains. This flexible volume will increase or decrease based on the temperature of the prime and pressure of the volume in the tubing and oxygenator. If, after connecting the circuit to the patient, more blood spontaneously drains from the patient into the circuit to distend the tubing and fill the oxygenator, then the patient may become acutely and substantially hypovolemic. The venous control system does not protect against this spontaneous drainage, since it only assures that the rate of blood flow into the patient does not exceed the rate of drainage from the patient. After testing in an animal model, it has been shown by Cornish et al. that measuring post membrane pressures on a closed loop ¼" circuit, and adding volume until the pressure is 100 – 110 mmHg at a flow rate of 200 mL/min assures that the ECMO circuit is filled to capacity. When this pressure is achieved, there is no detectable net volume loss, and there may actually be a slight volume push into the patient, with circuit connection and initiation of bypass. This practice, also known as "hyperpriming", lacks specific evidence of benefit, but anecdotally aids in decreasing the hypotension seen with initiation of either VA or VV ECMO.[6]

Some centers advocate double infusions of inotropes and vasopressors for the initial on-bypass procedure with separate infusions of these vasoactive medications infusing into the patient and into the ECMO circuit. The reasoning behind this has been the potential recirculation of the agents through the ECMO circuit. This practice is not necessary if the circuit prime has been perfected. Most centers that perform ECMO routinely are able to wean pressor support within an hour or two of initiation of bypass.[2, 5]

Initiating Blood Flow

Initiating ECMO blood flow is specific to each technique. VA ECMO should be started slowly to assure slow mixing of an oxygen rich prime blood with a potentially devastated, anoxic patient. VA blood flow is started at 20 mL/kg/min and slowly increased over 20 – 30 minutes to a maximum calculated flow of 120 mL/kg/min.

Initiating VV ECMO flow is similar to initiating VA ECMO. The practitioner should start at 20 mL/kg/min and slowly increase over the next 10 to 15 minutes to a maximum calculated flow of 150 mL/kg/min. The rate of increase is slightly faster than for VA ECMO since concerns for reperfusion injury and cardiac afterload do not exist.

Ventilatory support may be weaned almost immediately with initiation of flow. Within the first hour, on most patients, the ventilator may be weaned to complete rest settings. Rest settings vary from institution to institution and within patient populations.

Management of ECMO Blood Flow

Once the patient is on ECMO and the maximum calculated flow is achieved, the specialist must define the amount of flow required for each individual patient. Most patients do not require this much flow to maintain their oxygenation needs. Once the ventilator has been weaned to rest settings, and the pressor support has been weaned to desired levels or off, the patient is assessed. In VV ECMO, the recirculation curve should be defined. In VA ECMO, pre-membrane saturations are measured and ECMO flow is maintained at a level to achieve 65 – 75% saturation. It is not unusual to find that a neonate has been weaned within the first 24 hours to a flow of 200 – 250 cc/min. This patient may then spend the next 3 – 5 days on that flow until true signs of improving lung function begin to show.

Throughout the ECMO run, the oxygenation variables are continuously monitored. The pre-

oxygenator saturation value, taken in combination with an arterial saturation reading can yield information about the changing balance of recirculation and systemic oxygen delivery. For example, in VV ECMO, if the pre-oxygenator saturation rises and the patient's arterial saturation falls, the recirculation fraction must have increased. Alternatively, if the pre-oxygenator saturation falls and the patient's arterial saturation rises, the recirculation fraction must have decreased. This minute-to-minute management demonstrates the necessity of continually redefining the patients' recirculation curve.

Increases in the patient's saturation with no change or a slight increase in pre-oxygenator saturation generally marks improvement in the patient's lung function. The pre-oxygenator saturation increases because the patient's mixed venous saturation is increasing (generally an indication of improvement on VA ECMO.) The patient's arterial saturation improves because the respiratory system is adding oxygen to the pulmonary blood and because the mixed venous saturation is higher. This indicates that the patient is able to begin weaning.

Weaning and Trialing Off ECMO

The decision of timing to start weaning a patient is a difficult one. It involves the objective assessment of the patients' chest radiograph, arterial and mixed venous saturations, and response to decreases in total ECMO flow. The decision is also based on the caregivers' experience in the particular disease process and "knowing" that the patient should be ready to wean towards decannulation. The discussion below regarding weaning and trialing off refers to respiratory support ECMO. More detail regarding the management of the cardiac ECMO patient will be given in a separate chapter in this manual.

Weaning

Weaning is a term that refers to slowly decreasing the total ECMO flow over time and assessing the patient's response. The point at which weaning may begin usually follows a period of an elevation and stability of arterial and cephalad saturations, as well as improvement in the chest x-ray. Generally, the amount of flow that is weaned is 10-20 mL/min for neonates and 100-200 mL/min for larger pediatric patients. Response to flow weans should be evaluated for 15 minutes up to an hour after changes have been made. The patient will ultimately drive the speed at which the flow can be decreased.

When the majority of patient blood flow is being diverted through the lungs (~ 50 mL/kg/min of ECMO pump flow); ventilator settings should be increased to support the patient. This increase in settings is not extreme, especially in the neonate, and may already be in effect for the pediatric patient lungs that are being "recruited." The important item to remember is that eventually the patient will need the support of the ventilator. Do not assume that the patient's negative response to weaning is due to not being ready, when it may be due to lack of ventilator support.

VV and VA ECMO require somewhat different approaches to weaning. With VV ECMO the caregiver may be able to wean more quickly, with less time between changes and not see any affect on the patient. In VA ECMO, the patient will usually need to be weaned more slowly, with more time between weaning maneuvers to recover. This may be due to the additional cardiac support that VA ECMO offers. Also, complete weaning or "idling" flow is reached at 10-20 mL/kg/min in the VA patient. This level of flow ensures that a majority of blood flow is going through the lungs. While on VV ECMO, idling may be reached at 40-50 mL/kg/min.

The caregiver must also be aware of the minimum flow that is recommended for the size of the ECMO circuit being used. If the patient is weaned to 10 mL/kg/min, equaling 30 mL/min for a 3-kg neonate, that level of flow may lead to gross clot formation in the circuit. Generally, maintenance of minimum flow is required. For example, 100 mL/min is the minimum flow for a 1/4" neonatal circuit, 200 mL/min for a 3/8" pediatric circuit, and 500 mL/min for a 1/2" adult circuit. One must also consider the length of time the circuit will be at the minimum flow before decannulation. It is not unusual to increase the flow to 200 mL/min awaiting arrival of the surgical team and planned decannulation. Flow may then be weaned back to idle in time for the procedure.

The 100 Percent Oxygen Challenge

The 100 percent oxygen challenge is an additional tool used to assess the level of function of the lungs. It may be performed on both VA and VV ECMO patients. The timing of this test may vary from patient to patient. Most often the oxygen challenge occurs when the patient has weaned significantly, allowing a majority of blood to flow through the lungs. This is usually when ECMO flow is 30-50 mL/kg/min.

The test itself is simple. Ventilator inhaled oxygen concentration is increased to 1.0. Patient arterial saturations are assessed for 10-15 minutes, and a patient arterial blood gas is drawn. Optimal results include an increase in oximetry saturation during the test, and an increase in the patient's PaO_2 A result that encourages continued weaning, as well as progression towards decannulation is a $SaO_2 > 96$ % and a $PaO_2 > 150\text{-}200$ mmHg.

Trialing off ECMO

The trial off procedure is the last test prior to decannulation. The response of the patient once removed from all ECMO support without actually removing the cannulas is an important one. It allows the caregiver an opportunity to fine tune ventilator settings, pressors, and other supportive measures. The final determination can then be made if the patient is suitable for decannulation.

In VA ECMO, the patient must be separated or removed from the support of the ECMO circuit in order to assess the ability of the lungs and heart. The practitioner will begin by increasing the ventilator settings to levels felt to be acceptable for the post-bypass period, such as a PIP of 25-30, a PEEP of 5-6, a rate of 30, and 30-40% FiO_2 for the neonate. The pediatric patient may require more or less support depending on their disease process. Move all intravenous fluids to the patient, except for the heparin drip. Ensure that all monitoring devices are functioning. This should include a cuff blood pressure, arterial pressure monitoring, and pulse oximetry. An $ETCO_2$ monitor is beneficial in the pediatric patient to allow for minute-to-minute ventilator manipulations without frequent blood gas sampling.

VV ECMO also provides the unique situation where you do not have to wean to flows since all flow is in the right atrium. You can "cap" off the membrane, leave the flows high and basically be off ECMO. This can be done for 30-45 minutes to determine if the patient is going to require a marked increased in the ventilator support. If stable on low setting, the patient is ready for decannulation.

Remove the patient from bypass by clamping the venous line near the neck cannula, opening the bridge, and clamping the arterial line. Increase the flow to approximately 200 mL/min for neonatal circuits or maximum obtainable flow through the bridge for pediatric circuits.

Closely observe oxygenation. In VA ECMO, if the patient does not tolerate the trial off procedure you may see an immediate drop in SpO_2, blood pressure and/or heart rate. If the patient decompensates dramatically, do not prolong the procedure any further and return the patient to bypass. If the patient is tolerating the procedure, remain off bypass for 10-15 minutes and draw a patient arterial blood gas. If the results are acceptable, the trial off may be discontinued, and decannulation scheduled. If the results are marginal and the physician makes a ventilator adjustment, remain off bypass and repeat the arterial blood gas in 10-15 minutes. The specialist must assure patency of the ECMO cannulas during this procedure by "flashing" the cannulas every 5-10 minutes. This protects the cannulas from clotting due to stagnation. To "flash" the cannulas, return the pump flow to its previous setting, place the patient back on bypass, count to three, and then remove the patient from bypass again. Return to recirculation flow. Additionally, during prolonged trial off procedures, patient ACTs should be monitored every 30 minutes and managed according to parameters and heparin drip may be moved from pump to patient.

The trial off procedure for VV ECMO is dramatically different from VA ECMO. Because there is no direct cardiac support, it is simply a matter of removing the ability to ventilate and oxygenate through the ECMO circuit. This is known as "capping the membrane." The gas line is disconnected from the gas source and attached to the gas egress port of the oxygenator. This effectively 'strangles' the membrane, by preventing any gas exchange to occur, although approximately 10 to 15 minutes is required for a return to true mixed venous blood concentration. A patient arterial blood gas should

then be drawn for evaluation. This evaluation may continue for another 15 minutes or for as many hours as necessary. In pediatric or adult patients, with the use of an $ETCO_2$ monitoring, the physician may manipulate the ventilator settings while the patient is off ECMO in order to determine the optimal level of support required for the patient. This may take 2 to 4 hours in order to give the patient time to stabilize and/or react to changes made. Because the circuit is never clamped off as in VA ECMO, there is no concern for clot formation within the cannulas.

Note that some ECMO centers do not trial off their neonatal respiratory cases unless they have had a very questionable idle period. Idling with normal blood gases for 4-6 hours for the meconium aspiration or idiopathic pulmonary hypertension infant indicates that they are ready to come off ECMO and do not require a trial off period. The congenital diaphragmatic hernia patient may have an unstable idling period and require a trial off period before decannulation.

Decannulation

The decannulation procedure is scheduled once the patient has met criteria defined by the institution and is ready to be removed from ECMO support. The patient cannulae must be clamped in the traditional method during the process. Additional tubing clamps are needed on any secondary venous cannulas if they are present. The surgeon will remove the cannula(s), and the ECMO run is complete.

Summary

In the provision of extracorporeal life support, VV and VA are widely used techniques that are available for use. Choosing VV or VA requires the practitioner to appreciate the advantages and disadvantages and indications for each method. Understanding the concepts of oxygenation, recirculation and the use of the appropriate oxygenation monitors is crucial to the successful application of these practices.

Acknowledgment: The authors acknowledge Dr. Devn Cornish for his contributions to this chapter and for his role in the development of VV ECMO. Additionally, the authors would like to recommend further reading of this subject in Chapter 5 in the 3rd Edition of the ECMO "Red Book".

References

1. Kolobow T, Zapol W, Pierce J. High survival and minimal blood damage in lambs exposed to long term (1 week) veno-venous pumping with a polyurethane chamber roller pump with and without a membrane blood oxygenator. Trans Am Soc Artif Intern Organs. 1969; 15:172-177.

2. Andrews AF, Zwischenberger JB, Cilley RE, Drake KL. Venovenous extracorporeal membrane oxygenation (ECMO) using a double lumen cannula. Artif Organs. 1987; 11:265-268.

3. Klein MD, Andrews AF, Wesley JR, et al. Venovenous perfusion in ECMO for newborn respiratory insufficiency. A clinical comparison with venoarterial perfusion. Ann Surg. 1985; 201:520-526.

4. Kolobow T, Borelli M, Spatola R, Tsuno K, Prato P. Single catheter venous-venous membrane lung bypass in the treatment of experimental ARDS. ASAIO Trans. 1987; 33:561-564.

5. Zwischenberger JB, Toomasian JM, Drake K, Andrews AF, Kolobow T, Bartlett RH. Total respiratory support with single cannula venovenous ECMO: double lumen continuous flow vs. single lumen tidal flow. Trans Am Soc Artif Intern Organs. 1985; 31:610-615.

6. Cornish JD, Heiss KF, Clark RH, Strieper MJ, Boecler B, Kesser K. Efficacy of venovenous extracorporeal membrane oxygenation for neonates with respiratory and circulatory compromise. J Pediatr. 1993; 122:105-109.

7. Golej J, Winter P, Schoffman G, et al. Impact of extracorporeal membrane oxygenation modality on cytokine release during rescue from infant hypoxia. Shock 2003; 20:110-115.Short BL, Walker LK, Gleason CA, Jones MD, Jr., Traystman RJ. Effect of extracorporeal membrane oxygenation on cerebral blood flow and cerebral oxygen metabolism in newborn sheep. Pediatr Res. 1990; 28:50-53.

8. Fukuda S, Aoyama M, Yamada Y, et al. Comparison of venoarterial versus venovenous access in the cerebral circulation of newborns undergoing extracorporeal membrane oxygenation. Pediatr Surg Int. 1999; 15:78-84.

9. Hunter CJ, Blood AB, Bishai JM, et al. Cerebral blood flow and oxygenation during venoarterial and venovenous extracorporeal membrane oxygenation in the newborn lamb. Pediatr Crit Care Med. 2004; 5:475-481.

10. Pettignano R, Labuz M, GauthierTW, Huchkaby J, Clark RH. The use of cephalad cannulae to monitor jugular venous oxygen content during extracorporeal membrane oxygenation. Crit Care. 1997; 1:95-99.

11. Martin GR, Chauvin L, Short BL. Effects of hydralazine on cardiac performance in infants receiving extracorporeal membrane oxygenation. J Pediatr. 1991; 118:944-948.

12. Strieper MJ, Sharma S, Dooley KJ, Cornish JD, Clark RH. Effects of venovenous extracorporeal membrane oxygenation on cardiac performance as determined by echocardiographic measurements. J Pediatr. 1993; 122:950-955.

13. Martin GR, Short BL, Abbott C, O'Brien AM. Cardiac stun in infants undergoing extracorporeal membrane oxygenation. J Thorac Cardiovasc Surg. 1991; 101:607-611.

14. Ingyinn M, Rais-Bahrami K, Evangelista R et al. Comparison of the effect of venovenous versus venoarterial extracorporeal membrane oxygenation on renal blood flow in newborn lambs. Perfusion. 2005; 19:163-170.

15. Meliones JN, Moler FW, Custer JR, Dekeon MK, Chapman RA, Bartlett RH. Normalization of priming solution ionized calcium concentration improves hemodynamic stability of neonates receiving venovenous ECMO. ASAIO J. 1995; 41:884-888.

16. Zwischenberger JB, Nguyen TT, Upp JR, Jr., et al. Complications of neonatal extracorporeal membrane oxygenation. Collective experience from the Extracorporeal Life Support Organization. J Thorac Cardiovasc Surg. 1994; 107:838-849.

17. Swaniker F, Kolla S, Moler F, et al. Extracorporeal life support outcome for 128 pediatric patients with respiratory failure. J Pediatr Surg. 2000; 35:197-202.

18. Roy BJ, Cornish JD, Clark RH. Venovenous extracorporeal membrane oxygenation affects renal function. Pediatrics. 1995; 95:573-578.

19. Andrews AF, Klein MD, Toomasian RI, Roloff D, Bartlett RH. Venovenous extracorporeal

membrane oxygenation in neonates with respiratory failure. J Pediatr Surg. 1983; 18:339-346.

20. Anderson HL, Snedecor SM, Otsu T, Bartlett RH. Multicenter comparison of conventional venoarterial access versus venovenous double-lumen catheter access in newborn infants undergoing extracorporeal membrane oxygenation. J Pediatr Surg. 1993; 28:530-535.

21. Osiovich HC, Peliowski A, Ainsworth W, Etches PC. The Edmonton experience with venovenous extracorporeal membrane oxygenation. J Pediatr Surg. 1998; 3:1749-1752.

22. Heiss KF, Clark RH, Cornish JD, et al. Preferential use of venovenous extracorporeal membrane oxygenation for congenital diaphragmatic hernia. Pediatr Surg. 1995; 30:416-419.

23. Kugleman A, Gangitano E, Pincros J, Tantivit P, Taschuk R, Durand M. Venovenous versus venoarterial extracorporeal membrane oxygenation in congenital diaphragmatic hernia. J Pediatr Surg. 2003; 38:1131-1136.

24. Dimmitt RA, Moss LR, Rhine WD, Benitz WE, Henry MC, Vanmeurs KP. Venoarterial versus venovenous extracorporeal membrane oxygenation in congenital diaphragmatic hernia: the Extracorporeal Life Support Organization Registry, 1990-1999. J Pediatr Surg. 2001; 36:1199-1204.

25. Pettignano R, Fortenberry JD, Heard ML, et al. Primary use of the venovenous approach for extracorporeal membrane oxygenation in pediatric acute respiratory failure. Pediatr Crit Care Med. 2003; 4:291-298.

26. Van Meurs K, Lally KP, Peek G, Zwischenberger JB, ECMO: Extracorporeal Cardiopulmonary Support in Critical Care, 3rd Edition, Ann Arbor, Extracorporeal Life Support Organization, 2005.

Chapter 7 Questions

1. Name the four factors affecting recirculation during VV ECMO.
   a) Pump flow, cannula size, cardiac output, volume status
   b) Pump flow, cannula position, FiO_2 level, patient diagnosis
   c) Pump flow, right atrial size, cannula position, cardiac output
   d) Pump flow, cardiac status, patient size, patient diagnosis

2. When assessing a patient's oxygenation status on VA ECMO, which of the following is the best indicator of adequacy of oxygenation?
   a) Cephalad saturation
   b) Patient arterial saturation
   c) Patient PaO_2
   d) Pre membrane saturation

3. Increasing ECMO blood flow in response to a low patient arterial saturation in VV ECMO may cause a decrease in oxygen delivery.
   a) True
   b) False

4. What is the purpose of an Oxygen Challenge Test?
   a) To determine patient oxygenation ability
   b) To determine pulmonary status
   c) Whenever the physician feels like performing the test.
   d) To be able to wean the patient

5. The major difference between trialing off VA and VV ECMO is that the cannulas must be clamped in VV ECMO.
   a) True
   b) False

Chapter 7 Answers
   1. C
   2. D
   3. A
   4. B
   5. B

8

ECMO Equipment and Devices

William E. Harris CCP, FPP, Edward M. Darling MS, CCP and D. Scott Lawson MPS, CCP, LP

Objectives

After completion of this chapter, the participant should be able to:

- Discuss the general principles of the general principles of an ECMO circuit design
- Discuss the pro/con for catheter selection
- Discuss the pro/con for membrane and pump selection

Introduction

The current devices used for Extracorporeal Life Support (ECLS), commonly referred to as ECMO, continue to undergo progressive modifications by their respective manufacturers. Historically, disposable products and non-disposable hardware were borrowed from the Cardiac operating room utilized in cardiopulmonary bypass (CPB). Because these devices were generally designed to be used for relatively short time intervals of 2-4 hours associated with the open heart procedure, the ECLS clinician was presented with many challenges when this same equipment was incorporated for the longer days and weeks of the ECMO procedure. Because ECMO procedures were limited to only a handful of centers exploring its merits, manufacturers showed little initiative in equipment research and development that would better suit this unique procedure. Fortunately, as the medical community continues to report and accept the merits of ECLS in the various patient populations, the increased usage has prompted entrepreneurs and larger medical companies to develop better applicable products. Biocompatible circuits, new gas exchange devices, improved pumps, sophisticated computer controlled

and servo-regulated pump systems are just a few examples of these efforts to provide safer patient care and to improve outcome. As clinicians, we must continue to acquaint ourselves with this new technology and more importantly, strive to fully understand how these devices work when deciding to incorporate them in our individual systems. This chapter will attempt to explain many of the devices currently available but should NOT be substituted for the knowledge that the clinician can gain from specific product manuals, company- hired clinical specialists, and in-vitro laboratory testing.

General principles of ECMO systems

ECLS systems provide temporary support in patients with compromised heart or lung function. Often, both organs are compromised due to their inherent interaction and ECMO will deliver

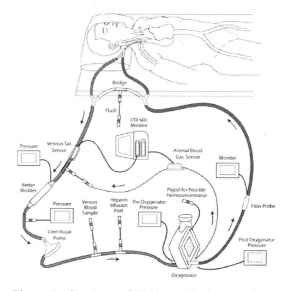

Figure 1. Courtesy of Ochsner Medical Center, New Orleans

adequate tissue perfusion through blood circulation and tissue gas exchange. The system does this by mechanically pumping blood through the patient's systemic vasculature delivering oxygen and removing carbon dioxide. Figure 1 shows one example of an ECLS circuit on an adult patient but one must note that there can be many variations of the circuit dependant on patient size, pathology of organ dysfunction, and the an institution's specific philosophy on circuit design.

However, a few simple rules should be considered when designing or revising the ECMO circuit.[1]

1. The shorter the better. Resistance through tubing increases as length increases and this can cause undo stress on the blood elements through excessive turbulence.

Increased circuit length also exposes the blood to additional foreign surfaces which can promote deleterious inflammatory reactions in the blood. This can lead to increased capillary leakage and associated extravascular tissue edema. Longer tubing length also increases priming volume with bank blood or crystalloid and increases the area for heat loss to the atmosphere. Hence, the circuit should be designed as short as possible but adequate to allow for patient movement and transport.

2. The fewer connectors, the better. Although the plastic tubing connectors manufactured today are far superior to historical ones, excessive connectors can still cause an increased incidence of turbulent blood flow in the ECMO circuit. Turbulence can will cause blood element damage and develop areas of stagnation inducing clot formation. Minimizing

straight connectors by utilizing double leur connectors (Figure 2a) when possible, and eliminating as many Y-connectors (Figure 2b) as possible should be strongly considered. One example of minimizing connectors might be the consideration to eliminate the traditional A-V bridge or the "diamonds" incorporating the oxygenator in some circuits. In addition, connectors and circuit tubing can be commercially put together and bonded which will reduce the incidence of inadvertent disconnections especially under circuit high-pressure conditions associated with common ECMO flows.

3. Keep ECMO circuits simple. Many circuits contain an excessive amount of tubing and stopcocks. One should evaluate on an individual basis if the circuit can be simplified to minimize complexity without sacrificing patient safety. A simpler circuit may have fewer complications and offers the clinician a system that can be better understood and maintained during the ECMO procedure. This is especially important considering the constant training of new ECMO clinicians in the field.

Cannulas:

Vascular cannulas used for ECMO

Proper cannula size and location are critical to the support of patients who require ECMO therapy. The size of the cannula in relation to the patient's body size must be considered when preparing for ECMO support. The cannula used to divert blood from the patient to the ECMO circuit is the venous

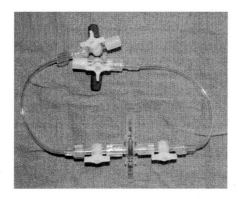

Figure 2a.

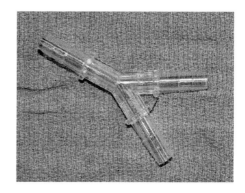

Figure 2b.

cannula. Access for venous cannulation is commonly the internal jugular vein (IJ). The cannula is inserted via the IJ and positioned down into the center of the right atrium. If trans-thoracic cannulation is preferred, direct cannulation of the right atrium can be achieved via a median sternotomy. In larger patients, a second venous cannula may be warranted for optimal venous drainage by accessing the femoral vein. Arterial cannulation is commonly achieved via the carotid artery to return the patient's blood back to him/her after gas exchange has occurred via the ECMO circuit. If trans-thoracic cannulation is preferred the surgeon can cannulate the ascending aorta directly via a median sternotomy. An alternative arterial cannulation site which can be used is the femoral artery. Dual lumen catheters are also available for use from Origen Biomedical, (see Figure 3 & 4) Avalon Laboratories and Maquet Cardiovascular when venovenous ECMO is employed. The venous lumen of an Origen dual lumen catheter has approximately twice the area as the arterial lumen. The dual lumen catheter is advantageous because a single cannulation site is used, the internal jugular vein and cannulation of the carotid artery can be avoided.

Alternative cannulation strategies can be employed in larger patients. The femoral artery and veins are possible sites for cannulation. Ichiba, et al. described a modified venovenous ECMO circuit which may reduce recirculation.[2] This brief article described the cannulation of the right IJ vein and the right femoral vein for drainage out of the patient and cannulation of the left femoral vein for reinfusion of the oxygenated blood from the ECMO circuit.

Cannula sizes are generally measured on the outer diameter (O.D.) of the cannula and termed as "french" size. One millimeter of length is equivalent to a 3 french (i.e. 7 mm = 21 fr.). Cannulas from different manufactures often have different flow and pressure drop characteristics even though they may be of the same french size.

Commonly used pediatric cannulas:

- Medtronic DLP (www.medtronic.com/card-surgery/arrested_heart/cannulae)
- Edwards Lifesciences (www.edwards.com/products/cardiac)

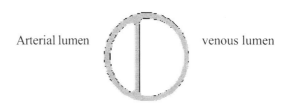

Arterial lumen   venous lumen

Figure 3. Dual lumen VV ECMO catheter design:

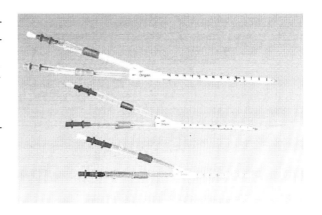

Figure 4. Dual lumen VV ECMO catheters -courtesy of Origen Biomedical

- Maquet Cardiovascular (www.maquet.com)
- Terumo Cardiovascular (www.terumo-us.com/doc/815427_TenderflowBrochure_July2006.pdf)
- Origin Biomedical (www.origen.net/catheter.html)
- Avalon Laboratories (www.avalonlabs.com/html/pulmonary_support.html)

See Table 1 for catalog numbers for some cannulas commonly used for ECMO

Servoregulation

The ECMO circuit is considered a closed circuit design such that the only blood that is pumped to the patient is that which is consistently drained from the patient's venous circulation. This is in contrast to cardiopulmonary bypass during heart surgery which employs a large reservoir which can collect variable amounts of venous blood and possibly fully drain the circulatory system regardless of pump flow. Be-

Table 1.

Company		Arterial cannulas				
		carotid			**aortic**	
	size	Cat. # coated*	Cat. # uncoated		Cat. # coated*	Cat. # uncoated
Medtronic	6 fr				CB77006	77006
	8 fr	CB96825-008	96820-008		CB77008	77008
	10 fr	CB96825-010	96820-010		CB77010	77010
	12 fr	CB96825-012	96820-012		CB77012	77012
	14 fr	CB96825-014	96820-014		CB77014	77014

Company		Venous cannulas				
		IJ			**right atrium**	
		Cat. # coated*	Cat. # uncoated		Cat. # coated*	Cat. # uncoated
Medtronic	8 fr	CB96835-008	96830-008		CB66108	66108
	10 fr	CB96835-010	96830-010		CB66110	66110
	12 fr	CB96835-012	96830-012		CB66112	66112
	14 fr	CB96835-014	96830-014		CB66114	66114
	16 fr				CB66116	66116

Company		**Dual Lumen for V-V**	Patient range
		Cat. #	(kg)+
Origen	12 fr	VV12F	2 - 5
	15 fr	VV15F	4 - 8
	18 fr	VV18F	7 - 12

*heparin coating - Carmeda   + recommendations courtesy of www.Origen.net

Product	Order Code	Size	Lead Diameter	Insertable Length	Connector Size
	10013	13 Fr. (4.3 mm)	11 Fr. (3.7 mm)	4" (10 cm)	1/4"
	10016	16 Fr. (5.3 mm)	14 Fr. (4.7 mm)	5" (13 cm)	1/4"
AVALON ELITE™ Bi-Caval DLC	10019	19 Fr. (6.3 mm)	16 Fr. (5.3 mm)	7.75" (20 cm)	1/4"
	10020	20 Fr. (6.7 mm)	17 Fr. (5.7 mm)	11.5" (29 cm)	3/8"
	10023	23 Fr. (7.7 mm)	20 Fr. (6.7 mm)	11.5" (29 cm)	3/8"
	10027	27 Fr. (9.0 mm)	24 Fr. (8.0 mm)	11.5" (29 cm)	3/8"
	10031	31 Fr. (10.3 mm)	27 Fr. (9.0 mm)	11.5" (29 cm)	3/8"

cause of ECMO's closed circuit design, a relatively sophisticated mechanism of communicating to the pump whether venous drainage is adequate or not for a given pump flow must be used. If the venous drainage becomes inadequate for a given flow, such as in the case of hypovolumia or a kinked cannula just to name a few, complications can occur by creating an overly negative suction pressure within the venous tubing. This could cause an inadvertent collapse and associated injury of the vessel wall on to the cannula or cavitation (the action of air being pulled out of solution). Servoregulation is the mechanism utilized for this communication between adequate venous return and roller pump flow. The traditional servoregulation system consists of a compliancy chamber (bladder) and a bladder box which houses the bladder and sends an electrical signal to either communicate to the pump to continue with current pump flow or abruptly stop due to inadequate venous drainage. This stoppage has been referred to as "chirping" due to the audio alarms that occur in these associated alarm states.

Pressure servoregulation has recently become a popular way to perform servoregulation.. Although the compliancy chamber is often still utilized, the electrical servoregulating bladder box can be eliminated and replaced with a pressure transducer which can then communicate to the pump information through the sophisticated pump console. In this manner, the clinician can set pressure limit parameters to adjust servoregulation action. Instead of an abrupt stoppage of pump flow, the newer consoles allow a gradual slowing of the pump flow which may be more physiological and less deleterious to the ECMO patient.

The use of servoregulation with centrifugal pumps remains controversial at this writing although recent studies suggest there may be beneficial reasons to do so.[3] As with roller pumps, excessive negative pressure and cavitation are concerns when utilizing centrifugal pumps. Fortunately, some of the newer consoles have taken this into account and incorporated servoregulation with centrifugal pump usage as well.

Compliance chambers:

A compliance chamber or ECMO bladder is an essential component of the ECMO circuit. This device acts as a reservoir from which the blood pump draws blood. The bladder allows the ECMO Specialist to better diagnosis low volume states within the patient. If a patient is losing fluid via bleeding or any other source, the bladder will not fill adequately and an increasing negative pressure will become evident. In this case, the ECMO Specialist may have to either lower the flow transiently until the low volume state is remedied or add volume to the patient. The flexible design of the bladder allows for relatively small fluid shifts within the circuit without affecting the patient's right atrium directly. This is where negative sided pressure servo-regulation or the use of a mechanical bladder box can be utilized. When an increasing negative pressure is sensed by a pressure transducer at the site of the bladder, a pressure regulated pump will be electronically servo-regulated to slow or stop the blood pump. On a system in which a bladder box is used, the decreasing size of the bladder is sensed and this mechanically releases a trigger which sounds an alarm to warn the ECMO Specialist of low volume states. Both types of feed back may keep the blood pump from exerting an extreme amount of negative pressure on the venous line and right atrium. Extreme negative pressure exerted upon blood can create cavitation (pulling

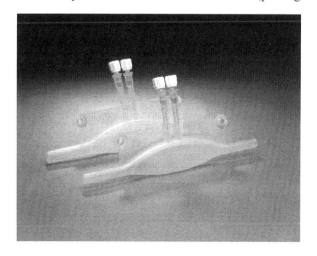

Figure 5. Courtesy of Medtronic

air out of solution) within the venous line which can lead significant hemolysis.[4]

Two companies utilize a horizontal design and can be used with bladder box or pressure servo-regulation. This design comes with dual luered ports located at the high point of the device to allow for air removal and/or pressure monitoring.

Medtronic
    R-14 - 30 ml prime volume, ¼ inch inlet and outlet ports
    R-38 - 3/8 inch inlet and outlet ports

Gish Biomed
    VRECMOB - 30 ml prime volume, ¼ inch inlet and outlet ports (www.gishbiomedical.com)

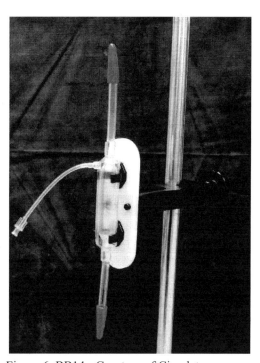

Figure 6. BB14 - Courtesy of Circulatory Technologies, Inc.

Another compliance chamber design is vertical and the makers claim better air trapping capability and better flow characteristics than horizontal ECMO bladders.[3]

Better Bladder™ (Circulatory Technology, Inc.) (www.cirtec.com)
    This device is FDA approved for use in ECMO. It can not be used with bladder box only pressure servo-regulation. One may shorten venous line by raising this compliance chamber higher in relation to the circuit. The Better Bladder may be heparin coated by companies which offer a heparin coating.
    BB14 – 20 ml prime volume, ¼ inch inlet and outlet ports (Figure 6)
    BB38 – 115 ml prime volume, 3/8 inch inlet and outlet ports

Bladder box
    Origen Biomedical (www.origen.net)

Available with electrical trigger that sounds an alarm if venous return is decreased.

Also available in two non-electrical versions (Bladder Holder & Bladder Carrier) will not alarm with low volume states.

The ECMO blood pump:

Roller or occlusive pump – Operates on the principal of positive fluid displacement. This pump has two rollers, which must be optimally occluded, placed 180° opposite of each other and pulls blood from the patient's right atrium, through a compliance reservoir and pushes the fluid forward in a fixed length and diameter of tubing to create pressure and flow into the oxygenator and then further into the

Table 2.

Tubing diameter	Prime volume ml/foot	Patient size range*
1/4 inch	9.65	up to 10 kg
3/8 inch	27	10 to 20 kg
1/2 inch	45	greater than 20 kg

* Duke University Health System

patient's arterial system. Flow is calculated based on the length and diameter of the tubing in the pump raceway and the pump RPM. The length of tubing used is fixed based on the length of the raceway of the specific pump manufacturer. However, the diameter of the tubing in the raceway is easily altered to best suit the needs of the patient needing support. Larger diameter tubing has more priming volume but needs fewer RPMs than smaller diameter tubing to achieve the same flow. The higher RPMs lead to increased wear on tubing in the raceway and a greater rate of hemolysis, so one should try to balance the need for fewer RPMs with an increase in prime volume. See Table 2.

The roller pump may be operated manually in the event of power failure by using a hand crank. Newer models of roller pumps are equipped with internal battery backup modes to operate for limited time periods during external power disruptions.

Advantages include; lower cost, less prime volume than centrifugal pumps and flow is not dependant upon after-load conditions. Also, an increased experience level exists with this pump as it has been the pump most commonly used for ECMO over the past 20+ years.[5] A recent study showed that a properly occluded roller head pump was statistically less hemolytic than the Medtronic BP-80 (Medtronic, Inc., Minneapolis, MN) centrifugal pump but statistically equal to the Sorin Revolution (Sorin Group, Mirandola, Italy) and Jostra Rotaflow (Maquet, Inc. Bridgewater, NJ) centrifugal pumps.[6]

Disadvantages include; spallation, the liberation of plastic particles from the tubing in the pump raceway which may embolize in the patient. The roller head blood pump must be servo-regulated either with a bladder box or pressure servo-regulation due to the fact that the roller pump can create massive positive and negative pressure conditions. The occlusion of the roller against the tubing and the raceway is critical as too little occlusion will give falsely elevated flow calculations and may lead to malperfusion. Too tight of an occlusion may lead to increased spallation, hemolysis and raceway rupture. It is highly recommended that Super Tygon® tubing be used in the raceway (S-65) as it is more resistant to wear than ordinary tubing. Super Tygon® tubing is in limited supply and being replaced by ECMO Tygon® (S-95-E) (Saint-Gobain Performance Plas-

tics, Courbevoie, France) tubing which has the same superior peristaltic pump life and is a non-DEHP polymer. Limited availability of both products may result in centers converting from roller pumps to centrifugal pumps in the future."

Roller head/occlusive blood pumps:

Sorin (www.soringroup-usa.com)

CAPS- historical, no longer in production, some still in use

Cobe- historical, no longer in production although some still in use

S3- currently, most widely used roller head pump

S5- newer model beginning to be used for ECMO applications

The Jostra HL30, Terumo System 1, Sarns, & Century have are all roller head blood pumps that have been reportedly used for ECMO applications as well.

Centrifugal pumps – Also known as a constrained vortex or non-occlusive pump. This pump works on the principle of a constrained vortex where; as an object spins in a fluid environment, an area of low pressure is generated at the center of the vortex and high pressure is generated at the periphery of the spinning fluid. A centrifugal pump has a plastic housing to constrain the vortex fitted with a single inlet and outlet. Fluid enters the pump at the center were the area of low pressure is created and exits at the outlet located on the outside of the housing where higher pressure is located. This outlet is where the pressure exerted on the fluid is transformed into flow. The faster the object spins, the higher the pressure and flow that is generated, so that the flow can be manipulated by altering the RPMs of the device. Flow is dependant upon pre-load and after-load conditions. This means that if the patient's volume status is reduced then this type of blood pump will remain at the set RPM but the flow will reduce automatically without exerting extreme negative pressure on the atrium. And in the face of an increased after load such as moderately increased blood pressure, flow will automatically drop without altering RPMs and without generating extreme levels of positive pressure. Centrifugal pumps may be operated manually using a hand crank although they are equipped with battery backup modes which will operate the pump for limited time periods in the case of external power loss.

Centrifugal pumps used in ECMO:

> Medtronic Biomedicus
> > BP-50 -Pediatric
> > > Prime volume 48 ml
> > > Max Flow 1.5 lpm
> > Biopump plus- adult
> > > Prime volume 86 ml

> Sorin Revolution
> > Prime volume -57 ml
> > Max flow -8 lpm

> Jostra Rotaflow
> > Prime volume -32 ml
> > Max flow -10 lpm

> Levitronix (www.levitronix.com/Home.php)
> > Magnetically levitated centrifugal pump with no bearings or seals

Oxygenators:

The oxygenator is a critical component of the ECMO circuit. As the blood leaves the blood pump it enters into either the oxygenator or heat exchanger depending upon which type of device is used. For oxygenators with integral heat exchangers, the blood will enter the heat exchanger first. The size of a patient requiring ECMO support is important to know so that one may correctly select the correct size ECMO circuit and oxygenator for that size patient.

See Table 3 for oxygenator specifications on several commonly used oxygenation devices used for ECMO support.

Silicone rubber oxygenation devices-

The Medtronic ECMO oxygenator line does not have integral heat exchangers so that a separate heat exchanger needs to be added into the circuit distal to the oxygenator. It is important to note the Medtronic ECMO oxygenators are the only oxygenation devices which use silicone plastic. These devices are the only oxygenators approved by the US FDA for long term use. These devices utilize a series of thin silicone sheets wrapped around a plastic screen wound around a polycarbonate core. Blood passes on one side of the silicone and a blended sweep gas flows through the silicone sheaths to obtain gas transfer. The silicone plastic offers no direct blood to gas interface and therefore

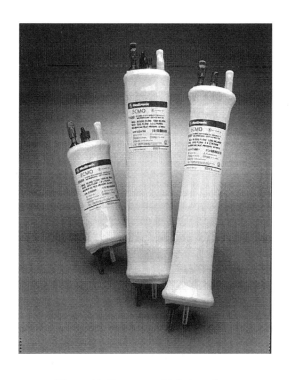

Figure 7. Courtesy of Medtronic

Table 3.

Oxygenators reportedly used for ECMO

	silicone	Surface area (m²)	prime vol (ml)	max Qb (lpm)	max Qg (lpm)
Medtronic	0600	0.6	90	1	1.8
	0800	0.8	100	1.2	2.4
	1500	1.5	175	1.8	4.5
	I-2500*	2.5	455	4.5	7.5
	I-3500*	3.5	575	5.5	10.5
	I-4500*	4.5	665	6.5	13.5

	polypropylene (miroporous) hollow fiber				
Medtronic	Minimax plus*	0.8	149	2.3	
	Affinity NT*	2.5	270	7	
Terumo	RX 05*	0.5	43	1.5	

	polymethylpentene hollow fiber				
Jostra	Quadrox D*	1.8	250	7	
	Quadrox iD Pediatric**	0.8	81	2.8	
Medos	Hilite LT 800**	0.32	55	0.8	
	Hilite LT 2400**	0.65	95	2.4	
	Hilite LT 7000*	1.9	275	7	

*Devices approved for 6 hours of continuous use by the FDA

** Devices not currently available in the
USA

the device can remain efficient for long periods of time. This design is relatively difficult to prime and ready for use and silicone rubber can not be coated with heparin. It also has a relatively large pressure drop across the membrane and poor flow characteristics. See Figure 7.

Polypropylene (micropourous) hollow fiber oxygenation devices-

These oxygenation devices were originally designed for short term use in the operating room environment. It employs a large number of polypropylene hollow fibers which have micro-tears throughout the fiber length. Generally, blood passes around the fibers and gas flows through the fibers. Gas exchange occurs at the points where the micro-tears are. So, this type of device has a direct blood to gas relationship where gas exchange occurs. This design allows for remarkable efficiency and very low pressure drop across the fiber bundle, however, the areas where direct blood to gas interfaces occur also allows for protein leakage over time. This protein leakage or 'wetting out' causes a decrease in gas exchange and ultimately failure of the device. The primary reasons why this type of device has been increasing used for ECMO applications are that it is very quick and easy to prime and ready for use and that it's surfaces can be coated with different types of heparin coatings. This type of design is advantageous for rapid response scenarios and for use with cardiac patients who are experiencing a significant amount of bleeding. See Figure 8.

Polymethylpentene (PMP) hollow fiber oxygenation devices-

The PMP material has been referred to as a 'closed' fiber, but this is a misnomer due to the fact that the material does have microscopic pores. However, these micro pores are much smaller than the polypropylene fibers and do not 'wet out' over time. The material retains the characteristics of other hollow fiber designs in that it is easily primed and readied for use, can be coated with heparin and has a very low pressure drop across the membrane bundle.

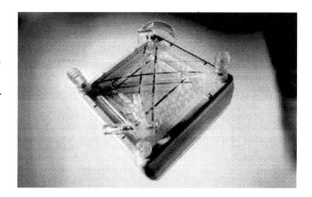

Figure 9a. Maquet Quadrox D

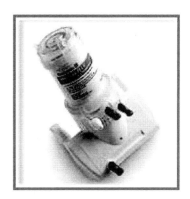

Figure 8. Courtesy of Medtronic

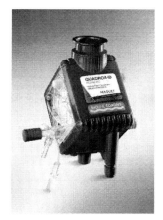

Figure 9b. Maquet Quadrox iD* Pediatric

Courtesy of Maquet Cardiovascular

*Not currently approved for use in the US

It also has the beneficial characteristic of silicone devices in that it will not lose function over time due to protein leakage. However, currently, the one PMP device available in the US is only approved for six hours of continuous use due to the reluctance of the manufacture to seek long term approval through the FDA. The Medos Hilite LT (Medos Medizintechnik AG, Stolberg, Germany) series of PMP oxygenators are not available in the US at the time of this writing. However sources from Medos Medizintechnik AG have informed the authors that these products are currently being reviewed by the US FDA and may be available to US customers by the end of 2009. See Figures 9a and b.

The ECMO Bridge

ECMO circuits have traditionally used a 'Bridge' in-between the arterial and venous lines to allow the ECMO Specialist to recirculate fluid when the patient has been taken off ECMO. In this way the ECMO circuit can be kept viable if the patient fails to remain stable off of ECMO support. By simply clamping beyond the Bridge on both the arterial and venous sides of the circuit and then opening the Bridge, one may flow through the circuit to decrease the incidence of thrombus formation in the circuit during the time that the patient is be trialed off of ECMO support. The traditional design of the ECMO Bridge is to place a relatively short section of tubing, often ¼", in-between the arterial and venous lines which is kept clamped during the ECMO run. This type of Bridge needs to be 'flashed' approximately every hour to keep thrombus from forming in the Bridge tubing. To 'flash' the Bridge one need only open the clamp briefly to allow blood flow through the tubing replacing the stagnant blood. However, Liem, et al. and De Mol, et al. both described an alteration in cerebral hemodynamics related to flashing of the Bridge.[7,8] To avoid these cerebral disturbances some ECMO centers have re-evaluated the need of a Bridge or redesigned it so that flashing is no longer necessary. One option is to keep the same Bridge design utilizing a Hoffman screw clamp to maintain a constant yet limited amount of blood flow through the Bridge. This eliminates the need to 'flash' the Bridge thereby avoiding possible changes in cerebral conditions. Another option is the use of

smaller diameter tubing, often 1/8", and stopcocks at either end of the Bridge. With this design the Bridge is filled with only crystalloid fluid during the ECMO run and no flow is allowed through it. This method, obviously, avoids 'flashing' since the Bridge is kept closed during ECMO support and only opened when the patient has been weaned from support. Yet another option is to have no Bridge connected to the circuit at all. This method avoids 'flashing' yet leaves the Specialist with no way of recirculating fluid through the circuit when off of ECMO support. If luered connectors are placed in the arterial and

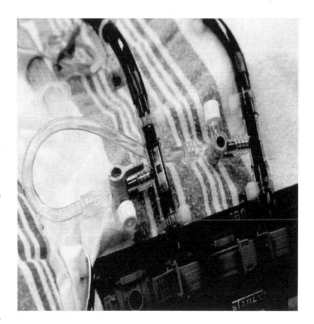

Figure 10. Stopcock Bridge

venous lines, a stopcock type of Bridge can be added once the patient has been weaned off of ECMO and used to recirculate the residual blood volume in the ECMO circuit. See Figure 10.

Heat Exchange and ECMO Heaters

The cells of the body produce heat as a by-product of their metabolism. Heat is then either stored in the tissue or eliminated to the external environment. If not affected by adverse conditions such as external temperature extremes, physical exercise, emotional distress or physical disease, the body will normally regulate itself to maintain a normal body temperature of about 37° Centigrade (98.6°F). Thermal regulation is accomplished by vasodilation or vasoconstriction of the body's circulatory system, thereby changing the blood flow patterns to the organ systems. Therefore, the various organ systems, including the skin, exhibit temperature variations within the body.[9]

Artificial heat exchangers are devices used in the conduct of ECLS and cardiopulmonary bypass (CPB). Their function is bidirectional and involves either adding or subtracting heat from the blood and hence, the body. Heat exchangers consist of stainless steel tubes or corrugated walls that separate the blood flowing through them from a circulating water source (Figures 11 and 12). Varying in design,

heat exchangers can be compared based on their efficiency of heat exchange or heat transfer coefficient, and this is:
Heat transfer coefficient =

inlet blood temperature - outlet blood temperature
/
inlet blood temperature - inlet water temperature

To improve efficiency of a given heat exchanger, the devices utilize the concept of counter current flow so that blood and water will flow in opposite direction. Care should be taken by the clinician to connect the heat exchanger correctly in order to guarantee this flow pattern.

Although hypothermia or cooling of the body to reduce metabolism is often used in cardiac surgery during CPB, the intent on ECMO or ECLS is to maintain normothermia. This is accomplished by regulating the water temperature slightly higher than the intended blood temperature in an effort to maintain desirable body temperatures. If a heat exchanger would malfunction, heat would be lost from the blood through the ECMO circuit to the considerably cool external environment. Even mild hypothermia can have an adverse effect of increased bleeding and a disruption in the body's normal physiological function. Therefore, the ECMO heat

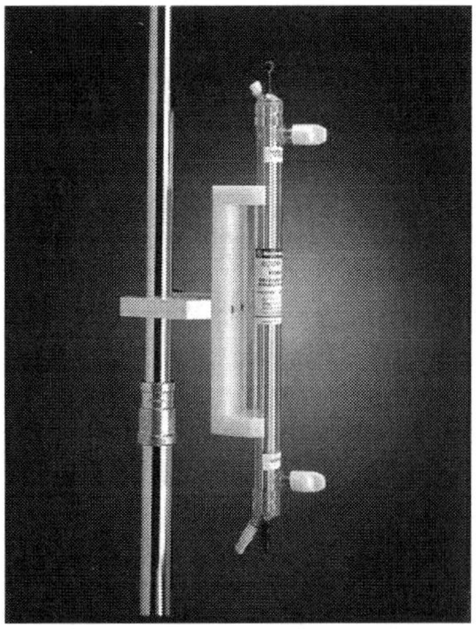

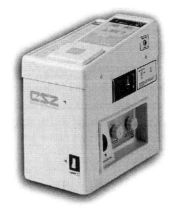

Figure 11. CMO Heat Exchanger

(courtesy of Medtonic Inc.)

Figure 12. Heater Thermal Unit

(courtesy of Cincinnati Sub Zero Inc)

exchanger is often the most distal component in the circuit to prevent ambient heat loss.

On the other hand, recent evidence has demonstrated that a mild drop in the body temperature to around 35° during resuscitation may have a salvaging effect on the brain until normal circulation from ECMO is established.

Conversely, hyperthermia can have a devastating effect on the brain and there is general acceptance that blood temperature not exceed 38.5°. Moreover, blood temperatures in excess of 42° have been associated with hemolysis and protein denaturation. Therefore, water heaters are regulated to avoid temperatures over 42°C to avoid such problems.

ECMO Safety and Monitoring Devices

Life threatening mechanical and patient complications can occur during long-term extracorporeal membrane oxygenation. Preventing, managing, and minimizing the impact of these complications and enhancing the overall safety of ECMO therapy is dependent on, (1) the well trained ECMO specialist and (2) the appropriate use of ECMO monitoring and safety devices. The following section will address the various monitoring and safety devices available.

The ECMO Console

The modern ECMO console provides the ECMO specialist with an integrated array of circuit monitoring and safety capabilities. This includes circuit pressure monitoring and bubble detection and, importantly, a comprehensive alarm system with automation and servo-regulation of the pump when abnormal conditions are detected.

Pressure monitoring:

Venous Line: With the advent of integrated pressure monitoring ECMO consoles it is possible to use a pressure-based system, rather than the historic mechanical bladder box for venous drainage servo-regulation. Mechanical bladder boxes, once the mainstay of ECMO servo-regulation is now only being used by 28% of ELSO center, being displaced by pressure-based venous control systems.[5]

Arterial Line: To prevent over-pressurization and tubing disconnect, the pressure of the arterial line of the ECMO circuit should be constantly monitored and set to alarm and stop the pump if pressure exceeds normal operating thresholds. Pressurization may occur if the arterial line is accidentally kinked or clamped.

Bubble detectors:

Air in circuit is a well described mechanical complication associated with ECMO. (ELSO Complications Report) Therefore, the use of a bubble detector during ECMO is considered essential to prevent accidental air embolism. Bubble detectors, most commonly use clamp-on tubing ultrasound transducers (Figure 13). The bubble detector should be set to alarm and immediately stop the pump if air is detected in the circuit. While it is encouraging that there has been progressive adoption of this important safety device in ECMO (Figure 14),[5,10,11] the use of bubble detectors on ECMO remain well below the rate used during pediatric cardiopulmonary bypass.[12]

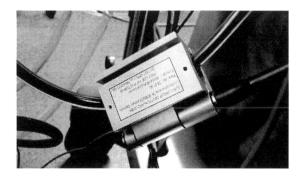

Figure 13. Bubble detector

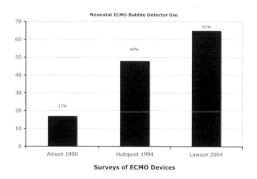

Figure 14.

Blood Flowmeter

The use of an ultrasonic blood flowmeter (Transonic, Ithaca, NY) has found several uses in ECMO applications (Figure 15).

Set/verification of pump occlusion: The flowmeter can be used to set pump roller occlusion upon initiation and to then continually verify flow rates over time when tubing compliance may change or occlusion settings slip.[13]

Flow rates in the setting of shunts: If A-V shunts are being used during ECMO to provide flow through a hemoconcentrator or an in-line blood gas cuvette the pump flow displayed on the by the pump will not be accurate. Placement of the flow sensor distal to a circuit shunt will display the actual blood flow rate to the patient.[14]

High/Low flow alarms & Bubble alarm: The flowmeter can provide low flow and high flow alarms if the pump flow rate is inadvertently turned up or down. The bubble alarm provides back-up to the integral console bubble detector.

Cephalic drainage flow measurements: The flowmeter can also be effective at measuring cephalad jugular venous drainage providing data on the patency of the cephalad cannula.

In-line Oxygen Saturation / In-line Blood Gas Monitors

For real-time assessment of adequacy of perfusion and oxygenator function, it is important to augment the periodic arterial and venous blood sampling with in-line monitors. These monitors are commonly used during cardiopulmonary bypass procedures and considered by many to be a standard of care essential for patient safety and prevention of malpractice suits.[15] Recent survey data indicates that 60% of neonatal ECMO centers use some form on inline blood monitoring.[5]

Oxygen Saturation Monitors: Devices using optical technology can accurately and non-invasively measure oxygen saturation in the blood traveling through the venous and arterial lines of the ECMO circuit. In VA ECMO, the majority of ECMO centers will monitor venous line oxygen saturation as reflective of the patients mixed venous saturation (SVO_2). Decreasing venous line saturations can alert the ECMO specialist of changes in oxygen delivery/consumption and allow for early interventions, eg. pump flow adjustments, red cell transfusion, increased sedation, removal of stimuli. Additionally, arterial line oxygen saturation monitoring will confirm that fully oxygenated blood is exiting the oxygenator. An added parameter commonly included in these monitors is hematocrit/hemoglobin providing the ECMO specialist with additional real-time data. See Figure 16.

In-line Arterial Blood Gas Monitoring: Approximately, 42% of neonatal ECMO programs will monitor in-line measurements of pH, pO_2, pCO_2, BE, $K+$ using a CDI 500 device (Terumo Cardiovascular) (Figure 17). This device used a flow through sensor and fiber optic technology to determine the blood gas parameters. This device can also simultaneously monitor venous saturations and hemoglobin/hematocrit. While the manufacturer makes no claims for the use of this device in long-

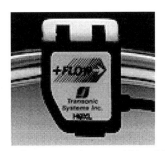

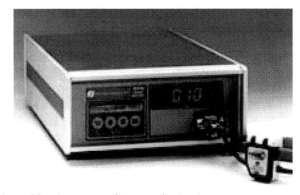

Figure 15. Ultrasound blood flow probe and monitior (courtesy of Transonic, Inc.)

term applications like ECMO, the ability to continuous monitor circuit pO2 and acid-base parameters, pCO2 provides valuable data to the ECMO specialist for patient and circuit troubleshooting.

Cerebral Oximetry Monitors

Near infrared spectroscopy (NIRS) has recently emerged as an effective technique for neurologic monitoring during extracorporeal circulation.[16] These devices (Figure 18) work on the fundamental principle that hemoglobin undergoes characteristic infrared absorption shifts based upon bound oxygen. Therefore, by placing a pad consisting of an emitter and detector on the patients forehead and emitting

infrared light into the brain and then detecting the resultant wavelength, a regional oxygen saturation can be determined. Recent use of NIRS technology in ECMO has shown to have potential as powerful bedside tool for cerebral monitoring.[17]

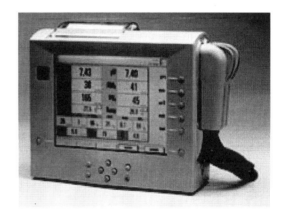

Figure 17. Extracorporeal In-line blood gas monitor (courtesy of Terumo Cardiovascular, Inc.)

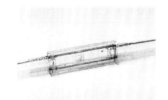

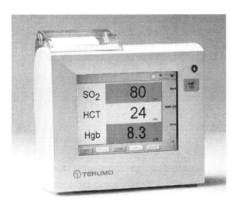

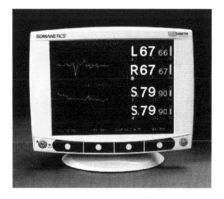

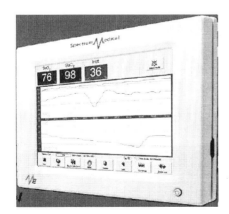

Figure 16. In-line oxygen saturation/hematocrit monitoring devices. (courtesy of Terumo Cardiovascular and Spectrum Medical, Inc.)

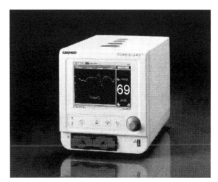

Figure 18. Two Cerebral Oximetry Devices that monitor trends in cerebral oxygen saturations (courtesy of Somenetics and Casmed)

Monitoring Recirculation during VV-ECMO

Recirculation, the fraction of oxygenated blood infused into the right atrium that is immediately pulled back into the venous line of the ECMO circuit during VV ECMO is a well-known limitation of the therapy.[1] As VV ECMO expands to more challenging patients, including congenital diaphragmatic hernia patients and babies requiring inotropic support, monitoring actual recirculation data may become important to identify changes and fully optimize the therapy.[18, 19] Using a technique called ultrasound dilution, it is now possible to monitor and measure recirculation during VV ECMO procedures. (Figure 19) Additionally, quantifying recirculation may allow for an accurate monitoring of patient mixed venous oxygen saturation and provide an additional index of perfusion adequacy.[20]

ACT Analyzers

The term hemostasis means prevention of blood loss by processes which inhibit blood flow through (out of) a ruptured vessel. Through a series of complex mechanisms including vascular spasm, protein and various enzymatic reactions, and platelet activation, blood will begin to clot when some type of stimulus (like an injury) is provided. ECMO, which requires blood to be diverted from the normal blood vessel circulation through a series of artificial extracorporeal (outside the body) components including tubing, oxygenators, and other disposables in the ECMO circuit also provides this stimulus to activate the clotting system. To prevent the clotting of our ECMO circuits, various medications can be infused to prevent the chemical reactions of clot formation from occurring. The most well known, heparin is the anticoagulant of choice as the drug has a rapid effect and can be administered in a bolus form, IV infusion, or slowly to the ECMO circuit. In addition, heparin's anticoagulant effect on the blood can be measured and adjusted to prevent clot formation but minimize excessive bleeding. The activated clotting time (ACT) is the most common bedside measurement utilized in the ECLS clinical setting. Measured in seconds, the ACT can be affected by a number of factors but in a given setting will change based on the blood's concentration of heparin. Therefore, the astute clinician alters the heparin infusion based on an institution's acceptable ACT range to obtain the desired effect.

There are several available devices on the market that measure the ACT (Table 4). Because the functional testing methods vary between these devices, the derived ACT ranges cannot be substituted when comparing or switching machines. In other words, ACT ranges must be tested when an individual ECMO program decides to change devices in their clinical practice. The acceptable range for ACT has been reported to be anywhere between 160 and 250 seconds although most programs will narrow this range to 180-220 seconds. An actively bleeding patient might require this range to be lowered but the risk of intra circuit clot formation then exists.

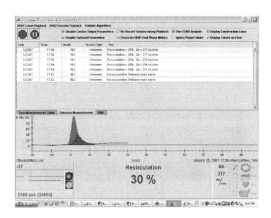

Figure 19. Screen Shot of VV-ECMO Recirculation Monitor (courtesy of Transonic, Inc.)

Table 4.

DEVICE	MANUFACTURER
Actalyke XL	Helena Laboratories
Actalyke Mini II	Helena Laboratories
Hemochron Signature Elite	International Technidyne
Hemochron J. Signature+	International Technidyne
Hemochron Response	International Technidyne
Hemochron 401	International Technidyne
ACT Plus	Medtronic
HMS Plus	Medtronic
I-Stat ACT	Abbott

Generally, the ACT test is performed every hour. The clinician pulls a small sample of blood from the ECMO circuit, infuses the blood to a disposable cartridge, and performs the necessary steps to initiate the ACT device timers (Figure 20). At the completion of the test, the heparin drip may be adjusted to maintain the desirable ACT range.

Thromboelastography (TEG)

Establishing the blood's inherent ability to clot without heparin can also be an effective tool in patient management. Often, the clinician may experience excessive bleeding from the ECMO patient despite minimal to no anticoagulant used. Reasons for excessive bleeding can vary but include low platelet count or poor viability or an inadequate concentration of proteins of the clotting cascade. The Thromboelastograph (TEG®) shown in Figure 15 is one device that has gained acceptance for determining this abnormal functionality. The TEG utilizes a sophisticated mechanism that monitors the clot formation and displays the results in a graphical form.[21] Results can determine if the patient's blood requires platelet, fresh frozen plasma, or cryoprecipitate infusion to normalize clot formation. Once normal function is assessed, the clinicians can then rely on ACT measurement and heparin infusion to sustain a normal ECMO run. See Figure 21.

Surface Coatings

Blood contacting a foreign surface will trigger a variety of activation processes involving numerous blood components. As is the case with our ECMO circuits, this contact activation of platelets, complement, neutrophils, and endothelial cells produces a number of vasodilatory substances which all play a role in an inflammatory response of the body. This response is exhibited by increased vascular permeability and hypotension or vasoconstriction and can cause an increase in morbidity and mortality.[22] One example of this reaction is the dramatic opacification that occurs on a chest x-ray a short time after a patient is placed on ECLS. Often referred to as "white out", the lungs lose free water thru increased alveolar permeability resulting in a reduction of pulmonary gas exchange. This deteriorating state on ECMO often requires an increase in pump flow to accommodate the further compromise of lung function.

In an attempt to minimize the effect of blood contact activation, scientists and manufacturers of CPB and ECMO equipment and disposables have invested significantly in developing several surface coatings (Table 5). Some coatings utilize the heparin molecule in various forms bonded covalently or ionically to minimize blood surface reactions, while others have developed a protein coating to

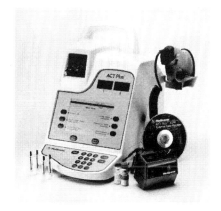

Figure 20. An example of an ACT machine (courtesy of Medtronic Inc.)

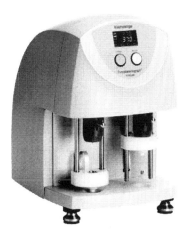

Figure 21. TEG machine

accomplish similar tasks. Another approach is to synthesize copolymers and blend to the plastics of the disposable which create a hydrophobic reaction to the blood elements repelling blood proteins away form the surface area.

The degree of biocompatibility to which each of these coatings present remains debatable, but the objective of minimizing the total body inflammatory response is common. As an ECLS community, we must continue to investigate and evaluate the various methods of surface coating available and determine those that will promote the best patient outcomes.

Table 5.

X Coating (PMEA)	Terumo
Carmeda	Medtronic
Trillium	Medtronic
Smartx	Cobe/Sorin
Phosphorylcholine (PC)	Cobe/Sorin
Bioline	Maquet
Safeline	Maquet
Softline	Maquet
GBS	Medos/Gish

References

1   Hansell, DR. ECMO Equipment and Devices. In. ECMO Specialist Manual 2nd edition. Ed. Krisa Van Meurs. Extracorporeal Life Support Organization 1999; 67-84.

2. Ichiba, S, Peek, GJ, Sosnowski, AW, et al. Modifying a Venovenous Extracorporeal Membrane Oxygenation Circuit to Reduce Recirculation. Ann Thorac Surg 2000;69:298-299

3. Tamari Y, Lee-Sensiba K, King S, Hall MH. An improved bladder for pump control during ECMO procedures. J Extra Corpor Technol. 1999 Jun;31(2):84-90.

4. Chambers, SD, Ceccio, SL, Annich, GA, Bartlett, RH. Extreme negative pressure does not cause erythrocyte damage in flowing blood. ASAIO J 1999;45:431-435

5. Lawson, DS, Walczak, R, Lawson, AF, et al. North American Neonatal Extracorporeal Membrane Oxygenation (ECMO) Devices: 2002 Survey Results. J Extracorp Tech 2004;36:16–21.

6. Lawson, DS, Ing, R, Cheiftez, IM, et al. Hemolytic characteristics of three commercially available centrifugal blood pumps. Pediatr Crit Care Med 2005;6:573–577.

7. Liem KD, Kollee LA, Klaessens JH, Geven WB, Festen C, De Haan AF, Oeseburg B. Disturbance of cerebral oxygenation and hemodynamics related to the opening of the bypass bridge during veno-arterial extracorporeal membrane oxygenation.Pediatr Res 1995;38(1):124-9.

8. De Mol AC, Van Heijst AF, Van der Staak FH, Liem KD. Disturbed cerebral circulation during opening of the venoarterial bypass bridge in extracorporeal membrane oxygenation. Int J Artif Organs. 2008;31(3):266-71.

9. Austin, JW, Horner, DL. The Heart-Lung Machine and Related Technologies of Open Heart Surgery. Phoenix, Arizona, Arrowhead Press Inc., 1990

10. AllisonP, Kurusz M, Graves D, Zwischenberger J. Devices and monitoring during neonatal ECMO: Survey results. Perfusion. 1990, 5:193-201.

11. Hultquist KA, Sussmane JB: ELSO Equipment Survey 1993-94. *ECMO Talk* 6:15, 1994

12. Groom RC, Froebe S, Martin J, et al. Update on Pediatric Perfusion Practice in North America: 2005 Survey. JECT 2005;37:343-350.

13. Snyder, E.J., Harb, H.M., Cullen, J.A., McElwee, D.L., "Setting Roller Pump Occlusion with the Transonic HT109 Flowmeter," ASAIO JOurnal, Vol. 43, p. 60-64, 1997. (517A)

14. Berube, M.C., Brink, L.W., "Ultrafiltration in the Cardiac ECMO Patient: Use of the Transonic HT109 Flowmeter to Determine Hemofilter Shunt and Actual Flow," Presented at the 12th Annual CNMC Symposium on ECMO & Advanced Therapies for Respiratory Failure, Keystone, CO, February 25-29, 1996. (715A)

15. Rubsamen DS. Continuous blood gas monitoring during cardiopulmonary bypass--how soon will it be the standard of care? Cardiothorac Anesth. 1990 Feb;4(1):1-4

16. Cook DJ. Neurologic Effects of Cardiopulmonary Bypass In:Gravlee GP, Davis RF, Stammers AH, Ungerleider RM eds. Cardiopulmonary Bypass: Principles and Practice, 3rd Ed, Philadelphia, PA, Lippincott Williams & Wilken.

17. Rais-Bahrami K. Walton DM. Sell JE.et al. Improved oxygenation with reduced recirculation during venovenous ECMO: comparison of two catheters. Perfusion. 17(6):415-9, 2002 Nov.

18. Darling E, Crowell T, Searles B. Rapid, bedside quantification of recirculation during venovenous ECMO. JECT 2006;38:100

19. Darling E, Crowell T, Searles B. Use of dilutional ultrasound to detect changes in recirculation during venovenous extracorporeal membrane oxygenation. ASAIO J, 2006;52(5):522-524

20. Walker J, Primmer J, Searles B, Darling E. The potential of accurate SVO$_2$ monitoring diuring venovenous extracorporeal membrane oxygenation: An in-vitro model using ultrasound dilution. Perfusion. 2007 Jul;22(4):239-44.

21. Navickas I, Cohen E. Eds. Haemoscope News. Issue 5.

22. Schiel, L, Burns S, Nogawa A, Rice R, Anzai T, Tanaka M. X coating; A new biopassive polymer coating. In. Canadian Perfusion 2001;11:8-9.

Chapter 8 questions

1. The advantages of a polymethylpentene (PMP) hollow fiber oxygenator are:
   a) Low trans-membrane pressure drop
   b) It can be heparin coated
   c) It will not 'wet out' over time
   d) All of the above

2. Which type of oxygenator has been approved by the US FDA for long term use?
   a) Maquet Quadrox D
   b) Terumo RX 05
   c) Medtronic ECMO 0800
   d) Travenol membrane oxygenator

3. Which type of oxygenator can be heparin coated?
   a) Silicone rubber
   b) Polypropylene
   c) Polymethylpentene
   d) B & C
   e) A, B & C

4. Which type of blood pump uses positive displacement to create pressure and flow?
   a) Centrifugal pump
   b) Roller head pump
   c) Non-occlusive pump
   d) A green one

5. An advantage of a dual lumen venovenous ECMO cathether is _____ .
   a) It is easier to insert
   b) It eliminates the need for carotid artery cannulation
   c) It is green
   d) It is longer and therefore may reach the right atrium with greater ease

6. Tubing length should be considered when designing an ECMO circuit. Longer length will cause the following:
   a) Lower resistance
   b) Increased heat loss
   c) Increase priming volume
   d) B & C
   e) A, B & C

7. Cavitation of the blood can be caused by:
   a) Roller pump continues without proper venous drainage
   b) Centrifugal pump continues without proper venous drainage
   c) Pulling blood on a syringe through a stopcock quickly
   d) Improper servoregulation with venous cannula collapse
   e) All the above of

8. Heat exchanger efficiency can be calculated and is dependent on which of the following:
   a) Outlet water temperature
   b) Outlet blood temperature
   c) Inlet blood temperature
   d) B & C
   e) All of the above

9. Heat exchangers can be used to do which of the following:
   a) Cool the patients blood
   b) Warm the patients blood
   c) Maintain normothermia
   d) Add necessary gases to the blood concentration
   e) A, B, and C
   f) A. B, C, and D

10. Bubble detectors identify air in the ECMO circuit using
    a) Bioimpedance
    b) Ultrasound
    c) Infrared light
    d) Turbulent vibrations

11. Recent survey data indicates that in-line blood gas monitoring is used by _____ of ECMO centers
    a) 20%
    b) 40%
    c) 60%
    d) 80%

12. Recirculation, a complication in VV ECMO can be quantified and monitored using:
    a) Ultrasound dilution
    b) Infrared spectrophotometry
    c) Diffusion osmosis
    d) Recirculation cannot be quantified

13. The average activated clotting time (ACT) on ECMO range from:
    a) 90-140s
    b) 180-220s
    c) 240-300s
    d) None of the above

14. ACT values define the which of the following:
    a) Level of anticoagulation of the blood
    b) The amount of heparin in the blood
    c) Normal underlying clotting mechanism of blood
    d) None of the above.

15. Surface coatings of the disposable plastics may do all of the following except:
    a) Prevent surface adhesion of clot formation
    b) Minimize systemic inflammatory reaction of the immune system
    c) Prevent blood clotting in the circuit
    d) Maintain circulating platelet viability

Chapter 8 Answers

1. d
2. c
3. d
4. b
5. b
6. d
7. e
8. d
9. e
10. b
11. c
12. a
13. b
14. a
15. c

9

ECMO Mechanical Complications

Micheal L. Heard, RN, James E. Lynch, BS, RRT, Joseph B. Zwischenberger, MD

Objectives

After completion of this chapter, the participant should be able to:

- Describe the role of the ECMO Specialist in emergency management.
- Discuss the assessment of an ECMO circuit and the environment for management of emergencies.
- Describe the importance in preventing emergencies.
- Perform the off bypass procedure.
- Describe the various component failures and how they may present.
- Describe how to intervene with various component failures for a successful conclusion.

Introduction

Mechanical complications are not an unusual occurrence on ECMO. A recent review of the ELSO Registry database found that component failures occur in 14.9% of ECMO runs.[1] The reason that catastrophic complications occur is due to the fact that ECMO consists of long-term use of disposable parts and high-tech equipment. The Air Force pilots who fly the B-52 bombers for long hours at a time say flying that aircraft consists of "hours and hours of boredom interspersed by moments of stark terror." ECMO can also be that way. It is critical that the ECMO Specialist not be lulled into a false sense of security by periods of relative calm. A rise in the circuit pressure, a slow leak of blood from the gas exhaust port of the membrane, or the development of air in the arterial line are examples of the numerous

brief warning signs of impending disaster during ECMO. It is imperative, therefore, that either the ECMO Specialist or the ECMO physician be at the bedside at all times because the prompt recognition and management of the situations as they occur will hopefully prevent disaster. The purpose of this chapter will be to familiarize the reader with the assessment of common mechanical emergencies that may occur and how to manage them successfully.

The ECMO Specialist

The one constant between all ECMO programs is the use of an individual who has been trained to assess, manage and intervene with the ECMO circuit. Referred to in this chapter as the ECMO Specialist, this individual can be a physician, perfusionist, registered nurse or respiratory therapist. The ECMO Specialist is considered the front line in the management of an emergency event. The management of emergencies can be universally applied despite the differences that exist in ECMO circuits, such as equipment and disposables, number of stopcocks, pigtails, types of pump heads and even oxygenators. Although these things are unique to each center, emergency management techniques remain constant.

Every ECMO Center must have a comprehensive education plan for both the original certification of personnel as well as continuing annual education. The importance of hands-on practice during water drills or animal labs cannot be underestimated. A consistent approach when teaching the ECMO Specialist to perform procedures on the ECMO circuit is a key component of water drill exercises. Many centers are using a simulator to demonstrate certain skills in a real time environment.

There are a few important tenets that should be taught. The first and most important aspect of emergency management is how to take a patient off bypass. Upon recognition of an emergency, the patient must be separated from the ECMO circuit to eliminate further detriment to the patient. In the case of a patient on a roller head pump, place a clamp on the **V**enous line first, open the **B**ridge, and then lastly clamp the **A**rterial line. The acronym V-B-A stands for Very Bad Accident and will help everyone remember the proper procedure in a time of stress. The blood flow is then stopped which allows correction of the problem. Discussed later in this chapter, clamping the arterial line first will be necessary in the event of an air embolus. After stopping ECMO, the patient will then require hand-bagging or emergency ventilator settings to ensure adequate respiratory support.

Another important principle to teach new Specialists is how to quickly recognize emergencies and intervene in a way that allows the most successful outcome of the emergency. The ability of the Specialist to proceed in a timely manner with emergency procedures is invaluable and may prevent secondary emergencies from occurring during a real patient experience. While advocating the usefulness of a timer during practice drills may be hard for some centers the educator must have a sense of whether or not the Specialist is performing up to standards and is incorporating the status of the patient at all times

Additionally, teaching the use of 'eye checks,' which reinforces the thought that the ECMO Specialist is constantly reviewing and assessing the circuit, is extremely significant. Eye checks include monitoring circuit pressures, patient vital signs, and looking for untoward signs on the ECMO circuit, such as "Air In" or "Blood Out." This concept is very helpful for determining how to react. If the Specialist sees air traveling through or blood leaking from, any component, anywhere on the circuit, the immediate reaction is to take the patient off bypass. In fact, because of the position of the ECMO Specialist in front of the pump, actually stopping blood flow *first* as they reach for tubing clamps may prevent the air from traveling further, or the blood from being pumped out under pressure. This immediate action may prevent the emergency from becoming much worse and improve the overall outcome for the patient.

The ECMO Circuit Check

Most events can be prevented with early recognition and the appropriate use of the technology available. The ECMO circuit check is a main responsibility of the Specialist and has the primary goal of preventing emergencies. It is a comprehensive check of all circuitry, equipment, system alarms, fluids and the patient. It is to be completed at the beginning of every shift, and with every hour of the shift. It consists of the following:

- A close scrutiny of the circuit components from arterial to venous for clots, air, leaks, and fibrin strands. Assessment of the function and integrity of the arterial filter, heat exchanger, oxygenator, and raceway or pump head. The security of connectors will be assessed as well as appropriate placement of tie bands. The cannulae will be intact and secured to the patient with sutures and to the bed with towel clamps or other means.

- The alarms on all equipment and their appropriate function will be verified. The bubble detector, if present, should be attached appropriately and functioning.
- The pressure monitors will be appropriately connected to the circuit and alarm limits set as per policy.
- The heater will be appropriately connected to the heat exchanger, the temperature probe will be connected to the appropriate site, and the water level will be full. The temperature set-point will be maintained as per policy.
- The gas module will be connected to the appropriate wall sources and/or tank sources. The gas line will be secure and without leaks to the oxygenator gas inlet port.
- All power cords will be securely plugged into the appropriate receptacle, usually an emergency red power outlet.
- The ECMO pump cart and the patient bed will be in "braked" position.

Additionally, the Specialist must assure that they have everything at close hand that might be useful during an emergency situation. While replacement disposables are inherently easy to think of, the idea of the environment that the patient is in must also be incorporated. Items that should be carefully considered include:

- Tubing clamps, preferably guarded, must be available on the pump cart. The number of clamps may vary but at a minimum there should be six.
- An ECMO supply cart or a room available within a short distance. This should be fully stocked with all disposable parts that may need to be replaced.
- A second ECMO pump cart or individual pieces of equipment available for replacing a failing piece of equipment should be available nearby.
- A volume expander, such as 5% albumin or normal saline, should be available on the pump cart at all times.
- An emergency blood product supply should be maintained in the Blood Bank or in an appropriate refrigerator that is nearby.
- Additional supplies for performing procedures collectively referred to as an 'Emergency Kit,' should be readily available (Table 1).

Table 1. Emergency Kit Components

- Sterile scissors or #10 blade
- Sterile tubing clamps
- Betadine swabs or Chlorhexidine Gluconate (CHG) prep swabs
- 18 gauge needles or other needle
- Various sizes of syringes
- Sterile and non-sterile 4 x 4 gauze pads
- 1-liter bag normal saline at bedside
- 1-60cc syringe with 60cc NS-changed q 24 hours-dated, timed and initialed
- Hand crank in pump cart drawer
- Safety goggles or mask with shield
- Sterile and non-sterile gloves

- Back-up personnel in the event of the emergency that requires extra hands should be available. This may be someone in-house or on-call, and may include physicians, perfusionists, coordinators, or other ECMO Specialists.

Basic Emergency Management

Each ECMO Center should have specific procedures for changing out every component of the ECMO Circuit. While there are differences in preparing disposable parts for replacement, the general approach to changing out parts should be similar for every procedure, as follows.

- A 'Time Out' should be done prior to beginning any procedure. This is done to review every participant's role in the emergency procedure. It is to assure that the correct supplies are available, that every step of the procedure is covered, and that there are no missing components.
- The patient and circuit are prepared for the procedure, such as prepping a sterile field.
- The patient is taken off bypass as per protocol (Table 2), and blood flow is stopped.
- The component is clamped out, using a 'double clamp' method (Table 3).
- The damaged component is cut out and removed.
- The new component is placed airlessly, using a saline drip method to assure all air bubbles are removed from the connection.
- All clamps are removed from the component.
- Blood flow is re-established, and circulation occurs through the circuit to assure there are no leaks, clamps, or other identified problems.
- The patient is returned to bypass as per protocol.

Teaching every Specialist how to double clamp, cut tubing, and fill tubing airlessly are invaluable skills. Tubing clamps can be difficult to manipulate the first time an inexperienced person handles them. Practicing opening and closing clamps securely on

Table 2. Off - Bypass Procedure

Roller head system:

Taking a patient off bypass (V-B-A)
- Clamp Venous line above the bridge
- Open Venous then Arterial bridge stop-cocks, or
- Open bridge clamp
- Clamp Arterial line above the bridge
- If necessary, stop flow (or decrease to < 200cc/min)

Returning a patient to bypass (A-B-V)
- Open Arterial line clamp
- Turn Arterial then Venous bridge stopcock off to circuit
- Open Venous line clamp
- Return to previous ECMO flow rate

Centrifugal system:

Taking a patient off bypass
- lace 1st clamp after oxygenator (must be post-shunt)
- Clamp patient off bypass- arterial and venous lines above the bridge
- Open bridge and remove first clamp post-oxygenator
- Resume flow through bridge

Returning a patient to bypass
- Place first clamp post-oxygenator (must be post shunt)
- Close the bridge
- Unclamp the venous and arterial lines
- Ensure RPMs are increased to 1500
- Remove first clamp post-oxygenator; increase RPMs as needed
- Clear bridge

tubing of various sizes will ensure a secure occlusion of the tubing, thus preventing fluid loss. The use of heavy duty scissors or a scalpel requires practice to assure that the cut is sure and even and that ragged edges do not occur. And finally, knowing how to make an airless connection takes practice, practice, practice! Learning to hold the two open ends while having a second person drip saline into them and then making the connection without air bubbles is very hard to do, but it is an absolutely necessary skill that must be accomplished.

Thrombosis

Clots in the ECMO circuit are the most common mechanical complication during ECMO.[2,3] The correct management of anticoagulation for the ECMO circuit cannot completely prevent clots from forming. In fact, the presence of 'normal' clots should be recognized and taught to the ECMO Specialist. These clots are small in size and usually have no potential to cause harm to the patient or circuit. Normal clots occur wherever there is stagnation that is not preventable, such as at the dependent side of the bottom of the Medtronic Oxygenators. (Medtronic, Minneapolis, MN) This area will often show dark clots after a few hours or days into the ECMO run. As long as the clots do not encroach upon the blood inlet or gas outlet, or cause pressure changes within the membrane, they are not considered dangerous.

Clot assessment can be difficult for the ECMO Specialist. The use of a bright halogen flashlight will assist in the visualization of the clots. Also, the ECMO Specialist will need to assess the ECMO circuit with a 3-dimensional approach. The 'top' of the tubing may be clear, but the 'bottom' or dependent side can be riddled with clots. Clot formation within tubing and connectors is often very easy to see and can be defined as dark clots or white, fibrin strands.

Turbulence, the spinning and tossing of blood cells, causes lysing of cells, and either red blood cells or white platelets are often the victims. Depending on which cells are present, the clots will be colored accordingly. Fibrin strands, which are most often seen streaming from connectors, result as an effect of having fibrin wrap around the lysed cells and attempting to form a solid clot. As discussed in Chapter 10, the clotting cascade is activated with any exposure to biomaterials. This causes the initiation of the extrinsic side of the cascade and an attempt to 'clot off' the ECMO circuit. Dark clots often form where there is stagnation, such as the earlier example of the oxygenator. Other areas of concern may include the bladder, the centrifugal pump head, arterial filter, and heat exchanger. It is the ECMO Specialist's responsibility to find these clots and monitor their presence throughout the ECMO run.

Stagnation in the traditional bladder (Medtronic or Gish Biomedical, Ranchos Santa Margarita, CA) may occur in circuits with lower blood flows. The bottom half of the bladder may not be within the blood stream flowing through it. Blood may become static and swirl within the space and form a dark clot. The consequence of this may be that the clot moves to the outlet side of the bladder where it can occlude blood flow, or travels further downstream to where it can block the blood inlet of the oxygenator. Prevention of these clots requires diligence on the part of the Specialist, including the assessment and removal of them. Some centers advocate 'massaging' the bladder, using a gentle squeezing of the bladder every hour to prevent these clots from even beginning to form.

Other components may become occluded with clots. The judicious use of pressure monitoring will aid in the assessment of these forming clots and prevent them from completely occluding the component. For example, the post membrane pressure module is useful in monitoring any occlusion downstream from the oxygenator. If the heat exchanger (Medtronic) were to develop clots, the pressure would increase. The same would be true for an arterial filter. Ruling out other areas of occlusion or increased pressure would need to be taken into account, such as kinking or movement on the patient side which may cause a back pressure in the return cannula. Clot formation within the oxygenator may result in occlusion of blood flow, causing increased

Table 3: Double Clamp and Cut Procedure

- If it is a large component to be removed, such as an oxygenator:
  - o   Using 2 clamps for above the component, place 1st clamp closest to the component to be removed, then the 2nd clamp ~ 2 – 3 inches distally from the 1st clamp.
  - o   Using 2 clamps for below the component, repeat as above.
  - o   Using heavy scissors or a scalpel blade, cut closest to the clamp that is nearest to the component being removed. This will assure that there is ample tubing left to make a new connection.

- If it is a small component to be removed, such as a connector or pigtail:
  - o   Only using 2 clamps, place each clamp on either side of the component.
  - o   If only a pigtail is to be removed, the distance of the two clamps from the site should only be such that blood loss is prevented.
  - o   Once the clamps are in place, the pigtail can be safely removed, and a new one placed airlessly.
  - o   When removing a connector, assure that each clamp is positioned far enough away from the connector to allow ample room to make a cut and then a connection. The primary purpose of these clamps is to prevent blood loss.
  - o   Cut closest to the connector, leaving as much tubing as possible on the side to be connected to the new connector.

- Follow the saying "Cut closest to the thing you want to get rid of". This will assure that you always have enough tubing to make new connections.
- Maintaining aseptic technique and cleaning the tubing prior to cutting should be incorporated into all policies pertaining to circuit procedures.
- Prior to placing 2nd clamp, if you squeeze the tubing, then place 2nd clamp, it will cavitate the tubing and decrease the likelihood of blood spray when the tubing is cut.

pre-membrane pressure or failure of the function of the membrane as noted by decreased oxygen and carbon dioxide transfer.

Once clot formation has been identified as causing failure of the component, occlusion of tubing, or is in imminent danger of moving into the patient, the Specialist must proceed with removing or changing the component. This may be done electively, before complete failure occurs, and will be a more controlled situation.

Air Embolism

Air in the circuit represents 4% of all complications reported to the ELSO Registry.[1] These can range from small bubbles visualized in the venous side of the circuit to a massive air embolus to the patient. The ECMO circuit has both negative and positive pressures within the system. Negative pressure is measured on the venous drain side of the circuit, from the venous cannula through the bladder. Positive pressure is measured from that point at which the blood starts to move forward though the pump head and into the oxygenator and the arterial return cannula. The appropriate placement and use of pressure modules that servo-regulate the pump and/or a bladder box are excellent preventive measures that should be employed for increased safety for the patient.

Without a bladder box, servo-regulated pressure. or with the alarm overridden if a kink or occlusion were to occur on the venous limb of the ECMO circuit or loss of venous return occur, the pump will generate significant negative pressure. This will result in air being pulled out of solution, known as cavitation. Without mechanisms to stop the pump in the event of loss of blood flow, serious amounts of air can travel through the circuit and may infuse into the patient.

Positive pressure may also become excessive and contribute to the failure of a component (i.e., the oxygenator) or may cause separation of tubing. Again, without a servo-regulated pressure to monitor pressures within the membrane and distally to the patient, if an occlusion were to occur, the back-pressure may cause a tear within the membrane oxygenator. This will allow blood to leak into the gas path of the oxygenator. Blood leaks in the gas

path may eventually occlude the gas egress and consequently cause excessive gas phase pressure. When that occurs, the gas phase pressure exceeds the blood phase pressure and will cause an additional tear within the membrane. Air will enter the blood phase and move towards the heat exchanger. The gas trapping capacity of the heat exchanger and an arterial filter is finite and may be rapidly exceeded. The air embolus will flow towards the arterial return cannula and into the patient.

Another potential source of air is when the partial pressure of oxygen in the blood is very high or supersaturated, as measured by post oxygenator blood gas. This may result in oxygen being forced out of solution. Hitting the membrane or operating the circuit in a low ambient pressure environment (such as in-flight in a non-pressurized cabin) may produce foam at the top of the oxygenator. Prevention of this phenomenon is easily achieved by keeping the post membrane pO_2 < 600 mmHg.

Additionally, the gas egress or exhaust should never be occluded during the ECMO run. While the Specialist is encouraged to assess for a condensate as well as for signs of pink-tinged fluid, they should *never* fully occlude the port with their finger. Even this brief occlusion can cause a precipitous rise in the gas phase pressure and risk a membrane rupture.

The hourly checks the Specialist performs will permit the prompt recognition and appropriate response to an air embolus. It should be noted that the chance of an air embolus happening at the exact moment the specialist is actively assessing the circuit would be incredibly rare. The continuous 'eyeing' of the circuit is an activity at which every Specialist should become an expert. The visualization of air moving through tubing can be seen and immediate action can be taken. Stopping pump flow first will immediately stop the air from traveling with flow. The next step of clamping the arterial side tubing close to the patient is imperative to prevent further movement of air upwards and into the patient. The bridge is opened, the venous line clamped and the patient is off bypass. If, however, air has already entered the patient, additional protective measures should be taken. Once the patient is off ECMO, the head is lowered relative to the body as much as possible in order to move any air away from the cerebral circulation. Once the patient has been stabilized, the use of a hyperbaric chamber for decompression should be considered. If air has entered the coronaries and caused acute cardiac decompensation, high dosages of inotropic drugs may be necessary.[4]

Air can also be found within the circuit and be considered benign. Air entrainment on the venous side from a loose connection or dislodgement of a side hole of a drainage cannula may result in air bubbles. These bubbles are small and easily moved by raising the tubing and allowing the air to rise and move downward with flow. Once the bubbles are isolated in the bladder, they can be easily removed. The bladder is considered one of the air traps that are available within an ECMO circuit. The next air trap would be the oxygenator. In the event that air bubbles continue to travel through the bladder or if air is accidentally infused through an IV line, it would become trapped on the post membrane side of the oxygenator. Most oxygenators have a pigtail placed to allow easy removal of air from this area. The use of a separate heat exchanger also provides an air trap. Small bubbles, which may come from platelet administration, are unable to force their way down a hydrostatic column and usually remain trapped at the top of the exchanger. While there may not be a pigtail present to easily remove the air, one

can remove the air safely by briefly stopping pump flow and aspirating from a pigtail positioned above the heat exchanger (Table 4). Some ECMO Centers have elected to use an arterial filter in-line after the heat exchanger or oxygenator. This would act as a last air trap for the circuit. Air is easily aspirated through a pigtail from the top of the filter.

Finally, the use of an air detector that servo-regulates the pump must be considered as the ultimate preventive measure. While air embolus is a rare complication, the use of this simple device on the tubing before the return cannula can easily prevent any air from entering the patient.

Membrane Oxygenator Failure

The majority of ECMO Centers use Medtronic membrane lung oxygenators, (74.3%), and only a fraction of them are reported as having failed (6%) during an ECMO run.[1] Hollow Fiber and Poly-methylpentene oxygenators are also employed at a number of ECMO centers, and it is reported that they have a failure rate of 18.3% and 0% respectively. Polymethylpentene oxygenators are relatively new to the U.S. market, and their use in ECMO is not wide spread, with only 19 of 13,782 cases collected

Table 4.: Heat Exchanger Air Removal Procedure

- Air is visible at the top of the ECMOtherm heat exchanger
- Attach a 60 cc syringe to a post membrane pigtail located in-between the membrane and the heat exchanger and hold upright
- While maintaining a thumb on the plunger of the syringe, open the stopcock
- Simultaneously stop pump flow and,
- Quickly and firmly aspirate the air into the syringe
- Continue to maintain control of syringe and,
- Restart pump flow and close stopcock
- Either remove syringe and de-air, or ensure air is not re-infused and,
- Return blood removed to patient through same stopcock
- This procedure should take <5 seconds, no need to take the patient off bypass
- If air bubbles remain in the heat exchanger, assure patient is stable, and then repeat the procedure
- If air bubbles go past the syringe towards the membrane, ignore them, restart the pump and allow them to return to the heat exchanger, repeat procedure
  - o Always identify the cause for the air. Air is not normal in the circuit.
  - o The best way to slow or stop air travel is by slowing or stopping the pump flow.
  - o Remember, air rises and moves with flow!

between 1997 and 2006. Recently, there are anecdotal reports that they have significantly less complications resulting in failure than do the silicone membrane oxygentators. Hollow Fiber oxygenators have also been improved in recent generations, but plasma leakage is still a potential problem.

Although the exact criteria used for documenting oxygenator failure from each center are not well defined, the report of failure to the ELSO Registry database usually includes the need for changing the component. Several reasons that oxygenators may fail include gas exchange alterations, such as when oxygen or carbon dioxide transfer is diminished. Pre-membrane pressure measurements that increase significantly perhaps reflecting clot formation within the membrane, are another reason that the oxygenator may need to be changed. Blood leaks from the gas exhaust port are another troublesome sign and usually warrant the removal of the oxygenator.

Many centers use a double-diamond configuration (often referred to as the Galveston Diamond), which allows in-line replacement of the oxygenator without interrupting ECMO flow. Generally, this is considered an advanced procedure due to its low frequency of occurrence. It may be beneficial to have a core group of Specialists or Perfusionists trained to perform the procedure. The bedside Specialist would be responsible for recognizing the signs and symptoms of failure and alerting the team. A planned change out procedure would occur, instead of an acute emergency. Every ECMO center must design their specific policy for identifying oxygenator failure and indications for change. The procedure should also be individualized for the center encompassing the type(s) of oxygenators employed.

Tubing Rupture

Tubing rupture is a rare mechanical complication (0.3%)[1] due to the diligence of the Specialist, as well as the development of Super Tygon (S95E or S65HL) (Norton Performance Plastics, Inc., Akron, OH) raceway tubing. However, polyvinyl chloride tubing (PVC), used for all other tubing requirements aside from the raceway, may become damaged or cracked. The Specialist is responsible for assessing the entire ECMO circuit, assuring that tubing is not caught under wheels, excessively kinked or worn. The use of guarded tubing clamps, which do not allow tubing to become 'bitten' within the jaws, will decrease the damage that may be done to the bridge and other tubing pieces. Careful use of non-penetrating towel clamps will also prevent accidental piercing of tubing.

Tubing connectors are used throughout the ECMO circuit. It is recommended that every connection be tie-banded, even manufactured connections. This will prevent the leakage of blood from any weak points that may occur in the event of over-pressurization of the blood path. The use of a servo-regulated system will also prevent the accidental increase in pressure, preventing accidental tubing separation.

Raceway rupture in a roller head circuit is a potential emergency, and every Specialist should be trained to change a raceway in a timely fashion. The prevention of rupture is easily accomplished by routine 'walking of the raceway.' This procedure involves advancing the section of raceway tubing that has been in the pump head out of the pump head. Each ECMO Center should have a defined policy for the frequency of this procedure. Most policies take into account the size of the raceway tubing as well as the RPMs it is subjected to. Neonatal circuits with ¼-inch raceway tubing may be walked every 6-14 days, while larger pediatric and adult circuits with $^3/_8$-inch or ½ inch, which may be exposed to higher revolutions and wear, may be walked every 4-6 days.

In the event that a raceway accidentally ruptures, the procedure for changing it out is straight-forward. This is one instance where having all supplies readily available is a necessity. The rupture will occur suddenly and without warning. The patient must be removed from ECMO immediately and emergency ventilation and patient management strategies employed. The actual procedure for changing out the damaged section of tubing may vary from institution to institution, but an example of how to perform it is provided in Table 5.

Cannula Problems

Cannulas are inserted during a sterile surgical procedure and care must be undertaken to avoid

Table 5: Raceway Rupture Procedure

Equipment
- Sterile section of 1/4" or 3/8" or 1/2" raceway tubing (Super Tygon-S95E or S65) with connectors attached of appropriate size
- Sterile scissors or sterile scalpel blade #10
- 4 tubing clamps
- 60cc syringe filled with Normal Saline
- Betadine or CHG swabs

Management
- Turn off pump (using speed control knob). Call for help.
- Come off bypass as per protocol
- Clamp inlet and outlet tubing of pump head
- Open tubing gate clamps and remove raceway from pump head
- Double clamp each side of the raceway section out leaving 2" between clamps
- Ideally, wipe tubing between clamps with Betadine or CHG swab briskly and allow to dry
- Using sterile scissors or scalpel blade, cut between double clamps and remove raceway
- The new raceway section should first be connected to end of circuit tubing closest to bladder
- Release clamp on circuit tubing closest to bladder and allow volume from bladder to fill tubing by gravity. (drop tubing level down to fill)
- Once the tubing is filled, clamp tubing on fluid filled section
- Using a 60cc syringe with needle, fill remaining raceway section with normal saline
- Tap gently as it fills to remove air bubbles
- Make airless connection to other end of circuit tubing on the pre-membrane side.
- REMOVE ALL CLAMPS
- Place tubing into pump head, clockwise, following lay of tubing
- Secure the inlet side tubing gate first.
- Turn pump head forward several turns and ensure adequate seating of the raceway, then secure the outlet tubing clamp.
- The bladder and/or pre and post pressure readings will be alarming!
- Give volume (saline, albumin or pRBCs) until bladder alarm is not sounding.
- Turn on pump flow and recirculate through bridge, check for clamps, air, etc.
- Bladder alarm may sound again as pressure equalizes.
- Go on bypass as per protocol
- Check ACT, Hct, replace volume if necessary
- Tighten connections and tie band
- Check occlusion with the Transonics Flowmete

vascular injury. The potential vascular injuries during cannula insertion include tearing of the internal jugular vein and/or superior vena cava with loss of venous control resulting in massive intrathoracic bleeding as well as intimal dissection of the common carotid artery preventing proper cannula placement and potentially leading to lethal aortic dissection. Even after appropriate venous cannula placement, cannula obstruction due to kinking is a common problem; therefore, adequate flow is extremely dependent on patient neck positioning and cannula fixation. Caution must be used by the surgeon as sutures have been known to kink a cannula.

After insertion, venous and/or arterial cannula position can be assessed by chest radiograph or echocardiogram. Initially, the practitioner will be able to determine effective placement by the ability to achieve calculated flows ranging from 120–150 cc/kg/min. An inability to achieve full flow on ECMO may be due to a misplaced venous cannula and may sometimes be remedied by the surgeon at the time of cannulation. High arterial return pressures may indicate a problem with the arterial return cannula.

Difficulties with arterial cannulation can also arise from the catheter being inserted too far into the ascending or descending aorta which may compromise coronary and cerebral oxygenated blood flow, or from being misplaced into the subclavian artery. If the returned blood flow can selectively enter the right subclavian artery, the right upper extremity can be infused with hyper-oxygenated blood flow, while the rest of the body is hypoxic and cyanotic. A cannula in the ascending aorta can cause increased afterload to left ventricular outflow and may contribute to left ventricular failure and cardiac stun. In addition, the cannula can be improperly placed across the aortic valve, causing aortic insufficiency. Finally, the cannula can be inserted against the left ventricular endothelium with the potential for left ventricular disruption or perforation.

Assuring proper suturing technique will lessen the chance of accidental kinking. The Specialist may also use a blanket or towel bundle placed underneath the cannula to support the weight of the tubing connections and maintain their integrity.

Accidental Decannulation

Accidental decannulation is an uncommon complication and one that is usually preventable. Inadvertent decannulation can have devastating consequences, involving the amount of hemorrhage that may occur as well as the loss of ECMO support.

The preventative measure that must be undertaken by all ECMO Specialists is appropriate securing of the cannulas to a fixed object, i.e., the mattress or side of the bed. Relying on sutures and/or tape on the surgical site is ill advised as these can become loose with time on ECMO. One way to assure the placement of the cannulas is for the ECMO Specialist to observe and record the depth of insertion of each neck and/or groin cannula, in centimeters, at the incision site. Comparing measurements with those from previous shifts, the Specialist will be able to identify placement changes and notify the ECMO physician. The use of towel clamps, unique tubing holders made for ECMO tubing, and other methods must be carefully evaluated by each center for their efficacy.

Additionally, the ECMO Specialist is responsible for protecting their environment at all times. Parents, nursing staff and other personnel must be made aware of the placement of cannulas and the attached tubings and warned against any touching or movement of such tubings. The Specialist also assures that the ECMO pump is appropriately braked into position in addition to the bed to prevent inadvertent moving of these objects away from each other.

Finally, the nursing staff must assure that patients are restrained in order to protect themselves from harm. Sedation, paralytics, and extremity restraints are all practices that may be utilized to prevent the patient from dislodging cannulas.

Even with all precautions in place, accidental decannulation still may occur. Tissue fatigue may contribute to the loss of the vessel and sutures. High pressure situations without a servo-regulated system may cause back pressure into the vessel. During transport, the bed may become separated from the ECMO pump by too much distance. Every ECMO program must consider the potential for this emergency and have a policy in place to manage it. An example of a policy for this emergency is in Table 6.

Equipment Failure

The potential for malfunctioning equipment is equatable with household items. If a microwave can malfunction, so can a piece of medical equipment. Each manufacturer describes a troubleshooting regime in their equipment manuals that every Specialist should know and have access to. In the event of complete failure, there must be a readily available replacement. Once again, the ECMO Specialist is responsible for appropriately managing such a change-out procedure.

One particular failure that every practitioner should know how to deal with is electrical or power loss. While it is unlikely that complete loss of power would occur within the hospital, there have been many accounts of this occurring during a natural disaster, such as Hurricane Katrina in New Orleans. There are components that are non-essential, such as the saturation monitors or heater. There are also components that must be dealt with quickly. The loss of power to the pump head can be managed with an uninterruptible battery source. The battery should engage immediately with any power loss and will ensure that pump flow is maintained until

Table 6: Accidental Decannulation Management Procedure

- Diagnosis:
    o Air in venous limb of circuit for venous decannulation
    o Venous bladder alarm, pump stopped
    o Blood loss at cannulation site
    o Cannula visible out of incision site

- Management:
    o Turn off pump flow first! Call for help, including surgeon!
    o Take patient off bypass as per protocol and circulate through the bridge
    o Have bedside RN place direct pressure on site
    o Prepare to immediately give available volume (NS). Call for emergency blood from Blood Bank
    o Stop ECMO flow
    o Attach volume to side of bridge pigtail opposite of decannulated site, OR,
    o Attach volume to pigtail closest to arterial return cannula or on venous limb
    o Clamp bridge, and unclamp line of remaining cannula
    o Push volume
    o Continue to give volume as necessary
    o Every 5 minutes, stop pushing volume, clamp line, unclamp bridge and recirculate briefly
    o The first recirculation will require removal of air in venous limb through bladder
    o If volume is still required, return to procedure, otherwise, recirculate

- In the event of an accidental decannulation on a patient with a double lumen catheter, the patient will have to be managed without the benefit of ECMO catheters to give volume.

- Volume should not be administered through a cephalad catheter.

- These management techniques are to be only used with two cannulation site VV ECMO or VA ECMO.

the situation is remedied. However, in the event that the battery fails or is fully discharged, manual hand cranking must be done. Every Specialist should practice this procedure during their water drills and be familiar with assessing the efficacy of their hand cranking when there are no patient monitors available. This may include feeling for bladder capacity or visually assessing the patient's color and pulse.

Miscellaneous Circuit Components

There are many different components in the many varied ECMO circuits that are available. Heat exchangers, as a separate disposable item, may fail. After redesign of the exchanger many years ago, the primary way these will fail now will be by thrombosis and occlusion of blood flow, temperature probe cracking and blood leaks. These heat exchangers are easily changed out and each center should have a procedure in place for this emergency. The heat exchanger is not essentially life supportive, so in the event of failure the Specialist may remove it and provide temporary heat support through the use of an overhead warmer or warming blanket until the new heat exchanger is primed and placed.

The arterial filter is another disposable that some ECMO centers may use. The failure of this component occurs with excessive clotting. Post membrane pressure monitoring will reflect the increasing obstruction and additionally, will prevent over-pressurization of the circuit. As with the heat exchanger, the Specialist may easily and quickly remove the filter and return the patient to bypass safely. The filter may then be replaced according to department policy.

Centrifugal pumps have a disposable pump head and may fail in a variety of ways, although the newest generation of centrifugal pumps has minimized many of the risks of failure. Some signs and symptoms may include the presence of a consumptive circuit coagulopathy which may indicate that the pump head has clots located within. The sudden increase in noise from the pump head may indicate that one of the bearings has failed. Hematuria is a sign that the heat generated within the pump head is excessive and is causing hemolysis. Most ECMO centers have a prophylactic procedure in place to change pump heads on a routine basis to avoid any

acute failure of the pump head. If an acute failure does occur, the ECMO Specialist must be well versed in the change out procedure.

Individual pieces have also been known to crack or fail from frequent use and fatigue. These include the pigtails and stopcocks. Prevention is the best method to prevent emergent failure. Avoiding over tightening of stopcocks onto pigtails, and pigtails onto connectors will lessen the chance of cracking the luer connections. Using gauze to protect pigtails when clamping them will prevent the tubing clamps' 'teeth' from indenting and cracking the miniature tubing. Additionally, a routine of changing frequently used stopcocks, such as the venous sampling port, will prevent the stopcock from becoming 'sticky' or stiff with use and eventually cracking. Stopcocks that are used on the Stopcock Bridge may also fail with improper positioning of the bridge, causing torque and stress on these parts. Assuring that the bridge is secured without inadvertent twisting and tension will minimize the potential of this part failing.

Summary

Mechanical complications are a possibility for any ECMO circuit at any time. The Boy Scouts' motto, "Be Prepared," is a fitting one for any ECMO Specialist to embrace. The better prepared and educated the Specialist is, the more likely that any emergency that occurs will be handled quickly and safely, with the best possible outcome for the patient. Every ECMO center should have comprehensive policies and procedures for managing every potential circuit and equipment failure possible.

References

1. Fleming GM, Gurney JG, Donohue JE, Reme-napp RT, Annich GM. Mechanical component failures in 28,171 neonatal and pediatric extra-corporeal oxygenation courses from 1987 to 2006. Ped Crit Care Med. 2009; 4:1-5.

2. Upp JR Jr, Bush PE, Zwischenberger JB. Com-plications of neonatal extracorporeal membrane oxygenation. Perfusion. 1994; 9:241-253.

3. Zwischenberger JB, Nguyen TT, Upp JR Jr, et al. Complications of neonatal extracorporeal mem-brane oxygenations. Collective experience from the Extracorporeal Life Support Organization. J Thorac Cardiovasc Surg. 1994; 107:838-848; discussion 848-849.

4. Van Meurs K, Lally KP, Peek G, Zwischenberg-er JB ECMO: Extracorporeal Cardiopulmonary Support in Critical Care, 3rd Edition, Ann Arbor, Extracorporeal Life Support Organization, 2005.

5. Van Meurs K, Rhine W, Derish P. ECMO Spe-cialist Training Manual, Second Edition, Ann Arbor, Extracorporeal Life Support Organiza-tion, 1999.

Chapter 9 Questions

1. The following are signs and symptoms of oxy-genator failure.
   a) Increased Pre membrane pressure
   b) Decreased oxygen and carbon dioxide transfer
   c) Hematuria
   d) Blood leak from the gas egress

2. What are 3 potential air traps in the ECMO Circuit?
   a) Bladder
   b) Raceway
   c) Oxygenator
   d) Cannulas

3. What is an indicator of clot formation within the neonatal heat exchanger?
   a) Deceased venous return
   b) Decreased pre membrane pressure
   c) Increased post membrane pressure
   d) Loss of heat exchanger function

4. Tubing clamps should be guarded to protect the tubing from cracks.
   a) True
   b) False

5. The proper technique for taking a patient off bypass in the even of arterial air should have the venous line clamped first.
   a) True
   b) False

Chapter 9 Answers

1. a, b, d
2. a and c
3. c
4. a
5. b

10

Management of Anticoagulation and Blood Products during ECMO

Laurance L. Lequier, MD and Patricia Massicotte, MD

Objectives

After completion of this chapter, the participant should be able to:

- Outline the routine heparin management of the ECLS patient
- Discuss the use of ACT measurements in coagulation management of the ECLS patient
- Discuss the risk associated with heparin treatment

Introduction

During extracorporeal life support (ECLS) there is continuous contact between circulating blood and the foreign surface of the circuit. When blood comes into contact with any non-endothelial surface, coagulation is initiated. Normally the vascular endothelium maintains the fluidity of blood via a complex interaction between blood cells and plasma factors resulting in a fine balance between procoagulant and anticoagulant activity. During extracorporeal circulation this fine balance is lost as procoagulant mechanisms are activated. In an attempt to minimize this procoagulant activity and prevent thrombosis in the extracorporeal circuit as well as in the patient, an exogenous anticoagulant is necessary. This anticoagulant use can result in bleeding in the systemic circulation. Bleeding and thrombosis occur regularly during the provision of ECLS and can result in significant complications.

Activation of the Coagulation System

When blood is exposed to the non-biologic surfaces of an extracorporeal circuit a complex inflammatory response is initiated.[1] ECLS activates multiple blood cells and plasma protein systems as part of this inflammatory response. This response includes platelets, neutrophils, monocytes, lymphocytes, and endothelial cells as well as the contact, fibrinolytic, and complement systems, along with the intrinsic and extrinsic coagulation pathways.[2] Platelets are activated by adherence to the foreign surface of the extracorporeal circuit leading to further platelet aggregation and activation of the clotting system. Platelet activation and consumption continues throughout the duration of ECLS. Cytokines produced by activated neutrophils contribute significantly to the inflammatory response to extracorporeal circulation.[3] The intrinsic coagulation pathway is likely the main stimulus of coagulation during ECLS, however in those patients who have had recent surgery, tissue factor and the extrinsic coagulation pathway play a major role as well. The binding of activated monocytes to the extracorporeal circuit also causes the release of tissue factor which can stimulate the extrinsic coagulation pathway. The alternative complement pathway, as opposed to the classic complement pathway, is mainly activated by ECLS. Activation of both the contact and fibrinolytic systems has been demonstrated by peak concentrations of Factor XIIa and fibrin degradation products early after the initiation of ECLS.[4] A number of other markers of activation of the clotting system including thrombin-antithrombin complex and d-dimer have been measured in patients after the initiation of ECLS. Such significant activation of the coagulation system results in a pattern of consumptive coagulopathy with demonstrated deficiencies in both platelets and coagulation factors soon after the initiation of ECLS. [5, 6]

Heparin Management

As a result of the activation of platelets and the coagulation system described above, anticoagulation is necessary to prevent clotting in the ECLS circuit. An ideal anticoagulant for this purpose would inhibit platelet and coagulation system activation in the extracorporeal circuit, but still allow enough activity to prevent bleeding in the patient. Such an ideal anticoagulant is not currently available and therefore heparin remains the default anticoagulant for ECLS. Heparin acts primarily by accelerating the action of endogenous antithrombin (AT) and ultimately inhibits thrombin and factor Xa.[7] Heparin inhibits thrombin after it is formed, but it does not inhibit thrombin formation nor does it inhibit thrombin already bound to fibrin.

Patients usually receive an initial bolus of heparin of between 50 -100 units per kg body weight at the time of cannulation for ECLS. The bolus dose can be adjusted based on clinical factors such as evidence of pre-existing bleeding, if for instance the patient has had recent surgery or cardiopulmonary bypass (CPB), and whether or not the heparin given during CPB has been completely reversed. A heparin infusion will be mixed and connected to the ECLS circuit immediately following initiation of ECLS. When the measured activated clotting time (ACT) drops to 300 second or lower, the heparin infusion can be started at or 10-20 units/kg/hr, unless there is excessive bleeding. Patients who are experiencing significant bleeding or who have just had cardiac surgery may not be started on heparin immediately.

Heparin infusion rates will be titrated by the ECLS specialist to maintain the ACT within the ordered daily parameters. The standard ACT parameter range will vary from center to center depending on local experience and the type of monitoring equipment being used.[8] Our own standard ACT range is 160-180 seconds, for a non-bleeding patient following initiation of ECLS using the ISTAT analyzer with Kaolin ACT cartridge. This is a starting guideline and will be adjusted based on specific patient condition and response to an-

ticoagulation therapy. Generally, a lower range of ACTs are desired for patients at increased risk for bleeding or who are having clinical bleeding, while higher ACT's are accepted when there appears to be clot developing anywhere in the ECLS circuit. Adequate ACTs are typically achieved with infusion rates of 20-40 units/kg/hour of heparin. Increased urine output, the use of renal replacement therapy, or the administration of platelets will usually result in an increased heparin requirement to maintain goal ACTs. Since heparin is dependent on circulating AT for most of its anticoagulant activity, it may be helpful to measure AT levels, particularly in the patient who has a high heparin requirement.[9] Pooled plasma and recombinant AT concentrate are now available and can be administered to patients with low levels (less than 50% of normal activity) and results in a significant decrease in markers of prothrombin activation.[10] The use of AT concentrate is preferred over the administration of fresh frozen plasma (FFP) for this purpose as giving standard bolus infusions of FFP does not easily achieve adequate AT levels in patients on ECLS.[11] Frequent boluses of FFP or continuous FFP infusions may be needed to ultimately achieve an increased AT level using FFP alone.

The ACT has been used for decades to monitor and guide heparin therapy in extracorporeal applications. It is a crude monitor of heparin anticoagulation requiring multiple serial determinations to improve accuracy, but it is a low cost, bedside test that is available around the clock.[12] However, the ACT has been shown to have poor correlation to the gold standard test, plasma heparin levels (anti-factor Xa activity), both in adults undergoing cardiopulmonary bypass and critically ill intensive care patients.[13, 14] The ACT alone was shown to be unreliable at predicting plasma heparin concentration in children undergoing cardiopulmonary bypass and more recently in a series of neonates on VA ECMO.[15, 16]. This may be due to lower physiologic levels of some coagulation factors in addition to the effects of hemodilution and hypothermia. More importantly, children have decreased levels of AT compared to adults, which may impair their response to heparin and result in inadequate anticoagulation when using ACT to guide heparin dosing.[17, 18, 19] The majority of ECLS centers use the ACT alone to dictate heparin dosage.[20] Unfortunately the ACT is not only affected by heparin but also platelets and other coagulation factors. A prolonged ACT, for example, may be due to a high heparin level and therefore indicate that the amount of heparin being given should be reduced. However, it may also be due to decreased fibrinogen, platelets, or other coagulation factors in which case the plasma heparin level and therefore heparin dose may be appropriate. The ACT has served the ECMO community well for over twenty years and will continue to be the most frequent measure of heparin anticoagulation during extracorporeal support. However, because of the potential shortcomings of heparin and the ACT discussed above, it may be useful to complement frequent ACT measurements intermittently with more elaborate tests like a plasma heparin (anti-factor Xa) level.[21]

Daily ACT parameters can be reviewed and adjusted based on the therapeutic effect of heparin as it relates to the bleeding and thrombosis status of the patient and ECLS circuit, as well as measured daily unfractionated heparin levels. We measure unfractionated heparin and serum antithrombin levels every morning as a routine. We then maintain a therapeutic heparin level of 0.25-0.50 units/kg and an AT level > 50% of normal activity. These levels can be measured more frequently if there is clinical bleeding or thrombosis issues if your laboratory is able to perform this service. As well, given that the ACT is more likely to overestimate heparin effect in children which may lead to inadequate anticoagulation and possible thrombosis, some ECLS programs adopt a minimum heparin dose of 10-20 units/kg/hour despite the ACT value. Pediatric hematology or pediatric thrombosis service consultants can be helpful to help tailor your individual anticoagulation protocols.

Clinical Consequences

Bleeding complications are frequently encountered during the provision of ECLS and are the principal cause of morbidity and mortality. In addition to the need for anticoagulation to maintain patency of the extracorporeal circuit, patients who require ECLS may be predisposed to bleeding in a number of ways. Infants are the most likely population to

receive extracorporeal support and are known to have, at baseline, lower levels of coagulation factors than do older children and adults.[22] Patients with cardiorespiratory compromise severe enough to require ECLS can demonstrate various degrees of disseminated intravascular coagulation (DIC). In one study, more than two thirds of infants and children demonstrated significant coagulation factor deficiencies prior to being placed on ECLS.[6] Over half of these patients continued to have coagulation factor deficiency despite factor replacement at the time of cannulation. Ongoing consumption of platelets and coagulation factors in the extracorporeal circuit during ECLS increases the chance of bleeding complications.

Surgical site bleeding, the most common source of bleeding, is reported in 6 – 32% of ECLS patients with the highest incidence occurring in patients who have had recent cardiac surgery.[23] Central nervous system hemorrhage, the most potentially devastating bleeding complication, occurs in 3 – 6% of patients who have received ECLS with neonates having the highest incidence. Hypoxemia, acidosis and cardiovascular instability prior to initiation of ECLS, prematurity, coagulopathy, and jugular vein/carotid artery ligation all increase the risk for intracranial hemorrhage.[24] The development of an intracranial hemorrhage may require discontinuation of ECLS.

In an effort to reduce the risk of bleeding complications and/or to treat clinical bleeding, significant blood product replacement may be required during the course of ECLS. Transfusions of packed red blood cells are given as needed to replace any blood loss and maintain a normal hematocrit (> 35%). Frequent platelet transfusions of 10 ml/kg, or 1 unit per 5 kg, are given to maintain a platelet count >100,000 cells/mm³ in most patients, particularly neonates. The threshold for platelet transfusion may be reduced in older patients with a lower risk of intracranial hemorrhage and a stable ECLS run. Fresh frozen plasma (FFP) is given in aliquots of 10 ml/kg as needed if the PT INR is > 2.0 and/or if there is significant bleeding. FFP may also be used, as previously described, in an effort to increase the serum antithrombin level. Cryoprecipitate can be given if the fibrinogen level is < 100 mg/dL.

Often the level of anticoagulation accepted may be reduced in the face of clinically significant bleeding. Surgical exploration with careful hemostasis may be required in some cases. Topical cryoprecipitate with thrombin glue can be used at the surgical sites to help control oozing. Additional agents, such as aminocaproic acid and aprotinin, both inhibitors of fibrinolysis, have been used successfully to manage significant surgical site bleeding.[25, 26] However, aprotinin has recently shown to be associated with renal dysfunction following cardiac surgery making its use controversial.[27] There are also several reports of using recombinant factor VIIa for severe intractable surgical site bleeding during ECLS with good effect at decreasing blood loss.[28, 29]

Novel Anticoagulation

There is a relatively new class of anticoagulants that bind to thrombin directly, independent of circulating AT.[30] These anticoagulants demonstrate more predictable pharmacokinetics and reduce thrombin generation to a greater degree when compared to heparin.[31] Two direct thrombin inhibitors, argatroban and lepirudin, have been used in ECLS, mainly in the context of pre-existing heparin induced thrombocytopenia (HIT).[32, 33] The advantage of acting independent of antithrombin, make these anticoagulants especially appealing for use in ECLS for infants and children, not just in cases of HIT. Dosing is adjusted by maintaining activated partial thromboplastin time (aPTT) ratios of 1.5-2.5. No reversal agent is currently available so care must be taken to avoid over anticoagulation.

An ideal anticoagulation strategy for ECLS would be to modify the extracorporeal circuit to make it as non-thrombogenic as vascular endothelium. Endothelial cells produce prostacyclin and nitric oxide (NO) which inhibit platelet adhesion and activation.[34] Both prostacyclin and NO added to extracorporeal circuits have been shown to reduce platelet consumption.[35, 36] Incorporation of NO releasing polymers onto the surface of extracorporeal circuits not only reduced platelet consumption, but also eliminated the need for systemic heparinization in an animal model.[37] Many centers are using heparin-bonded circuits in an effort to make their circuits more biocompatible and limit or eliminate the need for anticoagulation during cardiopulmonary bypass and ECLS. Some have shown that the use of these circuits reduces platelet activation, fibrinolysis and the inflammatory response.[38] Others have demonstrated decreased blood loss and need for blood product replacement when heparin-bonded circuits were used, however the useful effects of the coated circuits may be too short-lived to be of benefit in longer runs of ECLS.[39, 40] Some programs have experience with a "multi-system therapy protocol" to achieve both frequent and accurate heparin dosing including using dipyridamole to stabilize platelet function, aspirin to inhibit platelet aggregation, aprotinin to prevent excessive fibrinolysis, and pentoxiphylline to reduce blood viscosity.[41] This protocol resulted in reduced bleeding and was associated with improved survival in a group of ECLS compared to a group of historical control patients in which heparin therapy and ACT monitoring alone were used for anticoagulation.

Although there are several promising therapies on the horizon, clearly further investigation is needed to determine the optimal combination, duration, and dosage of coagulation inhibitors needed to limit bleeding and thrombotic complications in patients on ECLS. In the meantime, ACT-monitored heparin infusions will continue to be a mainstay of anticoagulation during the provision of extracorporeal support. Plasma antithrombin and unfractionated heparin levels are complementary tests that are now available to help guide heparin management and are increasingly being used in many ECLS centers.

References

1. Wan S, LeClerc JL, Vincent JL. Inflammatory response to cardiopulmonary bypass. *Chest* 1997;112:676-692.

2. Bowen FW and Edmunds HL, Jr. Coagulation, anticoagulation and the interaction of blood and artificial surfaces. In: Zwischenberger JB, Steinhorn RH, Bartlett, RH, eds. *ECMO: Extracorporeal cardiopulmonary support in critical care*. 2nd Ed. Ann Arbor, Mich ELSO 2000:67-96.

3. Fortenberry JD, Bhardwaj V, Niemer P et al. Neutrophil and cytokine activation with neo-

natal extracorporeal membrane oxygenation. *J Pediatr* 1996;128:670-8

4. Plotz FB, van Oeveren W, Bartlett RH et al. Blood activation during neonatal extracorporeal life support. *J Thorac Cardiovasc Surg* 1993;105:823-832.

5. Urlesberger B, Zobel G, Zenz W et al. Activation of the clotting system during extracorporeal membrane oxygenation in term newborn infants. *J Pediatr* 1996;129:264-268.

6. McManus ML, Kevy SV, Bower LK et al. Coagulation factor deficiencies during initiation of extracorporeal membrane oxygenation. *J Pediatr* 1995;126:900-904.

7. Samama MM, Bara L. Goulin-Thibault I. New data on the pharmacology of heparin and low molecular weight heparin. *Drugs* 1996;52:8-15.

8. Fleming GM, Gupta M, Cooley E et al. Maintaining the standard:a quality assurance study for new equipment in the Michigan ECMO program. *ASAIO J* 2007;53: 556-60

9. Shapiro A. Antithrombin deficiency in special clinical syndromes – Part I: Extracorporeal Membrane Oxygenation. *Seminars in Hematology* 1995;32:33-36.

10. Pollock ME, Owings JT, Gosselin RC. ATIII replacement during infant extracorporeal support. *Thromb Haemost* 1995;73:936.

11. Thureen PJ, Loomis M. Manco-Johnson M et al. Randomized trial of albumin versus plasma for correction of ATIII deficiency in neonatal ECMO. Second annual meeting of ELSO 1990 (Abstract 50).

12. Green TP, Isham-Schopf B, Steinhorn RH et al. Whole blood activated clotting time in infants during extracorporeal membrane oxygenation. *Crit Care Med* 1990;18:494-498.

13. DeWaele JJ, Van Cauwenberghe S. Hoste E, et al. The use of activated clotting time for monitoring heparin therapy in critically ill patients. *Intens Care Med* 2003;29:325-328.

14. Raymond PD, Ray MJ, Callen SN, Marsh NA. Heparin monitoring during cardiac surgery. Part 2: Calculating the overestimation of heparin by the activated clotting time. *Perfusion* 2003;18:277-281.

15. Nankervis CA, Preston TJ, Dysart KC et al. Assessing Heparin Dosing in Neonates on Veno-

arterial Extracorporeal Membrane Oxygenation. *ASAIO J* 2007; 53:111-114.

16. Gruenwald C, deSouza V, Chan AK, Andrew M. Whole blood heparin concentrations do not correlate with plasma antifactor Xa heparin concentrations in pediatric patients undergoing cardiopulmonary bypass. *Perfusion* 2000;15:203-209.

17. Male C, Johnston M, Sparling C, Brooker L, Andrew M, Massicotte P. The influence of developmental haemostasis on the laboratory diagnosis and management of haemostatic disorders during infancy and childhood. *Clinics in Lab Med* 1999;19:39-69.

18. Owings JT, Pollock ME, Gosselin RC, Ireland K, Jahr JS, Larkin EC. Anticoagulation of children undergoing cardiopulmonary bypass is overestimated by current monitoring techniques. *Arch Surg 2000;*135:1042-1047.

19. Baird CW, Zurakowski D, Robinson B et al. Anticoagulation and Pediatric Extracorporeal Membrane Oxygenation: Impact of ACT and Heparin Dose on Survival. *Ann Thorac Surg* 2007;83:912-20.

20. Graves DF, Chernin JM, Kurusz M, Zwischenberger JB. Anticoagulation practices during neonatal extracorporeal membrane oxygenation: survey results. *Perfusion* 1996;11:461-466.

21. Muntean W. Coagulation and anticoagulation in extracorporeal membrane oxygenation. *Artificial Organs* 1999;23:979-983.

22. Andrew M, Paes B, Johnston M. Development of the hemostatic system in the neonate and young infant. *Am J Pediatr Hematol Oncol* 1990;12:95-104.

23. Extracorporeal Life Support Organization. *Registry Report.* Ann Arbor: University of Michigan; January 2009.

24. Bulas D, Glass P. Neonatal ECMO: neuroimaging and neurodevelopmental outcome. *Seminars in Perinatology* 2005;29:58-65.

25. Downard CD, Betit P, Chang RW, Garza JJ, Arnold JH, Wilson JM. Impact of Amicar on hemorrhagic complications of ECMO: A ten year review. *J Pediatr Surg* 38:1212-1216.

26. Biswas AK, Lewis L, Sommerauer JF. Aprotinin in the management of life-threatening bleeding

during extracorporeal life support. *Perfusion* 2000;15:211-216.

27. Mangano DT, Tudor IC, Dietzel C, et al. The Risk Associated with Aprotinin in Cardiac Surgery. *NEJM* 2006 354;: 353-365.

28. Dominguez TE, Mitchell M, Friess SH et al. Use of recombinant factor UNA for refractory hemorrhage during extracorporeal membrane oxygenation. *Pediatr Crit Care Med* 2005;6:348-351.

29. Niebler, RA, Punzalan, RC, Marchan M et al. Activated recombinant factor VII for refractory bleeding during extracorporeal membrane oxygenation. *Pediatr Crit Care Med* 2009; 10; 1-5.

30. Bates SM, Weitz JI. The mechanism of action of thrombin inhibitors. *J. Invasive Cardiol* 2000;12:1-12.

31. Young G, Yonekawa KE, Nakagawa P, Nugent AJ. Argatroban as an alternative to heparin in extracorporeal membrane oxygenation circuits. *Perfusion* 2004;19:283-288.

32. Young G, Yonekawa KE, Nakagawa p, Nugent DJ. Argatroban as an alternative to heparin in extracorporeal membrane oxygenation circuits. *Perfusion* 2004;19:283-288.

33. Dager WE, Gosselin RC, Yoshikawa R, Owings JT. Lepirodin in heparin-induced thrombocytopenia and extracorporeal membrane oxygenation. *Ann Pharmacother* 2004;38:598-601.

34. Radomski MW, Palmer RMJ, Moncada S. The anti-aggregating properties of vascular endothelium: interactions between prostacycline and nitric oxide. *Br J Pharmacol* 1987;92:639-646.

35. Addonizio VR, Strauss J, Macarak EJ et al. Preservation of platelet number and function with prostaglandin E_1 during cardiopulmonary bypass in rhesus monkeys. *Surgery* 1978;83:619-625.

36. Jacobson J. Nitric oxide: platelet protectant properties during cardiopulmonary bypass/ECMO. *J Extra Corpor Technol* 2002;34:144-147.

37. Annich GM, Meinhardt JP, Mowery KA et al. Reduced platelet activation and thrombosis in extracorporeal circuits coated with nitric oxide release polymers. *Crit Care Med* 2000;28:915-920.

38. Palatianos GM, Foroulis CN, Vassili MI et al. A prospective, double-blind study of the efficacy of the bioline surface-heparinized extracorporeal perfusion circuit. *Ann Thorac Surg* 2003;76:129-135.

39. Marcolin R, Bonbino M, Pesenti A, et al. Venovenous ELS with heparin bonded circuits. *Int J Artif Organs* 1995;18:624-626.

40. Tayama E, Hayashida N. Akasu K et al. Biocompatibility of heparin-coated extracorporeal bypass circuits: New heparin bonded bioline system. *Artif Organs* 2000;24:618-623.

41. Glauber M, Szefner J, Senni M, Gamba A et al. Reduction of hemorrhagic complications during mechanically assisted circulation with the use of a multi-system anticoagulation protocol. *Artificial Organs* 1995;18:649-655.

Chapter 10 Questions

1. Which blood component is consumed and replaced most often during ECMO:
   a) red blood cells
   b) platelets
   c) fibrinogen
   d) plasma coagulation factors

2. What is the most significant bleeding site during ECMO:
   a) gastric
   b) surgical site
   c) cannulation site
   d) central nervous system

3. Heparin acts by accelerating the action of:
   a) prothrombin
   b) thrombin
   c) antithrombin
   d) fibrin

Chapter 10 Answers

1. b
2. d
3. c

11

Management of the Neonate on ECMO

Curt L. Shelley, MEd RRT-NPS AE-C and Nancy J. Rees, BSN RN

Objectives

After completion of this chapter, the participant will be able to:

- Describe the national trends for Neonatal ECMO
- List and explain the inclusion and exclusion criteria for Neonatal ECMO
- List and describe the diseases which respond to ECMO
- Delineate the steps taken to place a neonate on ECMO
- Describe the daily maintenance of a neonate on ECMO
- Describe the personnel and responsibilities each ECMO team member
- Describe the process of weaning from ECMO

Introduction

In 1973, Esperanza, an abandoned infant in Los Angeles, was treated for Meconium Aspiration Syndrome (MAS). The conventional treatment at the time was not working and it appeared that she was going to die. Utilizing a modified intraoperative cardiopulmonary bypass, Dr. Robert Bartlett was able to allow her lungs time to heal from the pneumonitis, inflammation and surfactant inactivation, which aspirated meconium causes.[1] Since then 22,867 Neonatal Respiratory ECMO cases have been reported to the Extracorporeal Life Support Organization (ELSO) Registry, with an overall 85% survival rate. However, in contrast to Pediatric Respiratory ECMO, Neonatal Respiratory ECMO

demand worldwide continues to decline.[2,3] At its peak, in 1992, 1516 Neonatal Respiratory cases per year were being reported to ELSO. Since then, the number of cases has dropped 58% to the 631 cases reported in 2008. A retrospective review of the ELSO database published in 2005 found that the use of inhaled nitric oxide (iNO), high frequency ventilation and surfactant all increased significantly. During the study period between 1996 and 2003, there was a marked decline in the total number of infants treated with ECMO for MAS, RDS and sepsis.[4] Confounding this finding though, is the fact that the ELSO database does not contain information on patients treated with these modalities, and subsequently did not require ECMO. However, the inference can be made that the lower number of reported ECMO cases is, at least tangentially, related to the use of iNO, HFV and surfactant.

As our knowledge of the disease processes and the technology of ECMO improve, varieties of processes have emerged from the many ECMO centers, all of which are equally effective. We are going to explore the most employed processes utilized to treat neonatal respiratory failure via ECMO.

Inclusion and Exclusion Criteria

The goal of each ECMO center is to identify patients who would benefit from ECMO while attempting to limit this patient population to those whose risks for undesirable complications is acceptable. Despite the advances noted earlier, the target population remains at the 50 to 75% mortality risk quartile, based on oxygenation index and PRISM scores, noted by Green in 1996 to be the one quartile that benefited from ECMO.[5] No other quartiles benefited above what was being offered by conventional treatments. The objective becomes how to identify this 50 to 75% quartile. The inclusion criteria consist of:

- Gestational age >34 weeks
  - o Intracranial hemorrhage risk increases dramatically with patients with less than 34 weeks gestation[6]
- Birth weight >2 kg
  - o A higher mortality is associated with birth weights less than 2 kg.[7] In addition, catheter size in this cohort will be a limiting factor to venous blood flow. Future thin-walled catheters, however, may improve blood flow.
- Reversible lung disease
  - o Chronic lung disease, more than 10 to 14 days of mechanical ventilation, and extended exposure to high oxygen concentrations are relative contraindications. Irreversible conditions, such as surfactant protein B deficiency, alveolar capillary dysplasia or pulmonary hypoplasia, may not be detected prior to placement on ECMO. However, once on ECMO, a definitive diagnosis can be made.
- The absence of uncontrolled bleeding or coagulopathy
  - o The heparinization needed to prevent clotting within the ECMO circuit will contribute to any coagulopathy and potentially create uncontrollable hemorrhage.[8]
- No intracranial hemorrhage ≥ grade III[9]
  - o While the risk for intracranial hemorrhage is large in a population of heparinized, previously hypoxic infants, Grade II IVH can be managed with judicious use of heparinization, limiting intravascular volume administration[10] and limiting the use of the bridge during VA ECMO.[11]
- No uncorrectable congenital heart disease
  - o A cardiac echo should be performed prior to cannulation.
    - o Unstable congenital heart patients may require ECMO prior to corrective surgery
- Failure of optimal medical management
  - o High frequency oscillator ventilation, surfactant and iNO have all been either utilized or determined to be not helpful.
- Lethal anomalies, such as Trisomy 13 or 18, would not benefit from ECMO. In addition, severe or irreversible brain injuries, as documented with a head ultrasound or CT, should be excluded.
  - o Decision to provide full support

Each of these criteria should be used as general guidelines, not absolutes. Erring on the side of caution and providing ECMO for borderline cases will allow for a conclusive diagnosis of abnormalities in a calm, composed manner. Rushed decisions to exclude ECMO may eliminate some patients who could benefit from ECMO and have productive lives. This inclusion threshold should be at the 80% mortality range. A study done by Green showed that the patients in the 50% to 75% mortality risk quartile had significantly better mortality compared to matched controls (29% vs. 71%, p< .05).[12]

The challenge is identifying patients who fall in the 50% to 75% mortality quartile. There are several calculations to evaluate the mortality probability. The oxygen index (OI) remains the most widely used due to its reliability to predict death or chronic lung disease.[13],[14] The indications for ECMO were determined over 25 years ago and subsequent research has proven that they are still as valid as they were 25 years ago. In a study published in 2006, Bayrakci found the mortality risk increases 16 times when OI > 33.2.[13]

Neonatal Diseases

Congenital Diaphragmatic Hernias

Of the 5721 Congenital Diaphragmatic Hernias (CDH) cases reported to ELSO from 1985 to 2008, 51% of the patients survived.[3] A prospective cohort study done in 2007 by the Congenital Diaphragmatic Hernia Study Group showed that survivability was indirectly related to the size of the defect.[15] Despite increased use of iNO, ECMO use in CDH cases remains high.[16] Accurate occurrence is difficult to determine because some severe CDH cases die in utero and are spontaneously aborted. However, it is estimated that 84% of all CDHs are left-sided, 14% are right-sided and 2% are bilateral.[17] Other anomalies are commonly associated with CDH, such as cardiac, gastrointestinal, genitourinary, skeletal or neural anomalies.[18] The compression of the fetal lungs by the herniated viscera in the chest cavity causes pulmonary underdevelopment and lung hypoplasia. The survivability of CDH cases is based mainly on the severity of the lung hypoplasia and the resulting persistent pulmonary hypertension (PPHN).[19]

Meconium Aspiration Syndrome

The most successfully treated disease, with a 94% survival rate, is Meconium Aspiration Syndrome (MAS). New therapies have prevented less sick neonates from requiring ECMO. Newer therapies being used to treat MAS are volume ventilation via synchronized intermittent mandatory ventilation (SIMV), high-frequency oscillatory ventilation (HFOV), surfactant and iNO.[20] However, there remains a population of MAS patients who do not respond to the new therapies, possibly due to outlying hospitals not transferring potential ECMO candidates in hopes of successful treatment with HFOV or iNO. Then when these non-responders have demonstrated that newer therapies have not worked, the continuing right-to-left shunting, progressing hypoxia and precarious transport to an ECMO center place these patients into a higher morbidity cohort. This finding is supported by the fact that the survival rate for MAS on ECMO has dropped and the time on ECMO has increased.[21]

The chemical pneumonitis, inflammation and pneumothoraces caused by ball-valve effect of meconium respond extremely well to treatment with VV ECMO.[22] A study done in 2007 found that MAS patients had a significantly lower number of complications per patient when compared to non-MAS patients. Therefore, by relaxing the entry

criteria more MAS patients would be treated with ECMO, thereby improving patient outcomes.[23] Delayed ECMO initiation, on the other hand, has been found to be a predictor of increased length of hospital stay, with no significant change in survival rates in infants with MAS.[22]

Persistent Pulmonary Hypertension of the Newborn

Persistent Pulmonary Hypertension of the Newborn (PPHN) cases requiring ECMO has decreased as the use of iNO has become prevalent.[24] PPHN is defined as a constriction of the pulmonary vasculature causing an increase in the pulmonary vascular resistance, failing to relax in response to increasing SaO_2 resulting in hypoxemia.[25] In utero, pulmonary vascular resistance (PVR) is greater than systemic vascular resistance. At birth, due to the negative intrathoracic pressure caused by the chest wall moving and the subsequent increase in SaO_2, the PVR decreases, the pulmonary blood flow increases and the right-to-left shunting which was present due to the open ductus arteriosus is stopped. However, if the patient remains hypoxic, the PVR will remain high and the right-to-left shunt will continue to allow deoxygenated blood to circulate to the body. PPHN can be caused by any condition which leads to hypoxia, thereby causing the ductus arteriosus to open and allow a right-to-left shunt. ECMO allows hyper-oxygenated blood to be circulated and thereby close the open ductus arteriosus and prevent the right-to-left shunt from occurring, while the underlying condition which caused the shunting, is resolved.[26] Of the 3721 PPHN cases reported to ELSO as of December 2008, 78% survived to discharge.[3]

Respiratory Distress Syndrome

A critical component leading to Respiratory Distress Syndrome (RDS) is the dysfunction and abnormal synthesis of surfactant.[27] Despite positive results from treatment with antenatal steroids, placental transfusions, immediate use of continuous positive airway pressure (NCPAP), early administration of surfactant, and gentle modes of ventilation to minimize damage to immature lungs, ELSO reports that 1470 RDS patients have required ECMO, with 84% survivability.[3]

Sepsis

Sepsis is a leading cause of infant mortality.[28] While use of intrapartum antibiotic prophylaxis has led to declines in perinatal sepsis caused by the bacteria group B streptococcus (GBS), interventions to prevent perinatal sepsis due to other causes have not yet been clearly defined.[28] GBS commonly is presented as overwhelming vascular collapse. The cardiovascular instability and coagulopathy caused by GBS, while complicating the patient management, is supported by the cardiac output and oxygenation provided by ECMO. The 2007 American College of Critical Care Medicine Clinical Practice guidelines call for ECMO in infant patients with refractory shock.[29] As of December 2008, 2580 patients have been reported to ELSO, with a 75% success rate.[3]

The ECMO Team

The ECMO Team is a collection of personnel with unique skills, knowledge and abilities to work as a team with a clear chain-of-command. According to the Joint Commission on Accreditation of Healthcare Organizations, ineffective communication is the most frequently cited root cause for sentinel events.[30] Therefore, the ECMO Team must be adept at giving and receiving information. Programs may be led by a senior surgeon, neonatologist, or pediatric intensivist but typically has the involvement of all these departments. During cannulation surgery, the surgeon is assisted by an OR team consisting of a surgical assistant, scrub nurse and circulating nurse. Other medical staff involved include the neonatologist, pediatric intensivist, or pediatric surgeon trained in ECMO management, who medically manages the patient.

Other subspecialty non-ECMO physicians, such as nephrology, radiology, or cardiology, may have input into the management of the patient; however, all orders should be communicated to and approved by the attending ECMO physician. Next in the chain-of-command is typically the ECMO Coordinator or Manager, usually a senior nurse or respiratory therapist with extensive ECMO training who has been designated as the non-physician team leadership. Perfusion staff may also have responsibilities for priming, and in some cases, sit shifts on the pump as a specialist.

The minute-to-minute care of the ECMO circuit is the responsibility of the ECMO Specialist, arguably the most important link of the ECMO chain as he or she is at the bedside every minute of every day. The ECMO Specialist is a perfusionist, RN, or respiratory therapist specially trained in ECMO management of the patient and the circuit. The bedside nurse is responsible for general patient care responsibilities, recording of events, and assisting the ECMO Specialist as needed. The bedside respiratory therapist is responsible for the ventilator and airway management.

ECMO Initiation

Prior to placing the patient on ECMO, a complete history and physical examination should be completed. Chest and abdominal radiographs, complete blood counts and differential, blood type and cross, coagulation studies, serum electrolytes, BUN and creatinine laboratory studies should be completed. Cranial ultrasound and a cardiac echocardiogram should be done to evaluate the existence of and extent of any intracranial hemorrhage and cardiac anomalies. The existence of a cardiac anomaly should not be considered an absolute contraindication. However, having noted that, there are several conditions that should be considered as absolute contraindications, such as incurable malignancy, advanced multi-system organ failure, extreme prematurity, and severe central nervous system damage.[31]

Once the decision to initiate ECMO is made, and consent from the parents has been obtained, a pre-set sequence of tasks have to take place quickly. The blood bank should be notified as early in the process as possible to begin washing and typing two units of CMV negative, irradiated, packed red blood cells for priming the circuit. Unless the ECMO medical leadership has made the decision to use unwashed O- PRBCs, the washing of the prime blood is the most time consuming factor of the cannulation. Due to this time delay, many centers now use unwashed, fresh RBCs and remove excess potassium via hemofiltration. An x-ray plate is placed under the patient so that when the patient is draped during cannulation, an x-ray can be taken to determine the placement of the ECMO cannulas. A Foley catheter should be inserted prior to heparinization.

Before this process begins, the following labs are drawn:

- Complete blood count, including hemoglobin, hematocrit and platelet count
- Disseminated intravascular coagulation (DIC) screen, including prothrombin time and partial thromboplastin time
- Blood type and screen
- Electrolytes, including potassium and ionized calcium
- Blood urea nitrogen, creatinine, and glucose concentrations

The surgery team is notified. As most cannulations are performed in an intensive care unit, the surgery team will need to provide instruments and supplies for the cannulation. Medical, nursing, and respiratory staff must attend to manage the patient prior to and during the placement of the patient onto ECMO.

The patient should be on a surgical warmer capable of elevating. If the patient is on HFOV with non-flexible tubing, the ventilator will have to be raised and placed on a stand so that it is level with the patient. It is preferable to replace the circuit of any patient on HFOV with a heated-wire, flexible circuit.

The pre-assembled ECMO pump and circuit, fluid primed, is brought to the bedside, along with the ECMO supply cart. Most ECMO centers use a balanced-salt solution such as Normosol or Plasmalyte A as the fluid primer, instead of normal saline, due to the approximation of normal electrolyte values of the solutions. Following is one institution's practice for circuit prime.

(1) 10 ml of 25% albumin is injected into the circulating clear fluid and allowed to circulate for five minutes, coating the internal diameter of the ECMO circuit with a protein layer that will help prevent platelet adhesion to the plastic surface.

(2) Once two units of packed red blood cells arrive at the bedside, medications are added to each unit prior to blood priming of the ECMO circuit. These medications are:

- 50 to 100 units heparin, depending on the patient's coagulation status
- 45 ml 25% albumin
- 25 ml THAM
- 10 meq sodium bicarbonate
- 50 ml of Fresh Frozen Plasma (FFP) per unit of blood has been added to this prime recipe by several centers with good results in preventing dilution of coagulation factors
- 300 mg calcium gluconate, added last to prevent premature clotting of the prime blood

(3) Using a blood filter, each unit of medicated PRBCs is spiked via the priming spike of the ECMO circuit and the clear fluid is slowly "chased" out of the ECMO circuit at a rate of 50 ml/min.

(4) After the blood has circulated in the ECMO circuit through the priming bag, the following labs are drawn on the circuit blood, prior to placement on the patient:

- ABG, to calibrate the in-line blood gas monitor, if base excess is less than -20 then add 10 meq $NaHCO_3$
- Hematocrit, using hemofiltration the hematocrit can be raised to >30%
- Potassium, and out of normal levels treated by either adding potassium or by quickly hemofiltering off excess potassium
- Ionized Calcium, again out of normal levels are treated prior to the initiation of ECMO
- Baseline Activated Clotting Time (ACT), in light of absence of clotting factors, the ACT should be elevated >500 seconds

As the ECMO circuit is being prepared, the patient is prepared for cannulation. As most cannulations are done in an intensive care unit, standard principles of preparation and infection control normally utilized in the operating room should be adhered to, including "Time Out." The bedside RN continues to be responsible for monitoring and care of the patient. The respiratory therapist is responsible for the endotracheal tube and ventilator circuit and prevention of an inadvertent extubation. A long extension medication line should be primed and attached to either a central (preferred) or a peripheral venous access to allow for administration of blood products and medications during surgery, while the patient is draped and inaccessible. The manual resuscitation device should be removed from the bed, but still immediately available, to prevent accumulation of oxygen under the surgical drapes as a possible fire hazard due to the electrocautery in use. Once the patient and all tubing, EKG leads, blood pressure transducers, and x-ray plate are all properly positioned, the patient can be draped with surgical drapes. During the actual cannulation, the bedside nurse or an MD will be called upon to administer these medications and blood products, so they need to be checked, drawn up in syringes and readily available.

Cannulation

Anesthesia for extrathoracic cannulation will include a narcotic for pain control and a short-term muscle relaxant. A local anesthetic is injected at the surgical site to provide additional pain control, but an anesthesiologist is not usually present for ECMO initiation. In the absence of an anesthesiologist, the ECMO physician is responsible for patient management and communication with the surgeon. If the ECMO physician is the surgeon cannulating, the neonatologist or intensivist is responsible for the patient management until the surgeon is able to direct the care. The surgeon, assisted by the bedside nurse and respiratory therapist, will position the patient, typically with the head rotated to the left and a shoulder roll hyperextending the neck to expose the right side of the ne

The anesthesia will include a narcotic for pain control, usually several doses of fentanyl (anesthetic doses of fentanyl are 20-40 mcg/kg). A local injection of 1 or 2% lidocaine may be injected at the surgical site to add to the pain control. A 0.1 mg/kg dose of pancuronium is administered after the narcotic, with extra doses available if one dose does not result in the desired effect. Once the neck vessels are isolated and prior to ligating, a loading dose of 50 to 100 units/kg of heparin is given to systemically anticoagulant the patient and allowed to circulate for five minutes. The dose is determined by the coagulation status, as measured by the PT and the fibrinogen levels. The goal should be to have an ACT higher than the normal range of 160 to 200 seconds, but not so high as to put the patient at risk of excessive bleeding as would be expected with an ACT of >500. Ranges of 200-250 seconds will prevent the catheters from clotting off during the procedure.

In the US, the historical overall preference has been for venoarterial ECMO (VA); however, that preference is changing toward venovenous ECMO (VV).[32] Venovenous ECMO is associated with higher survivability and lower morbidity, possibly due to the advantages of avoidance of instrumentation and ligation of the carotid artery, the avoidance of alteration of pulsatile arterial blood flow patterns, and the cerebral emboli protection VV ECMO provides.[43] VV ECMO is not an option for infants too small to instrument with a 12 fr. VV double-lumen cannula. Keeping Poiseuille's equation in mind, where a decrease in the radius of a tube by 50% results in a 4 times increase[4] in resistance to flow[33], the largest cannula allowable should be used.

After choosing either venoarterial or venovenous ECMO, cannulas of the appropriate size are passed to the surgical technician, while maintaining sterility. After instrumentation of the right internal jugular vein and possibly the right common carotid artery, the cannulas are allowed to fill with blood from the patient and clamped. Pressing on the liver will facilitate the blood priming of the cannulas.

The priming bag can be squeezed to raise the circuit venous pressure to 60 to 75 cmH$_2$O prior to clamping off the circuit immediately prior to placement on the patient. The resulting venous pressure, post ECMO initiation, will allow for good flows and possibly prevent the need for volume pushes to achieve target ECMO flow.

The person priming the ECMO circuit, usually a perfusionist, ECMO Coordinator, or Specialist, then pulls back the plastic covering of the sterile sections of the ECMO circuit and passes the tubing to the surgeon. The arterial and venous lines from the priming bag are attached to the appropriate cannulas, taking care to de-air the tubing prior to attaching. All tubing clamps are removed at this time via the VBA routine, and the bridge is clamped (if using a bridge with external clamp) or closed off if using a "bloodless bridge". This sequence should be done very quickly, within three seconds if possible.

The ECMO flow is initiated at 50 ml/min and over five to ten minutes the flow is slowly increased to 100 to 150 ml/kg/min flow, while monitoring the venous pressure. The ECMO flow is titrated to maintain a venous pressure greater than -25 cmH$_2$O and according to desired flows.

Once ECMO flow is stabilized, an ACT, and patient and arterial pump blood gas should be drawn. The ACT may be elevated and the patient blood gas should be approximating normal values. An ACT should be drawn every 15-30 minutes and once the value is <300 seconds, a heparin drip should be started at 20-50 units/kg/hour and titrated to maintain ACTs according to institutional guidelines . Because of the heparinization of the patient, all venopunctures and injections of any kind should be diligently avoided. Endotracheal suctioning should be only as aggressive as needed to clear the endotracheal tube. Nasopharyngeal bleeding is particularly difficult to staunch, so nasal suctioning should be avoided.

The ventilator settings are lowered to rest settings. Depending on which type of ECMO support (VA or VV) is being utilized, these settings can be either immediately implemented if the patient is on VA ECMO, or slowly weaned to if the patient is on VV ECMO. Nitric oxide, can be either turned off, if on VA ECMO, or weaned off over 8-24 hours, if on VV ECMO. The pump flow should be optimized to maintain PaO$_2$as ordered by the ECMO physician. PaCO$_2$ should be normalized via the sweep gas to maintain levels as ordered, usually beginning with a range that approximates the patient's current PaCO$_2$. Changes made to the sweep gas requires re-checking of an arterial pump gas in addition to a patient blood gas.. If the patient is on pressor infusions, once optimal oxygenation is obtained, the pressor can be weaned gradually. All fluids, such as TPN and analgesics, should be moved from the patient to the venous side of the ECMO circuit.

Daily Patient Management

Now that the patient has been heparinized and the ACT is elevated, no arterial or venous punctures or heel sticks should be performed.

Fluid, Electrolytes, Nutrition

Historically, enteral nutrition is withheld from the neonatal ECMO patient due to concern about the potential to develop necrotizing enterocolitis.[34] However, there have been some retrospective reviews that show that routine use of enteral feedings of neonates on ECMO is feasible.[35,36, 37] Whether a conservative or liberal approach is taken regarding enteral nutrition, catabolism (breaking down complex molecules into simple building blocks) is severe in the ECMO patient. Therefore, judicious use of carbohydrates, lipids, and particularly protein is needed to optimize lean body mass.[31]

Due to the systemic inflammatory response after initiation of ECMO, and fluid resuscitation prior to ECMO initiation, most patients become edematous, resulting in a 5 to 30% increase in birth weight.[38] Restricting daily fluid intake to 60-100 ml/kg/day and diuretics will facilitate diuresis. Natural diuresis will resume as cardiac output improves, capillary leak resolves and fluid mobilization happens.[31] If renal failure persists, despite aggressive diuretics, hemofiltration can be easily incorporated into the ECMO circuit (see Chapter 17). One component of fluid management that needs to be compensated for is the fluid loss inherent from the oxygenator. Depending on which oxygenator is in use, insensible water loss has been estimated from 48 to 82 ml/day/lpm of sweep gas,[39,40,41] with the Medtronic Minimax being the highest and the Jostra Quadrox D being the lowest.

Amino acids added to the TPN provide protein to the caloric intake. Some center restrict fat emulsion use because of concern for layering, agglutination, and clot formation in areas of flow stasis such as the bladder and the oxygenator and can cause cracked stopcocks.[42] Other centers use fat emulsions and have not seen this phenomenon. Use should be determined by your ECMO physician.

Serum electrolytes, BUN and TPN labs should be monitored at least daily. Sodium levels may become elevated if the patient is fluid restricted. Potassium levels commonly become depressed (mechanism not totally understood), necessitating adding 3 to 6 mEq/kg/day of potassium to the TPN. Ionized calcium levels should be maintained >1.1 mmol/L. Minerals and trace elements should also be added to the TPN.

Common labs and frequency (centers' preferences vary):

- ACT: every one hour, more frequently if either out of range or if heparin is turned off.
- If using the CDI blood gas monitoring system, blood gases: pre and post oxygenator should be done every 12 hours to calibrate the CDI
- Patient gases should be done every 4 to 6 hours. Some centers require patient gases every 1-2 hours to monitor lactic acid levels, CO_2 levels, and pH status.
- CBC with differential and platelet count: every 6 to 12 hours depending on the coagulation status.
- Na, K, Cl, HCO_3, iCa and glucose: should be done every 12 hours or as needed
- Coagulation studies: some centers monitor PT, PTT, fibrinogen, anti-thrombin III levels, and FSP, while others only monitor fibrinogen along with the ACT.
- Plasma free hemoglobin daily, or in some centers, only when significant hemolysis is suspected
- TPN, total protein and albumin: daily
- Bilirubin: as indicated
- Blood cultures: if sepsis is suspect or if WBC count varies

Cardiovascular System

Neonatal respiratory ECMO cases frequently have a compromised cardiac function due to myocardium hypoxia. Pre-ECMO, the mean blood pressure is maintained via volume infusions and pressors. Once ECMO has been initiated, the pressors can be weaned off. If the infant is on VA ECMO, the pressors can frequently be weaned quickly. In contrast, however, if on VV ECMO, the pressors have to be weaned more prudently due to the reliance on native cardiac output to maintain a normalized MAP. With

either type of support, the increase in myocardium oxygenation usually results in an increase in contractility and output.

One aspect of a depressed myocardium is cardiac stun. While the etiology of cardiac stun is undetermined, it transiently appears more often in patients who have suffered severe hypoxia or in whom the tip of the arterial catheter is placed too close to the coronary arteries and the retrograde flow prevents proper aortic valve function. It is characterized by a pulse pressure <10 mmHg or when the patient's PaO_2 is within 50 to 100 mmHg of the pump FiO_2.[43] Infants in whom cardiac stun develops appear to be more ill before ECMO and have a higher mortality.[44]

Hypertension (MAP > 65 mmHg) is a common complication after the initiation of ECMO[45] that should be aggressively treated. The risk for intracranial hemorrhage in the heparinized patient is high. The improvement of oxygenation of the previously depressed myocardium will dramatically increase the ventricular function, thereby reducing the need for pressors, which should be weaned off as quickly as possible.

Oxygen Delivery

The oxygen content equation is: $(1.36 * Hgb) * (S_aO_2 \div 100) + (0.0031 * PaO_2)$. Therefore, any change in the ECMO circuit's PaO_2 will have only a minimal impact on the oxygen content. Changes in the hemoglobin, however, have a tremendous impact. Each 1 gm increase in the hemoglobin increases the oxygen content by 1.224 ml/dl. Contrasting this, each 1% increase in SaO_2 only increases the oxygen content by 0.2 ml/dl and 10 mmHg increases in the PaO_2 increases the oxygen content by 0.031 ml/dl. Due to this, transfusing to raise the hematocrit to 35% and running the ECMO flow at 150 ml/kg/min will maximize oxygen delivery, while increasing the PO_2 delivered by the ECMO pump (membrane blood gas) from 200 to 300mmHg will have a negligible effect. In simplistic terms, to get more oxygen molecules to the tissues, filling the train cars past full will not deliver more oxygen to the tissue, but increasing the numbers of train cars and making them move faster will.

Pulmonary System

While on ECMO, gas exchange by the native lungs is not needed. Therefore, the ventilator is weaned to "rest" settings intended to allow the lungs to recover from the injury induced by high ventilator settings. In addition, the inflammatory response, which typically happens after the initiation of ECMO, is allowed to subside. With lower tidal volumes the impaired lung compliance, caused by inflammation and over stretching, can occur and with time subside without the additional injury of repeated overinflation.[46] The pace of the ventilator wean is dictated by the type of ECMO. If the patient is on VA ECMO, the lungs have been bypassed and complete gas exchange is done by the ECMO pump. Therefore, the ventilator can be quickly turned down to rest settings and if iNO has been utilized, it can be turned off. In contrast to this, if VV ECMO is utilized, the ventilator should be weaned more slowly. If the ventilator is quickly weaned while on VV ECMO, the lungs could rapidly consolidate and collapse, thereby causing cardiac distress and a drop in cardiac output. Therefore, the ventilator wean while on VV ECMO should progress more slowly, taking hours, rather than minutes. A final target ventilator rest setting is center/physician specific with most centers preferring a PEEP of 8 to 10 for respiratory cases and 4 to 5 for cardiac cases. A respiratory rate from 5 to 10 bpm is typical; however, each center's approach is different.[47]

Infection Control

After placement on ECMO, the instrumentation and exposure to the plastic tubing and sensors increases the probability for infection. This probability is especially acute for the neonate with an immature immune system. However, in spite of this elevated risk, only 6.2% of cases reported to ELSO listed a culture-proven infection as a complication,[3] which has been consistent since 2000.[31] An initial drop in white blood cells and platelets is usually encountered after placement on ECMO and circuit exchanges, due to the adhesion of these cells to the oxygenator and the plastic tubing. In addition, it has been demonstrated that cardiopulmonary bypass causes systemic inflammatory response, which can progress to an acute lung inflammation.[48]

Most, if not all, infants would have been started on antibiotics by the time ECMO was needed. Despite the contention that there is no definitive reason to continue antibiotics once the patient is on ECMO, most centers do continue ampicillin along with an aminoglycoside or a cephalosporin to provide a broad-spectrum antibiotic coverage. If a subsequent infection were documented, an antibiotic to which the infection is susceptible would be indicated. Keep in mind that studies have shown that vancomycin clearance is decreased and volume of distribution is increased in ECMO patients, therefore vancomycin levels should be closely monitored.[49]

Renal System

Transient renal dysfunction after placement on ECMO is commonly seen in the neonatal population. Hypoxia, hypotension, and fluid resuscitation efforts prior to ECMO and renal inflammatory response to the ECMO circuit are probable contributors to this phenomenon. In the majority of cases, the renal dysfunction spontaneously resolves within the first 48 to 72 hours of ECMO. Acute Renal Failure (ARF) is characterized by poor urine output and elevated BUN and creatinine levels. Furosemide, 1 to 2 mg/kg every 12 to 24 hours or 0.05 to 0.4 mg/kg/hr continuous infusion will facilitate urine output.[50] Chlorothiazide, 1 to 2 mg/kg every 12 hours or dopamine at 5 micrograms/kg/hr have also been shown to increase renal function.[51] In cases in which the urine output does not improve after 48 to 72 hours, the hypoxia and hypotension suffered prior to ECMO may have caused acute tubular necrosis (ATN). Each glomerulus has a tubule that is very dependent on oxygen delivery. Hypoperfusion of the tubules will cause dysfunction, which will subside within 7 to 21 days, once the underlying hypoperfusion is resolved.[52]

Hemofiltration can be utilized to accomplish rapid fluid and dissolved solutes removal, while retaining proteins and cellular components. Removing fluid, while retaining whole blood, platelets and plasma coagulation proteins, allows the hematocrit level to be optimized, thereby increasing oxygen delivery and preserving clotting ability.

Neurologic System

Patients placed on ECMO, as a rule, have suffered hypoxia, hypotension, acidosis, hypercarbia, possible CPR, repeated doses of inotropes, and blood loss from instrumentation. After placement on ECMO, the brain is subjected to blood flow disruption from the ligation of the jugular vein and possible right carotid artery, cerebral ischemia and reperfusion.[53] Surprisingly, despite the high number of invasive procedures and possible life-threatening situations, one study found that 88% of survivors at 11 and 19-month follow-ups were found to be developmentally normal.[54] Neurological exams should be done frequently, with pupil checks at a minimum, with each hourly circuit check. Seizure activity is reported in 11% of all neonatal cases reported to ELSO.[31] Phenobarbital is recommended as the first-line drug for anticonvulsant.[55]

A cranial ultrasound should be done prior to placement on ECMO to determine the existence of, and extent of, any intracranial hemorrhage (ICH). One study showed that 93% of ICHs occurred during the first five days of ECMO. In light of the expense of head ultrasounds, and the unlikelihood of an ICH occurring – absent any clinical suspicion – after five days of ECMO, some centers do not continue head ultrasound studies. Others continue every other day studies.[56]

Sedatives and anti-anxiety drugs, such as morphine and midazolam are commonly used, as they have been shown to not be absorbed as easily by the ECMO circuit. When sedatives that are more potent are required, as during surgery, fentanyl can be used if infused post-oxygenator. However higher than normal doses are usually needed. One study showed that 80% of fentanyl was absorbed in a circuit without an oxygenator, and 86% was absorbed when a Quadrox D was added.[57] The same study showed that as much as 40% of the circulating morphine was absorbed by the ECMO circuit.[57]

Although a 2004 study demonstrated that routine placement of a cephalad jugular cannula did not provide significant benefit[58] many centers use this catheter to augment flow on venovenous ECMO and monitor cerebral saturations. Tygon tubing has been shown, during prolonged roller pump use, to suffer from spallation, which is the release of microscopic plastic particles from the inside diameter of the raceway. However, it has been shown that after 72 hours of use, spallation falls to almost zero and there is no other alternative to Tygon tubing for raceways.[59] Therefore, while spallation remains a theoretical neurologic concern, studies have not shown any clinically observable impairment.

Hematology

Hemolysis is a constant challenge while on ECMO. Red blood cells are injured due to the shear forces caused by the pressure transitions through the cannulas. The platelets are consumed by the silicone membrane oxygenators, as are the clotting factors. Plasma free hemoglobin levels can be used to determine the level of hemolysis. Many centers follow these daily to determine the degree of hemolysis in the circuit, especially related to fibrin/clot formation. Maintaining a hematocrit >35% while on ECMO, and raising that parameter to >40% only prior to trial off, will help limit unnecessary blood administration and maximize oxygen delivery just before discontinuation of ECMO.

Communication

After placement on ECMO, the attending physician should conduct daily, bedside rounds with the Specialist, ECMO Coordinator and bedside nurse. During these rounds, any changes or events that occurred during the previous 24 hours should be discussed and the plan-of-care adjusted accordingly. The objectives for the day, the overall plan-of-care and the end-point for the run should be discussed and if needed, adjusted. ECMO is a team effort. That team effort is best focused when everyone is aware of the overall goal and daily objectives. Daily objectives, such as tests, ACT, blood pressure, blood gas, and coagulation parameters should be reviewed. Any out of range lab values should be discussed and addressed. Everyone should be aware of the daily plan-of-care and his or her part of the team's effort. An erasable white-board, at the bedside, could be used to list all the contact information for the ECMO Coordinator, ECMO physician on-call, and perfusionist on-call. The emergency ventilator settings should be posted so that minimal communication is necessary during an emergency

Additionally, shift change reports should also review the overall goal and the daily objectives. A written checklist facilitates a smooth transition between shifts. All ECMO pump settings, infusions, sweep gas, ventilator settings, lab values/parameters and medications due should be reviewed. Oncoming and offgoing Specialists, prior to the shift change, should assess the circuit. Each hour the circuit should be assessed, an ACT drawn, and the heparin titrated.

ECMO Weaning

The eventual wean off ECMO must be part of the discussion in each day's rounds. After the initial inflammatory response has subsided, the urine output has returned and the lung function has improved, the wean from ECMO can be attempted. Center wean off ECMO using varying techniques. Two methods are discussed:

1. Trial-off Technique: The wean from VA ECMO begins 12 hours, or more, prior to the trial off. To prevent immediately tasking a full load to the heart, an hourly wean of the pump flow by 10 to 20 ml/min is done with a concurrent increase in the ventilator support. The flow is slowly weaned down to a target idling flow. Some centers consider an idling flow of 100 ml/min to be sufficient, while others use a flow of 50 ml/kg/min. Prior to the trial, all infusions except the heparin, are moved to the patient. Once the target flow is achieved and the ventilatory support is increased to the settings to be used post-ECMO, the cannulas are clamped. The cannula clamping follows the standard sequence of Venous-Bridge-Arterial. To allow heparinized blood to flush the cannulas while trialing off, they are flashed every five minutes by opening the venous cannula, clamping the bridge and opening the arterial cannula for five to ten seconds, then reversing the sequence. A patient blood gas is taken every ten minutes while trialing off. The length of the trial off is not universally standardized. Due to concern that clots could form in the clamped cannulas, some centers limit the length of VA ECMO trials to 20 minutes, while others extend this time as long as two to three hours. If the trial lasts more than 5

minutes, the sweep gas to the oxygenator is turned off and the heparin infusion is stopped. If the trial lasts more than 20 minutes, a patient ACT should be checked. After the trial off, if the patient is not to be decannulated, the infusions are moved back to the ECMO pump.

2. No Trial Off: Some centers do not do a trial off unless it is a very unstable patient such as a CDH patient (See Chapter 15). In these centers after the lung function starts to return (improved X-ray), the ECMO flow is weaned by 10-20 mL per hour as the patient's blood gases allow until idling, usually 60 mL/min. This process usually takes 1-2 days. If the patient idles for 4-6 hours with good blood gases, the patient can be removed from ECMO successfully.

Trials off VV ECMO are much easier. Since there is not any true cardiac output support, the ventricular function should not suffer. The isovolumic property of VV ECMO allows for trials off without a weaning of the flow and for extended trial times. The ventilator support is increased from rest settings. If the patient is to be immediately considered for decannulation, all infusions except for heparin, are moved to the patient. The sweep gas tubing is disconnected from the source and reconnected to the exhaust port on the oxygenator, isolating the membrane and preventing any gas exchange. The heparin infusion is continued and ACTs are still followed as per protocol. The patient's SvO_2 can be continuously monitored with the inline blood gas monitor and a patient blood gas is taken after 20 minutes. This trial off can be maintained for several hours as the heparin continues to be infused and the ACTs are maintained. One of VV ECMO's benefits is the ability to extend the trial-off length so that ventilator management can be fine-tuned and the patient has the opportunity to demonstrate his or her ability to survive off ECMO for several hours.

Conclusion

After 35 years of experience with neonatal ECMO, the worldwide knowledge base has increased so that future patients will benefit from practitioners who have learned from the progenitors of the field. We now know more about what diseases respond best to ECMO as well as what complications occur and how to deal with them. In addition, with this improved knowledge, the patient selection will grow to include not just the moribund, but also the moderately severe respiratory and cardiac failure patients.

Future frontiers for neonatal ECMO will include circuits that prevent clotting, peristaltic pumps and miniaturized devices thereby increasing the potential patient population to those patients who presently cannot be heparinized. Despite declining use since 1992, future neonatal ECMO has bright prospects to benefit a large population whose options are limited once oscillator ventilators and iNO have been exploited.

References

1   Bartlett R. Keynote Address and Patient Presentation. "One Patient at a Time." Proceedings of the 15th Anniversary ELSO Conference in conjunction with AmSECT Pediatric Perfusion Conference; 2004 Sep 9-12; Ann Arbor, Michigan.

2   Beardsmore CS, Westaway J, Killer H, Firmin RK, Pandya H. How does the changing profile of infants who are referred for extracorporeal membrane oxygenation affect their overall respiratory outcome? Pediatrics. 2007 Oct;120(4):e762-8

3   Extracorporeal Life Support Organization. ECLS Registry Report, International Summary. 2009.

4   Fliman PJ, DeRegnier RO, Kinsella JP, Reynolds M, Rankin LL, Steinhorn RH. Neonatal Extracorporeal Life Support: Impact of New Therapies on Survival. The Journal of Pediatrics. 2006 May; 48(5):595-9.

5   Green TP, Moler FW, Goodman DM. Probability of survival after prolonged extracorporeal membrane oxygenation in pediatric patients with acute respiratory failure. Extracorporeal Life Support Organization. Crit Care Med. 1995; 23(6):1132-9.

6   Hardart GE, Hardart MK, Arnold JH. Intracranial hemorrhage in premature neonates treated with extracorporeal membrane oxygenation correlates with conceptional age. J Pediatr. 2004, 145(2):184-9

7   Revenis ME, Glass P, Short BL. Mortality and morbidity rates among lower birth weight infants (2000 to 2500 grams) treated with extracorporeal membrane oxygenation. J Pediatr. 1992;121(3):452-8.

8   Farrow KN, Steinhorn RH. ECMO, Extracorporeal Cardiopulmonary Support in Critical Care. 3rd ed. Van Meurs K, editor. Ann Arbor (MI): Extracorporeal Life Support Organization; 2005.

9   ELSO. Patient Specific Supplements to the ELSO General Guidelines. Extracorporeal Life Support Organization. 2009 April. Available from: http://www.elso.med.umich.edu/

WordForms/ELSO%20Pt%20Specific%20 Guidelines.pdf

10 De Mol AC, Gerrits LC, van Heijst AF, Straatman H, van der Staak FH, Leim KD. Intravascular volume administration: a contributing risk factor for intracranial hemorrhage during extracorporeal membrane oxygenation? Pediatrics. 2008;121(6):e1599-603.

11 De Mol AC, Van Heijst AF, Van der Staak FH, Liem KD. Disturbed cerebral circulation during opening of the Venoarterial bypass bridge in extracorporeal membrane oxygenation. Int J Artif Organs. 2008;31(3):266-71.

12 Green TP. The impact of extracorporeal membrane oxygenation on survival in pediatric patients with acute respiratory failure. Pediatric Critical Care Study Group. Critical Care Medicine. 1996; 24(2):323-9.

13 Bayrakci B, Josephson C, Fackler J. Oxygenation index for extracorporeal membrane oxygenation: is there predictive significance? J Artif Organs. 2007;10:6-9.

14 Trachsel D, McCrindle BW, Nakagawa S, Bohn D. Oxygenation Index predicts outcome in children with acute hypoxemic respiratory failure. Am J Respir Crit Care Med. 2005;172;206-211.

15 Congenital Diaphragmatic Hernia Study Group, Lally KP, Lally PA, Lasky RE, Tibboel D, Jaksic T, et al. Defect size determines survival in infants with congenital diaphragmatic hernia. Pediatrics. 2007 Sep;120(3):e651-7.

16 Lally KP, Lally PA, Van Meurs KP, Bohn DJ, Davis CF, Rodgers B, et al. Treatment evolution in high-risk congenital diaphragmatic hernia: ten years' experience with diaphragmatic agenesis. Ann Surg. 2006 Oct;244(4):505-13.

17 Langham MR, Kays DW, Ledbetter DJ, Frentzen B, Sanford LL, Richards DS. Congenital diaphragmatic hernia: epidemiology and outcome. Clin Perinatol. 1996; 23:671–688.

18 Kaiser JR, Rosenfeld CR. A population-based study of congenital diaphragmatic hernia: impact of associated anomalies and preoperative blood gases on survival. J Pediatr Surg. 1999; 34:1196–1202.

19 de Mello DE, Reid LM. Embryonic and early fetal development of human lung vasculature

and its functional implications. Pediatr Dev Pathol. 2000;3:439–449

20 Bhutani VK. Developing a systems approach to prevent meconium aspiration syndrome: lessons learned from multinational studies. J Perinatol. 2008; Dec;28 Suppl 3:S30-5.

21 Short BL. Extracorporeal membrane oxygenation: use in meconium aspiration syndrome. J Perinatol. 2008 Dec;28 Suppl 3:S79-83.

22 Kugelman A, Gangitano E, Taschuk R, Garza R, Riskin A, McEvoy C, Durand M. Extracorporeal membrane oxygenation in infants with meconium aspiration syndrome: a decade of experience with venovenous ECMO. J Pediatr Surg. 2005 Jul;40(7):1082-9.

23 Radhakrishnan RS, Lally PA, Lally KP, Cox CS Jr. ECMO for meconium aspiration syndrome: support for relaxed entry criteria. ASAIO J. 2007 Jul-Aug;53(4):489-91.

24 Soll RF. Inhaled nitric oxide in the neonate. J Perinatol. 2009 May;29 Suppl 2:S63-7.

25 Latini G, Del Vecchio A, De Felice C, Verrotti A, Bossone E. Persistent pulmonary hypertension of the newborn: therapeutical approach. Mini Rev Med Chem. 2008 Dec;8(14):1507-13.

26 Hansell DR. Extracorporeal Membrane Oxygenation for Perinatal and Pediatric Patients. Respir Care. 2003 Apr;48(4):352-62.

27 Carnielli VP, Zimmermann LJ, Hamvas A, Cogo PE. Pulmonary surfactant kinetics of the newborn infant: novel insights from studies with stable isotopes. J Perinatol. 2009 May;29 Suppl 2:S29-37.

28 Schrag S, Schuchat A. Prevention of neonatal sepsis. Clin Perinatol. 2005 Sep;32(3):601-15.

29 Brierley J, Carcillo JA, Choong K, Cornell T, Decaen A, Deymann A, et al. Clinical practice parameters for hemodynamic support of pediatric and neonatal septic shock: 2007 update from the American College of Critical Care Medicine. Crit Care Med. 2009 Feb;37(2):666-88.

30 2009 Critical Access Hospital Natioinal Patient Safety Goals. Joint Commission. Available at: http://www.jointcommission.org/PatientSafety/ NationalPatientSafetyGoals/09_cah_npsgs.htm. Accessed May 15, 2009.

31 Van Meurs K, Lally KP, Peek G, Zwischenberger JB, eds. ECMO: Extracorporeal cardio-

pulmonary support in critical care. Ann Arbor, MI; ELSO; 2005.

32 Karimova A, Brown K, Ridout D, Beierlein W, Cassidy J, Smith J, et al. Neonatal extracorporeal membrane oxygenation: practice patterns and predictors of outcome in the UK. Arch Dis Child Fetal Neonatal Ed. 2009 Mar;94(2):F129-32.

33 Determinants of blood vessel resistance. Available at: http://www.cvphysiology.com/Hemodynamics/H003.htm. Accessed May 27, 2009.

34 Ohri Sk, Bjarnason I, Pathi V, et al. cardiopulmonary bypass impairs small intestinal transport and increases gut permeability. Ann ThoracSurg. 1993; 55:1080-1086.

35 Hanekamp MN, Spoel M, Sharman-Koendjbiharie I, Peters JW, Albers MJ, Tibboel D. Routine enteral nutrition in neonates on extracorporeal membrane oxygenation. Pediatr Crit Care Med. 2005 May; 6(3):275-9.

36 Hanekamp MN, Spoel M, Sharman-Koendjbiharie M, Hop WC, Hopman WP, Jansen JB, Tibboel D. Gut hormone profiles in critically ill neonates on extracorporeal membrane oxygenation. J Pediatr Gastroenterol Nutr. 2005 Feb; 40(2):175-9.

37 Pettignao R. Food for thought. Pediatr Crit Care Med. 2005; 6(3): 371-2.

38 Anderson HL, Coran AG, Drongowski RA, Ha HJ, Bartlett RH. Extracellular fluid and total body water changes in neonates undergoing extracorporeal membrane oxygenation. J Pediatr Surg. 1992 Aug;27(8):1003-7

39 Lawson DS, Holt D. Insensible water loss from the Jostra Quadrox D oxygenator: an in vitro study. Perfusion. 2007 Nov;22(6):407-10.

40 Camacho T, Totapally BR, Hultquist K, Nelson G, Eawaz D, Sussmane JB, Wolfsdorf J. Insensible water loss during extracorporeal membrane oxygenation: an in vitro study. ASAIO J. 2000 Sep-Oct;46(5):620-4.

41 Alexander PJ, Lawson DS, Cornell J, Craig DM, Cheifetz IM. Insensible water loss from the medtronic minimax oxygenator: an In Vitro study. ASAIO J. 2006 Mar-Apr;52(2):206-10.

42 Buck ML, Wooldridge P, Ksenich RA. Comparison of methods for intravenous infusion of fat emulsion during extracorporeal membrane oxygenation. Pharmacotherapy. 2005 Nov;25(11):1536-40.

43 Short BL. Extracorporeal Membrane Oxygenation. In: Avery G, Mhairi G, MacDonald M, Seshia M, Mullett M, eds. Avery's Neonatology. 6th ed. Philadelphia, PA: Lippincott Williams & Wilkins; 2005: 622-33.

44 Martin GR, Short BL, Abbott C, O'Brien AM. Cardiac stun in infants undergoing extracorporeal membrane oxygenation. J Thorac Cardiovasc Surg. 1991 Apr;101(4):607-11.

45 Sell LL, Cullen ML, Lerner GR, Whittlesey GC, Shanley CJ, Klein MD. Hypertension during extracorporeal membrane oxygenation: cause, effect, and management. Surgery. 1987 Oct;102(4):724-30.

46 Hernandez LA, Peevy KJ, Moise AA, Parker JC. Chest wall restriction limits high airway pressure-induced lung injury in young rabbits. J Appl Physiol. 1989 May;66(5):2364-8.

47 Mugford M, Elbourne D, Field D. Extracorporeal membrane oxygenation for severe respiratory failure in newborn infants. Cochrane Database Syst Rev. 2008 Jul 16;(3).

48 Halter J, Steinberg J, Fink G, Lutz C, Picone A, Maybury R, et al. Evidence of systemic cytokine release in patients undergoing cardiopulmonary bypass. J Extra Corpor Technol. 2005 Sep; 37(3):272-7.

49 Mulla H, Pooboni S. Population pharmacokinetics of vancomycin in patients receiving extracorporeal membrane oxygenation. Br J Clin Pharmacol. 2005 Sep; 60(3):265-75.

50 van der Vorst MM, den Hartigh J, Wildschut E, Tibboel D, Burggraaf J. An exploratory study with an adaptive continuous intravenous furosemide regimen in neonates treated with extracorporeal membrane oxygenation. Crit Care. 2007;11(5):R111.

51 Bhatt Dr. Bruggman Ds, Thayer-Thomas JC, et al. Neonatal Drug Formulary. 5th ed. Fontana, CA: Neonatal Drug Formulary; 2002.

52 Acute Tubular Necrosis (ATN) – Overview, Causes, Symptoms, Diagnosis, Treatment. The nephrologychannel. Available at: http://www.nephrologychannel.com/atn/index.shtml. Accessed June 23, 2009.

53 Gazzolo D, Abella R, Marinoni E, Di Iorio R, Volti GL, Galvano F, et al. Circulating biochemical markers of brain damage in infants complicated by ischemia reperfusion injury. Cardiovasc Hematol Agents Med Chem. 2009 Apr;7(2):108-26.

54 Khambekar K, Nichani S, Luyt DK, Peek G, Firmin RK, Field DJ, et al. Developmental outcome in newborn infants treated for acute respiratory failure with extracorporeal membrane oxygenation: present experience. Arch Dis Child Fetal Neonatal Ed. 2006 Jan;91(1):F21-5.

55 Taketomo CK, Hodding JH, Kraus DM. Pediatric Dosing Handbook. 12th ed. Hudson, OHG: Lexi-Comp, Inc.; 2005.

56 Khan AM, Shabarek FM, Zwischenberger JB, Warner BW, Cheu HW, Jaksic T, et al. Utility of daily head ultrasonography for infants on extracorporeal membrane oxygenation. J Pediatr Surg. 1998 Aug;33(8):1229-32.

57 Preston TJ, Hodge AB, Riley JB, Leib-Sargel C, Nicol KK. In vitro drug adsorption and plasma free hemoglobin levels associated with hollow fiber oxygenators in the extracorporeal life support (ECLS) circuit. J Extra Corpor Technol. 2007 Dec;39(4):234-7.

58 Skarsgard ED, Salt DR, Lee SK; Extracorporeal Life Support Organization Registry. Venovenous extracorporeal membrane oxygenation in neonatal respiratory failure: does routine, cephalad jugular drainage improve outcome? J Pediatr Surg. 2004 May;39(5):672-6.

59 Peek GJ, Thompson A, Killer HM, Firmin RK. Spallation performance of extracorporeal membrane oxygenation tubing. Perfusion. 2000 Sep;15(5):457-66.

Chapter 11 Questions

1. Excess potassium in the prime blood can be treated with hemofiltration.
   a) True
   b) False

2. A decrease in the radius of a tube by 50% results in increase in resistance to flow by how much?
   a) 2 times
   b) 4 times
   c) 10 times
   d) 16 times

3. Why would the ACT of prime blood be elevated?
   a) Too much heparin
   b) Not enough Calcium
   c) No clotting factors
   d) Not body temperature

4. While doing a trial off with VV ECMO, the SvO_2 on the in-line blood gas monitor reads 72%. Is this a good thing?
   a) No, the patient's oxygenation is too low the patient needs to be placed back on ECMO
   b) Neither, the SvO_2 being displayed is not relevant
   c) Neither, the reading is not accurate
   d) Yes, the patient's oxygenation is adequate

5. According to the Joint Commission on Accreditation of Healthcare Organizations, what is the most frequently cited root cause for sentinel events?
   a) Wrong medication administration
   b) Surgical procedures
   c) Poor communication
   d) Infection control

Chapter 11 Answers:

1. True
2. D.
3. C.
4. D.
5. C.

12

Management of the Pediatric ECMO Patient

Jeffrey Sussmane, MD

Objectives

After completion of this chapter, the participant should be able to:

- Discuss the common pediatric lung diseases treated with ECMO
- Outline the contraindications to ECMO in the pediatric population
- Outline the coagulation management of the pediatric patient

Introduction

Pediatric ECMO is a unique application of a well tested clinical modality.[1-4] The intensive nature, expertise and long term clinical commitment required to safely and successfully offer this therapy, requires that it should be offered in regionalized ECMO centers. Teaching and research programs assist in maintaining this expertise. Early consultation and transport may also dramatically improve the opportunity for survival of the sickest of Pediatric ICU patients.

Common Pediatric Diagnosis

Respiratory diseases that are commonly considered for ECMO treatment when conventional treatment has failed include, ARDS or acute hypoxemic respiratory failure, pneumonia (viral, bacteria, aspiration), pulmonary embolus, post traumatic, asthma or bronchiolitis (commonly secondary to RSV or Influenza), acute chest syndrome (sickle cell), near drowning, "persistent air leak syndrome", and acute respiratory failure secondary to curable malignancy,.

Unique pediatric patients that receive chronic, very modest ventilation support and suffer severe acute "reversible injury" are occasionally considered. These children should be reviewed on a case by case basis with discussion with the family and the ECMO physician.

Children with primary or predominately cardiac dysfunction are candidates for ECMO (see chapter 13 for details). Common diagnoses include cardiogenic shock, septic shock, intractable arrhythmias, post cardiopulmonary bypass support, and reversible pulmonary hypertension.

Pediatric ECMO Respiratory Selection Guidelines

ECMO should be considered for any child with "acute, life-threatening, reversible cardio-respiratory failure" with unsuccessful applications of "maximum medical management". There are no widely accepted pediatric definitions of "life-threatening", "reversible pediatric cardio-respiratory failure" or "maximum medical management." Guidelines for patient selection are discussed below.

When considering whether a patient has reversible lung injury, one must consider the degree of ventilatory support and its duration. Concerns for irreversible lung injury are raised when a patient has been on mechanical ventilation for 10 days or more. Some do not consider ECMO if the patient has been on ventilatory support over 7 days. Each ECMO center must determine its limit based on outcome data at their institution.

The Oxygenation Index (OI) is commonly utilized for the pediatric population. An OI of greater than 40 for > 6 hours while on a ventilator from 12 hours to 7 days has been suggested to predict 70%

135

mortality.[5] A PaO_2 /FiO_2 < 50 mmHg or a P(A-a) O_2 > 600 mmHg may also suggest morbid respiratory failure. Patients with recalcitrant respiratory acidosis, pH < 7.15, with hypercapnia, a static lung compliance < 0.5 cc/cmH_2O/kg, as well as "persistent air leak syndrome", should also be considered for ECMO therapy.

Cardiac and Septic Shock ECMO Selection Guidelines

- Acute, life threatening, but potentially reversible cardiovascular decompensation which is unresponsive to maximal medical management including, when appropriate, vasodilator and/or vasoconstrictive agents, inotropic agents, antiarrhythmic agents, and cardiac pacing.
- Progressive hypotension < 2 SD for age.
- LA or RA pressure greater than 20 mmHg for more than 6 hours.
- Tachyarrhythmias or brady-arrhythmias and/or low cardiac output secondary to reversible toxic drug effects.
- SVO_2 < 60%.
- Persistent acidosis , pH < 7.15
- CI < 2.0 L/m
- Echocardiographic evidence of severe biventricular failure – Ejection Fraction < 30% if combined with other evidence of inadequate end organ perfusion.
- Oncology/ bone marrow transplant patients with maximal medical support and unresponsive acidosis, hypotension, cardiorespiratory failure. Accepted survival opportunity from primary cancer must be documented.
- Note: Decreasing renal function defined as urine < 1 ml/kg/hr for 6 hours in any of the above scenarios indicate a need for improved perfusion and need for ECMO.

Common Pediatric ECMO Exclusion Guidelines

- The Age of the patient / days of ventilation:
  o < 2 years > 10 days,
  o 2-8 years > 8 days,
  o > 8 years > 7 days.

- Iatrogenic lung injury from oxygen toxicity or barotrauma /volutrauma plays a major role in the development of irreversible lung injury. Most centers may agree that a PEEP greater than 15 cm H_2O, a mean airway pressure (MAP) greater than 25 cm H_2O, a peak inspiratory pressure greater than 45 cm H_2O for >7 days may induce irreversible injury.
- Major life threatening hemorrhage (excluding pulmonary hemorrhage) or severe coagulopathy that may likely be uncontrollable on Heparin
- Immunosuppressed is a relative contraindication. Prognosis would need to extensively discussed with the primary clinical team and family prior to consideration for ECMO.
- Acute or chronic severe central nervous system injury including encephalitis, persistent vegetative state, encephalopathy, meningitis, hypoxic ischemic encephalopathy or intractable seizures. Recent cerebral-vascular accident or severe traumatic brain injury are potential exclusions due to risk of intracranial hemorrhage. Worrisome physical exam findings include fixed and dilated pupils, or pupil asymmetry of 2mm or greater.
- Severe chronic lung disease (CLD) as the primary disorder. Patients with CLD who develop acute viral illnesses such as RSV bronchiolitis and are not responding to conventional therapy can be considered for ECMO therapy.
- Fixed elevated pulmonary vascular resistance.
- Severe chromosomal abnormalities (Trisomy 13 or 18). Trisomy 21 is not a contraindication.
- Patients with metabolic or oncological disease where the prognosis from the primary disease is poor
- All patients less than 1 year should have an echocardiogram and cardiology consultation to rule out major uncorrected cardiac malformations. While ECMO in some instances may be required, most patients will need repair of congenital heart disease

in order to wean off ECMO. Additionally, cardiac function or carotid branching pattern off of the aorta may influence the approach to cannulation (V-A versus V-V). Certain cardiac diseases such as severe aortic insufficiency and coarctation of the aorta are a relative contraindications to V-A bypass. Bypass of non-critical coarctations have been undertaken, but post-membrane pressures must be monitored closely and if increased, flow will need to be decreased.

- Uncontrolled septic shock should be assessed individually and in some circumstances ECMO may be appropriate.
- Uncorrected DIC should be assessed individually.
- Ongoing cardiac arrest unless there is an established ECPR program with predefined patient selection criteria and procedures for rapid initiation of ECMO. – see Chapter 16 for full discussion of use of ECPR for arresting patients
- Prolonged hypoxic ischemic insult

Patient Management Guidelines

Membrane Oxygenator – The selection of an oxygenator should be specifically tailored to the expected respiratory requirements, and the expected pump flow rates. These should be calculated by the "rated membrane flow." This is the flow rate at which the venous blood will be expected to reach the inlet of the oxygenator with 75% saturation and be fully saturated (100%) at the outlet of the membrane. The following guidelines may be useful. Most small pediatric patients utilize the silicone Medtronic ® 1500 that is rated for patients up to 19 kgs. The Medtronic ® 2500 is rated for patients up to 70 kgs but is generally utilized for patients up to 40 kgs.; and the Medtronic ® 4500 is rated for patients < 96 kgs but is generally reserved for patients < 60 kgs.. The Medtronic Minimax ® Hollow fiber is rated up to 20 kgs. And the Maxima ® Hollow fiber is rated to 100 kgs. The Quadrox-D ® membrane has recently had success over a broad weight range outside of the neonate.

General guidelines for clinical management of the pediatric patient include the following parameters.

1. ACT's between 160 - 220 (flow dependent) (note: represents ACT utilizing the I-Stat® System
2. VA ECMO – Patient PaO_2 between 60-80 mmHg
3. VV ECMO – Patient PaO_2 between 45 and 80 mmHg
4. pH between 7.35 - 7.45
5. VA ECMO – Hgb 13-15
6. VV ECMO – Hgb 15
7. VA ECMO Hct greater than 40
8. VV ECMO – HCT greater than 45
9. $PaCO_2$ between 35 – 45 mmHg
10. Platelet count 75,000 or greater if bleeding is a concern
11. Urine output $= \geq 2$ml/kg/hr
12. Heparin drip to maintain above ACTs; general range 25 to 50 units/kg/hr
    a. A child with poor renal function will most likely have a decreased heparin requirement (less than 30 units/kg/hr).
    b. Lasix will increase the heparin requirement
    c. A child with a hemofilter will have an increase heparin requirement
13. VA ECMO Flow (calculated) = 100ml/kg/min x .8 (80% of estimated cardiac output)
14. Regulate ECMO flow to maintain venous saturation of 70 - 75%
15. VV ECMO Flow = 80-120 ml/kg/min
    a. Regulate flow to maintain true mixed venous saturation 65-85%
    b. Monitor difference between "arterial' and "venous" circuit saturations (see included chart).
    c. Calculate "Recirculation Fraction"
    d. Calculate "Effective Flow"
    e. Manage pulse-oximeter saturation and true arterial blood gas measurements.
16. Fluid maintenance = 80-100 ml/kg/day
17. Caloric intake, 60 - 90/kg/day
18. Na 2 - 4 meq/kg/day requirements

19. K 2 - 3 meq/kg/day requirements
20. Ca++ 25 - 30 mg/kg/day requirements
21. Lasix (1-2 mg/kg) is often needed in the following circumstances:
    a. Decreased urine output (less than 1 ml/kg/hr)
    b. Elevated blood pressure
    c. Increased positive fluid balance
22. Narcotics as needed (refer to your unit protocols). Note, if fentanyl is used, the silicone membrane oxygenator absorbs fentanyl. This will prevent achieving therapeutic levels until the membrane is saturated. Remember this when changing a circuit out with a silicone membrane. At least 1 hour of sedation medications need to be added to the new circuit prior to change.
23. Sedative/anticonvulsant as needed (refer to your unit protocol).
24. Paralytic agents as needed

Special Considerations for the Pediatric ECMO Patient

The ECMO run is often longer and less predictable for the pediatric patient than the neonatal respiratory ECMO patient. In general, the more sudden or acute the decompensation the quicker the disease process may respond to appropriate therapy. The previously healthy pediatric patient placed on ECMO for a rapid deterioration may respond in a few days. If a child is placed on ECMO for respiratory failure that has not responded to aggressive maximal therapy for several days then the course may be very protracted. It is not possible to give firm guidelines, and successful pediatric ECMO runs may last many weeks. The length of time on the pump should be continually assessed with the clinical condition of the child. It is common to have a long run with very slow improvement. If multi-organ failure develops, then continuation of ECMO may not be warranted. Providing the family with the known limitations of ECMO therapy early in the ECMO course will help parents understand recommendations from the ECMO team on continuation or stopping ECMO when critical events occur during the ECMO run.

Lungs

It is important during extracorporeal support, to recognize that the ECMO circuit, not the ventilator, is maintaining the child's blood gases. The ventilator is set at minimum levels to allow the lungs to "rest", and prevent the development of ventilator associated complications such as barotrauma, and oxygen toxicity. The importance of good pulmonary care for the patient on ECMO cannot be over-stressed. Timely pulmonary recruitment must be attempted for any successful decannulation. Bronchoscopy may be very helpful in diagnosing and treating causes of lung collapse.

Central Nervous System (CNS)

The most significant, primary or secondary, complications in the ECMO patient may be CNS-related, either cerebral edema, infarction or intracranial hemorrhage. CNS problems seem to be related to pre ECMO disease, levels of hypoxia, acidosis, and/or hypercarbia. Accordingly, neurological checks must be incorporated into the routine care. Included in the neurological check are: pupil size and reaction, level of consciousness, reflexes, and movement. Careful observation of any seizure activity is important, as seizures require prompt treatment. CT scans of the brain may be influential in determining course of therapy. Ultrasound may be considered in younger patients with an adequate fontanel.

Hemofiltration

Initially, aggressive recognition and management of oliguria is important. In cases of persistent low urine output and hypervolemia, hemofiltration may be undertaken to maintain intake and output balance. In these cases, it is easily facilitated by the ECMO circuit (see Chapter 17 for details).

Dialysis

When a patient needs hemodialysis, despite hemofiltration, this process is also facilitated by use of the ECMO circuit (see Chapter 17 for details).

Apheresis Utilizing the ECMO Circuit

Apheresis is indicated when a clinical need to separate blood components arises from a patient's medical condition (see Chapter 18 for details).

Special Considerations for Clinical Care

Blood Product Administration

The pediatric ECMO patient has a greater risk for developing significant bleeding complications on ECMO, especially related to chest tubes and other invasive procedures, than the newborn on ECMO. Blood product administration recommendations are listed below.

Packed Red Blood Cells (PRBCs)

PRBCs may be administered into the circuit via a pre bladder pigtail. In cases of transfusion over an hour or more, an auto syringe or infusion pump set-up should be used. Once the transfusion is complete, the access port is flushed with sterile saline and capped. Great caution must be used to avoid air embolus for any pre-pump access for medications or blood products.
PRBCs may be administered in the following instances to:
   a. Maintain the hemoglobin 12-15 Hgb
   b. Maintain the hematocrit 35-45 Hct
   c. Maintain central venous pressure greater than 5 as a volume replacement if indicated by hgb/hct
   d. Maintain mean arterial pressure within age indicated ranges as volume replacement as indicated by hgb/hct
   e. Replace patient blood loss due to lab sampling or hemorrhage or circuit emergency
   f. Replace volume for hypovolemia if indicated by hgb/hct for low venous return pressure or pump "chatter"

   g. Increase oxygen delivery by ability to increase pump flow, to maintain physiologic needs in unstable patients

Fresh Frozen Plasma (FFP)

FFP is administered in the same manner as PRBCs. It may be given in the following instances:
   a. Volume replacement for hypovolemia with PRBCs in ratio of 1 FFP to 3 PRBCs
   b. Massive hemorrhage
   c. Persistent decrease in activated clotting times (ACT's) resulting in an increase in total units/kg/hr heparin administration or deficiency of antithrombin III (ATIII)
   d. Heparin administration less than 25 units/kg/hr (evidence of DIC)
   e. Persistent decreases in ACT's with an increase in heparin units/kg/hr (low heparin levels, from increased excretion, or immunologic intolerance).
   f. Massive transfusion reaction

Platelets

Platelets must **only** be given through a peripheral venous line or when necessary post-oxygenator. An access port with double stopcocks is positioned on the Y for this purpose. The access port is de-bubbled first and only 10 - 20ml luer tip syringes are to be used. Platelets may be given directly to the patient if they are pooled or centrifuged. Once the transfusion is complete, the access port is flushed with sterile saline.

The platelet level should be maintained high, greater than 100,000 if possible. This may be achieved by transfusing one or more centrifuged platelets (seven units of pooled platelets).

Cryoprecipitate

The administration of cryoprecipitate into the ECMO circuit is not recommended. If physician orders and patient status merit such use, the recommendation is to give via a peripheral IV directly to the patient and monitor ACTs accordingly, unless no other access is available.

Cryoprecipitate may be administered in the following instances:

    a. if the fibrinogen level is less than 200 mg/dl

    b. if the fibrin split products are greater than 40 mg/dl

    c. uncontrollable hemorrhage (fibrin glue)

Protocol for Platelet and Cryoprecipatate Administration

The infusion of platelets and occasionally cryoprecipitate is a necessary procedure during ECLS. Present ECLS technology describes an extreme thrombocytopenia related to extracorporeal circulation, particularly when using the silicone membrane oxygenator for gas exchange. The purpose of this protocol is to ease the complexity of this procedure, and insure stability in patient oxygenation and coagulation status. ACTs should be repeated every 15 minutes and adjustment of the heparin drip may be required to maintain ACTs in the desired range. Doubling the heparin infusion dose during platelets administration will maintain ACTs within desired range. The bridge must remain clamped during infusion. Previous therapeutic heparin dose can be resumed post infusion with ACT's monitored every 15 minutes for at least 45 minutes.

General guidelines:
- Maintain ordered parameters during administration. Transfusion may need to be slowed (5ml every 15 minutes) if difficulties arise.
- Platelets may be administered in the following instances:
  - To maintain a platelet count greater than 75,000
  - Uncontrollable hemorrhage
  - When the platelet count is desired to be at a higher level such as in the case of IVH or elective surgical procedure

Amicar®

Epsilon- Aminocaproic Acid (Amicar ®) inhibits the zymogen formation of plasmin from plasminogen. Plasmin is responsible for the breakdown of the fibrin clot. Amicar ® decreases levels of systemic plasmin thereby increasing the fibrin clot formation and inhibiting fibrinolysis. This decreases the amount of bleeding, particularly in peri-operative patients. If available, do a thromboelastogram (TEG) prior to Amicar ® administration. The most effective use of Amicar is to give it before a surgical procedure, e.g., chest tube placement and then maintain a drip for a period of time depending on the clinical state of the patient.

The dose is = 50 - 100 mg/kg bolus over one hour continuous drip of 10 - 40- mg/kg/hr. This drug will help attain hemostasis in the anticoagulated ECLS patient. It will also precipitate fibrin formation and clotting in the extracorporeal circuitry, so the length of treatment should be related to the risk for bleeding in the patient if not used. Amicar ® is indicated only for patients at high risk for hemorrhage. This includes all post-op patients, (i.e. congenital diaphragmatic hernia, post-op cardiac repair, etc.). Of note, Amicar is renally excreted, so if the patient has oliguria, the dose should be adjusted. Amicar ® therapy is regulated to maintain:

ACT	160-200 (flow dependent)
FDP	10-40
Fibrinogen	>200
Platelets	>150

Editorial

David C. Stockwell, MD MBA

Criteria for ECMO are not as refined as they are in the neonatal population because of the wider variety of lung disease, more diverse outcomes, the influence of chronic disease states, and difficulty in diagnoses irreversible lung disease in the pediatric population. This chapter outlines one centers approach to this difficult decision process. There are many areas of pediatric ECMO that need further investigation including blood product triggers, assessment of cardiac function and the proper use of pain control and sedation in this population. Our European colleagues use very low dose sedation &/or no pain medications resulting an awake/alert patient on ECMO with good outcomes. Further investigation into this approach will help determine recommendations in this area

References

1. Hill JD, O'Brian TG, Murray JJ, et. al Extracoporeal oxygenation for acute post-traumatic respiratory failure (shock-lung syndrome): Use of the Bramson Membrane Lung. N Engl J med 1972; 286:629-634.
2. Bartlett RH, Gazzaniga AB, Jefferies MR, et. al Extracorporeal membrane oxygenation (ECMO) cardiopulmonary support in infancy. Trans Am Soc Artif organs 1976; 22: 80-93
3. Zapol WM, Snider MT, Hill JD, et.al. Extracorporeal membrane Oxygenation in severe acute respiratory failure. JAMA 1979; 242:2193-2196
4. Barlett RH. Esperanza. Presidential address. Trans Am Soc Artif Intern Organs 1985; 31:723-726
5. Trachsel D., McCrindle BW., Nakagawa S. and Bohn D. Am. J. Respir. Crit. Care Med. Trachsel et al. 172 (2): 206.
6. Sussmane J. et. al ; Extracorporeal Life Support Manual (ECLS); Miami Children's Hospital, 2007

Chapter 12 Questions

1. A patient on ECMO has a platelet count of 80,000 and needs platelets. The patient has a CVL only, where should the platelets be given and why? You are giving the platelets post-oxygenator, why would you refrain from flashing the bridge?

2. A patient on ECMO has increasing ACT's and the Heparin drip is at the lowest allowable dose of 25 units/kg/hour, without effect on the ACT's. Describe possible reasons for this and your interventions.

3. You are at full flow when the bladder pressure begins to decrease and intermittently shuts off the pump. Describe the possible problems and your interventions.

4. The PaO2 is best regulated by adjusting:
   a) blood flow from the roller pump
   b) oxygen gas sweep
   c) blood volume to the ECMO circuit
   d) hemoglobin

5. Oxygen content refers to:
   a) amount of total oxygen carried in plasma
   b) amount of total oxygen bound to hemoglobin
   c) amount of total oxygen carried in blood
   d) oxygen concentration in the oxygenator membrane surface

6. Under what circumstances would you change the Sweep? Why?

7. How is the flow determined for Pediatric patient on ECMO?

8. How do you know that the oxygenator be used is the appropriate size for the patient ?

Chapter 12 Answers

1. Central venous catheters in small or newborn ecmo patients may be placed very close to the ecmo venous catheter. This increase the likelihood of membrane dysfunction with the infusion of platelets quickly into membrane via the central catheter. If this risk is high than the platelets should be given post membrane, with the assurance that the bridge remained clamped, to avoid recirculation and direct membrane exposure.

2. Heparin requires ATIII for it's clinical anticoagulation effect. Low levels of ATII are the most common scenario, especially in critical newborns and during long ecmo runs where FFP has not been given adequately.

3. : Decreased baldder pressure equates to decreased venous return from the patient. This may be physiologic with intravascular depletion, or mechanical with venous obstruction due to mechanical or structural changes. Catheter position, (critical in double lumen support), tension pneumo or hemothorax, pneumo or hemopericardium are also emergencies.

4. a

5. c

6. Sweep controls the patient pCO_2. Increased sweep decreases the patient pCO2. Decreased sweep increases the patient pCO_2.

7. The ECMO flow is determined by patient weight and metabolic condition. This is identical to newborns except the maximum flow for Pediatric patients is generally lower.

8. A careful determination of the manufacturer specifications that give the rated flow of the membrane to the patients size in kilograms is crucial for a successful ECMO support. Estimate of metabolic requirements based on disease and condition lead to an educated choice for the appropriate ECMO pump flow to support the patient.

Competencies [6]

	EQUIPMENT *Maintains and operates equipment within established guidelines.*		
TASK/TOPIC	**COMPETENCIES**	**Met Competency (Date& Initials)**	**Learning Contract (Date & Initials)**
ECMO Pump & Related Equipment - Routine Use	• States location, purpose and indication of use. • Cleans equipment per dept policies. • States equipment's limitations. • Identifies resources to troubleshoot. • States location of operator's manual. • Takes precautions to avoid damage. • Demonstrates start-up, operation, shut-down. • Takes precautions to avoid theft. • Locates/uses supplies for operating. • Documents as necessary. • Follows P&Ps for preventative & routine maintenance.		
ECMO Pump & Related Equipment- Emergency/Replacement Procedures	• If applicable, states procedures for protecting patient when equipment fails. • States procedures for obtaining replacement/back-up equipment. • States procedures for getting equipment serviced.		
Infusion Pumps -	• States location, purpose and indication of use. • Cleans equipment per dept policies • States equipment's limitations. • Identifies resources to troubleshoot. • States location of operator's manual. • Takes precautions to avoid damage. • Demonstrates start-up, operation, shut-down. • Takes precautions to avoid theft. • Locates/uses supplies for operating. • Documents as necessary. • Follows P&Ps for preventative & routine maintenance.		
Infusion Pumps—Emergency/Replacement Procedures	• If applicable, states procedures for protecting patient when equipment fails. • States procedures for obtaining replacement/back-up equipment. • States procedures for getting equipment serviced.		

	EQUIPMENT *Maintains and operates equipment within established guidelines.*		
TASK/TOPIC	**COMPETENCIES**	**Met Competency (Date& Initials)**	**Learning Contract (Date & Initials)**
ECLS Circuit	• Demonstrates the appropriate technique in assessing the ECLS circuit. • Performs a thorough patient assessment, (respiratory, neurological, cannualae site, and vital signs) and the interpretation of the assessment. • Discuss the interpretation of clinical signs and symptoms appropriately and communicates with physicians. • Demonstrates or describes the relationship of ECLS blood flow to oxygen delivery and oxygen consumption. • Reviews the relationship of sweep gas and carbon dioxide removal • Evaluates the interpretation of the patient arterial blood gas and the appropriate response with sweep and ECFR. • Identifies the correct interventions for laboratory values. • Reviews for the correct adjustments necessary for maintaining the prescribed saturation of venous blood. • Monitors the cumulative daily input and output fluid status of the ECLS patient. Maintains hourly I/O record status with the bedside nurse. • Performs the various interventions in the management of hemorrhage (i.e., cannulae site, IV sites, GI, etc.).		

13

Management of the Cardiac ECMO Patient

Ruth Ferroni, BSN, RN, CCRN, John Berger, MD and Jennifer J. Schuette, MD

Objectives

After completion of this chapter, the participant should be able to:

- review the criteria for using ECMO in the cardiac patient
- outline major differences between using ECMO for respiratory failure versus cardiac failure
- summarize the daily management of the cardiac ECMO patient, including potential complications, lab assessment, neurological evaluation, and weaning strategies
- discuss special coagulation issues related to the post-operative cardiac patient

- review special management strategies required for the cardiac patient with mixed pulmonary and systemic circulations

Introduction

Extracorporeal life support (ECLS), or extracorporeal membrane oxygenation (ECMO), is being increasingly used to support the circulation of patients with cardiac failure who are unresponsive to conventional therapies.[1] (Figures 1, 2, 3 and 4)

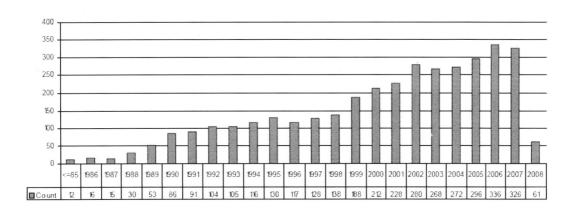

Figure 1. Annual cardiac runs world-wide in the neonatal population (age 0 to 30 days). (Source: ELSO registry, 2008; the 2008 data is incomplete.)

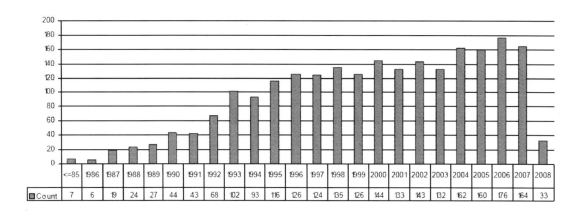

Figure 2. Annual cardiac runs world-wide in the infant population (age 31 days to less than one year). (Source: ELSO registry, 2008; the 2008 data is incomplete.)

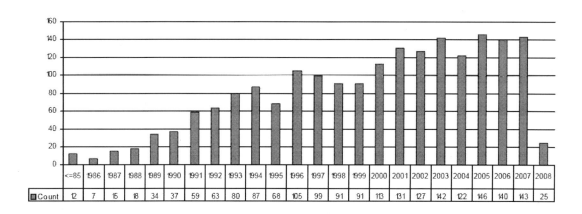

Figure 3. Annual cardiac runs world-wide in the pediatric population (age one to sixteen years of age). (Source: ELSO registry, 2008; the 2008 data is incomplete.)

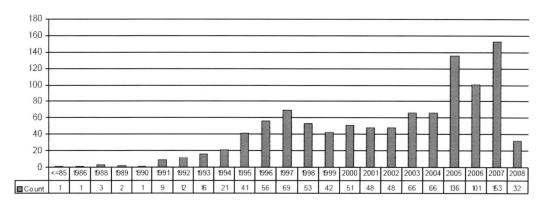

Figure 4. Annual cardiac runs world-wide in the adult population (over sixteen years of age). (Source: ELSO registry, 2008; the 2008 data is incomplete.)

146

The Extracorporeal Life Support Organization (ELSO) reports survival rates of 23-71% for patients placed on ECMO for cardiac indications, with variation based on age and the etiology of the cardiac failure. These indications can be broadly characterized into the following groups: congenital heart disease, cardiac arrest, cardiogenic shock, cardiomyopathy, myocarditis, and miscellaneous cardiac causes. (See Appendix for survival data based on age and etiology of cardiac failure.) At one time, patients with single ventricle physiology were not considered to be ECMO candidates, but this is no longer the case[2]; in fact, mechanical cardiac support is used electively in some centers during the immediate post-operative phase after Norwood Stage I surgery (the initial palliation for hypoplastic left heart syndrome and its variants).[3] Mechanical circulatory support can also be a useful strategy in the management of graft dysfunction after pediatric cardiac transplantation in both the early and late post-operative periods.[4]

Cardiac ECMO Indications

Each patient being considered as an ECMO candidate in the setting of cardiac failure should be carefully evaluated in terms of the following two issues: 1) the likelihood that his or her cardiac failure is due to a potentially reversible process and 2) his or her risk of mortality without ECMO versus the risks inherent in undergoing ECMO. A patient is considered a candidate for ECMO in the setting of cardiopulmonary failure that is refractory to maximal medical management and that has potentially reversible cause. Unfortunately, a prediction equation such as oxygen index has not been developed that reliably and quantitatively predicts the need for ECMO in the cardiac population. ECMO should be considered for support of pediatric cardiac patients in the following clinical scenarios[5]:
- pre-operative stabilization
- pre- or post-procedure stabilization for high risk cardiac catheterization procedures
- failure to wean from cardiopulmonary bypass
- progressive postoperative heart failure (i.e., low cardiac output syndrome)
- intractable pulmonary hypertension

- refractory dysrhythmias
- cardiac arrest in the post-operative setting
- myocarditis
- acute respiratory failure exacerbated by congenital heart disease
- dilated cardiomyopathy as a bridge to ventricular assist device or to evaluate for candidacy for a ventricular assist device

Contraindications to ECMO:

- end stage, irreversible, or inoperable cardiac disease unless the patient is a cardiac transplant candidate
- significant neurological or end-organ impairment
- uncontrolled bleeding within major organs
- extremes of size and weight
- inaccessible vessels during cardiopulmonary resuscitation
- family and/or patient directives to limit resuscitation

In patients with congenital heart disease who also have multiple other non-cardiac anomalies, such as genetic defects or dysfunction of other organ systems, a discussion with the family prior to operative cardiac repair should address the appropriateness of ECMO during the post-operative period.

Cardiac Versus Pulmonary ECMO

Cannulation

Vessel selection is according to the surgeon's preference. Patients undergoing rapid deployment (i.e., ECMO initiation with CPR in progress, or E-CPR) are frequently in the early post operative phase, and a transthoracic approach is the most efficient in the majority of these cases. Maintenance of good CPR, as evidenced by a good pulse tracing on the arterial line, palpable central pulses with compressions, and an end-tidal CO_2 reading of greater than 15-20 mmHg will likely improve outcome in ECPR patients.[6,7] Surface cooling by placing ice on the head is used in many centers during and immediately after the arrest phase to reduce neurological sequelae.[8] The remainder of the procedure is comparable to standard cannulation of an ECMO patient. Neck and femoral vessels may be used and may be preferred to reduce the risk of infection when time permits; transthoracic cannulation can also be transitioned to neck and/or femoral sites in the setting of prolonged ECMO support.

One clinical situation that merits particular attention at the time of cannulation is the patient with cavopulmonary connections, such as patients who have undergone bidirectional Glenn or Fontan repairs. A second venous cannula may be necessary to achieve adequate venous return to the ECMO circuit; whenever possible, the first venous cannula should be placed in the superior vena cava (SVC) or neck vessel in this subset of patients, allowing for adequate venous drainage of the head. If the upper venous circulation is not adequately drained, elevated SVC pressures in combination with low systemic arterial blood pressures place these patients at risk for inadequate cerebral perfusion pressure, possibly contributing to a poor neurological outcome.[9]

Oxygen Saturation Monitoring

Patients with two ventricle complete repair and no residual mixing of the pulmonary and systemic circulations should have an oxygen saturation of 95 to 100%. The systemic venous saturation (SvO_2) should also be in the normal range, or approximately 70 to 80%. Patients who are placed on ECMO for cardiac failure due to conditions such as myocarditis, cardiomyopathy, transplant rejection or dysrhythmias should also have oxygen saturations in the normal range since there is (in most cases) no anatomic mixing defect.

Patients with mixing of the pulmonary and systemic circulations, such as single ventricle patients who have not progressed to complete repair, are unable to physiologically produce a normal arterial saturation of 100%. When ECMO is first initiated, if patients are being essentially fully supported by the ECMO circuit, oxygen saturations may be quite high because the majority of the blood flow is bypassing the heart—where most if not all pulmonary and systemic mixing occurs. As the patient is weaned from ECMO and more blood flows through the heart, mixing will increase and the patient will return to

his or her expected oxygen saturation based on the cardiac anatomy. Patients with complete mixing lesions should be expected to have arterial oxygen saturations of 70-85% and a PaO_2 on an arterial blood gas of 30-45 mmHg when ECMO support is minimal.

The use of ECMO for the support of patients with aortopulmonary shunts (such as the Blalock-Taussig shunt) is another challenging clinical scenario for the ECMO specialist. ECMO pump flows may need to be increased to 150 to 200 mL/kg/min to provide adequate systemic flow because of run off into the pulmonary circulation through the shunt.[10,11] If inadequate systemic perfusion remains an issue in the patient with an aortopulmonary shunt, as indicated by persistent metabolic acidosis, pulmonary overcirculation on chest radiograph, and hyperoxemia, consideration may be given to partially clipping the surgical shunt to balance the two circulations (this requires a surgical procedure while on ECMO). There is no consensus on this intervention, however, and other authors suggest that altering shunt flow may worsen outcome.[12] If flow through the shunt is altered, shunt flow will need to be re-established as ECMO support is weaned to assure adequate pulmonary circulation. An alternative strategy is to remove the membrane oxygenator from the system; this takes away the pulmonary vasodilatory effects of the oxygen, potentially diminishing pulmonary overcirculation while improving systemic perfusion. This maneuver essentially converts the ECMO circuit to a ventricular assist device, however, and lung function must be adequate for this to be successful. If this maneuver is implemented, oxygen saturation goals should be adjusted accordingly.

Patients with healthy lungs should not have the ventilator adjusted to "rest" settings; if possible, ventilator settings should be manipulated to ensure that the pulmonary veins are delivering blood that is 100% saturated to the left atrium. This will maximize oxygenation to the coronary circulation, which is derived primarily from the left ventricle even during ECMO if there is any appreciable ventricular ejection. Providing adequate oxygenation to the heart will hasten myocardial recovery. The majority of ECMO-supported cardiac patients are maintained on ventilator settings of 30-40% oxygen,

16-20 breaths/min, 5 cm PEEP and a tidal volume of 6-10 cc/kg.

The postoperative cardiac patient may have shunting at the atrial level, the ventricular level, and/ or through a surgical shunt. In fact, there may be multiple shunt locations depending on the type of defect and the surgical repair. The ECMO specialist must be aware of the patient's cardiac anatomy, the location and direction of any anatomic or surgical shunts, and how the measurements from the arterial line and the in-line SvO_2 saturation monitor might be affected. Depending on the patient's anatomy and the presence or absence of a left atrial vent, the in-line SvO_2 monitor may not be a reflection of the adequacy of cardiac output.

Near-infrared spectroscopy (NIRS) is a non-invasive optical technique used to monitor regional oxygen saturation (rSo_2); these devices measure the concentration of oxygenated and deoxygenated hemoglobin, thereby determining the underlying tissue oxygenation.[13] The detectors can be placed on the forehead to assess cerebral oxygenation, as well as over splanchnic beds such as the abdomen and flank to measure tissue oxygenation in those areas. Most devices utilize two detectors, one measuring the total tissue oxygenation and the other measuring the superficial tissue oxygenation only; this allows for the contribution of the superficial tissues to be eliminated from the final rSo_2 read by the device. Although studies undertaken in pediatric post-operative cardiac patients comparing rSo_2 as measured by a NIRS device with saturations measured in the superior vena cava (SVC), right atrium (RA), and pulmonary artery (PA) have shown a statistically significant correlation between the two measurements, there is a such a wide range of agreement that using this number as an absolute surrogate for mixed venous saturation is probably not possible at this time.[14, 15] More research is ongoing utilizing this promising and non-invasive monitor of tissue oxygenation.

Daily Management of the Cardiac ECMO Patient

An understanding of the patient's cardiac anatomy is essential for the ECMO specialist; expectations regarding oxygenation and hemodynamics for a given patient can be clearly formulated only after the cardiac anatomy is well understood. One of the initial assessments that can be made on the ECMO patient is the degree to which the myocardium is recovering; this is reflected in the pulse contour and pulse pressure (i.e., a difference between the systolic and diastolic readings). Since the extracorporeal pump creates a flow that is essentially non-pulsatile, the more support being offered by the ECMO circuit, the flatter the arterial line tracing will be. As the patient recovers function and less support is being contributed by the pump, the arterial wave form will demonstrate an increasing pulse pressure. Some degree of ventricular ejection is preferred, even early on in the ECMO course, as this is usually the main source of coronary blood flow.

Atrial Decompression

There are times when the degree of myocardial failure is so significant that even a small amount of blood flow going to the lungs and returning to the heart may not be adequately ejected. This can result in atrial and ventricular distension and thus worsening function, a downward spiral that will not allow the heart to recover. Additionally, if left unchecked, this increase in pressure can be transmitted back into the pulmonary circulation, resulting in pulmonary edema and pulmonary hemorrhage. Echocardiography can be useful in detecting atrial and ventricular distension and to guide the need for intervention.

Options to decompress the heart include: 1) direct placement of an additional cannula (or "vent") into the left atrium (which requires an open chest); or 2) a transcatheter approach to create a connection between the left and right atria, or enlarge a connection if one exists but is inadequate (the latter approach allows for blood returning to the LA to flow into the RA and then the ECMO circuit rather than into the left ventricle.) Patients with single ventricle anatomy usually will have adequate communication between the atria, making decompression unnecessary—although if these patients do poorly even after ECMO is initiated, the atrial connection should be reassessed. The left atrial vent is then connected into the venous return line of the ECMO circuit. Since the vent will be contributing presumably 100% saturated blood flow coming from the pulmonary veins and then mixing with the systemic venous blood, the Svo$_2$ sensor may no longer be a reflection of the adequacy of oxygen delivery[16] and other measures to assess the adequacy of systemic perfusion are required.

Hemodynamic Monitoring

It is important for the ECMO specialist to monitor hemodynamic parameters along with ECMO pump flow rates to assess the adequacy of cardiac output. The venous pressures (central venous pressure [CVP], right atrial pressure [RAP], and left atrial pressure [LAP]) should be monitored; global increases in venous pressures despite adequate pump flows may suggest inadequate ventricular function or tamponade-type physiology. Discuss the optimal pressure ranges with the ECMO physician and pace volume resuscitation according to these parameters.

The arterial line waveform characteristics should also be monitored. A mean arterial range of 35-45 mmHg for neonates and greater than 60 -70 mmHg in larger children and adults is generally accepted. Although the failing ventricle benefits from ECMO to allow for recovery of function, completely "resting" of the ventricle by providing too much bypass flow (i.e., allowing essentially no ventricular ejection) may be detrimental to the heart. It is important that the heart regains normal contraction and conduction function as soon as possible to avoid involution of the myocardium and formation of ventricular thrombus. Inotropic support during ECMO for cardiac patients is usually substantially decreased compared to pre-ECMO levels. These patients are routinely maintained on low dose dopamine and vasodilator infusions; increasing inotropic support to aid ventricular ejection may be implemented earlier in other cardiac patients compared with those on ECMO purely for respiratory support. The successful outcome for cardiac patients has been shown to correlate with early return of contractile function[17], although survivors have been reported after prolonged support (over 250 hours).

A poorly functioning heart is susceptible to dysrhythmias, and any rhythm change should be reported promptly to the ECMO physician. AV synchrony should be re-established as soon as possible. Temporary pacing, antiarrhythmic agents and cardioversion/defibrillation have been used to return the heart to sinus rhythm during ECMO. While it may be possible to maintain adequate systemic perfusion and ECMO flows while not in sinus rhythm, the heart may overdistend in the presence of certain dysrhythmias (in particular ventricular fibrillation) and this may cause irreversible myocardial injury.

Anti-Coagulation Management

As with pulmonary ECMO, systemic anticoagulation with heparin is necessary to prevent clot formation in the ECMO circuit. It can be quite challenging to balance control of post-operative bleeding while minimizing formation of clots in the ECMO circuit in the immediate post-operative phase. The ECMO physician will often elect to give a smaller bolus dose of heparin (0-50 units/kg rather than the usual 50-100 u/kg in the non-post-operative patient) at the initiation of ECMO. A continuous heparin infusion is begun once the ACT result is less than 300 seconds; it is thought that post-operative bleeding is more commonly secondary to loss of clotting factors rather than heparin administration, so it is extremely unusual to manage a patient on ECMO without heparin even in the face of a documented coagulopathy. If it does become necessary to discontinue the heparin in the face of major and persistent bleeding, a second circuit should be primed and available due to the risk of sudden circuit failure resulting from clot formation.

ACT parameters will vary according to the ECMO flows being used; a patient with post-operative bleeding and high ECMO flows may have an ACT goal of 150-170 seconds, whereas a patient with minimal bleeding, on low flows and with some concern for clot formation in the circuit may require ACTs of 200-220 seconds. Blood product administration of platelets and clotting factors may rapidly decrease the ACT, so it should be monitored closely (every 15 minutes) during blood product administration. Bleeding on ECMO can usually be controlled with transfusion of clotting products while adjusting the heparin infusion to keep the ACT in a lower range. As ECMO flows are decreased and circuit clot becomes more of a risk, ACTs parameters must be adjusted accordingly.

Ventilator Management

Ventilator management is focused on adjusting the settings to achieve normal pulmonary vein saturation, thus providing richly oxygenated blood flow to the coronary circulation. This is fairly easy to accomplish with normal lung function and compliance. However, exposure to cardiopulmonary bypass can result in pulmonary endothelial injury; pre-existing pulmonary parenchymal disease can pose an additional clinical challenge. Thus, ECMO may be supporting both the heart and lung in some patients. Changes in ventilator settings are guided by physical assessment, lung volumes/compliance, blood gas results, and daily chest radiographs. In the patient with lung injury, a balance must be struck to minimize ventilator associated barotraumas while maximizing oxygen delivery to the heart to encourage recovery of function. Typical "rest" settings used in the respiratory failure ECMO patient can exacerbate myocardial ischemic damage and delay recovery, and therefore are rarely indicated.

Elevated pulmonary vascular resistance (PVR), either pre-existing or secondary to exposure to cardiopulmonary bypass and then to the ECMO circuit, may further hinder oxygenation in the patient relying in part on native pulmonary blood flow for oxygenation. Inhaled nitric oxide (iNO) or systemic vasodilators (such as milrinone) should be considered in these patients.

Sedation, Pain Management and Neurological Assessment

Sedation and pain management in the cardiac ECMO patient may differ somewhat from the respiratory failure ECMO patient. Older patients who are cannulated via the neck and/or via the femoral approach may be more awake, allowing for movement provided they are stable on moderate ECMO settings. Patients cannulated through a sternotomy incision usually require heavier sedation, and often paralytics, to maintain cannulae position and stable pump flows. Continuous intravenous infusion of a muscle relaxant may be warranted; however, once the patient has stabilized, it is preferable to use intermittent boluses to allow for a basic neurological assessment to be done.

The rate of intracranial hemorrhage in neonatal cardiac patients treated with ECMO has increased from 4 - 8% to 10 -18% since the 1990's (ELSO Registry data, 2008). Possible causes include repair of more complex congenital heart lesions resulting in added risk, changing strategies in anticoagulation, the increasing use of ECMO to assist in the resuscitation of patients in cardiac arrest, and other factors. If patient condition permits, a sedation "holiday" can be considered to better assess neurological function; it should be kept in mind that a patient who has received prolonged sedation and/or paralytic, especially in the setting of impaired hepatic or renal function, may have an unusually prolonged drug effect.

Routine head ultrasound should be done per institutional protocol in patients with an open fontanelle; further neurological studies (EEG, head CT) may be warranted based on the patient's clinical exam, but the benefits of obtaining this information should clearly outweigh the risks of undertaking the study. If a patient suffers a significant neurological injury while on ECMO, a discussion regarding the appropriateness of continued ECMO support should take place between the family and the medical team.

Fluid Management

Fluid overload is a common problem in the post-operative cardiac patient; causative factors include the need for post-operative fluid resuscitation, decreased urine output as a result of low cardiac output, and capillary leak associated with the inflammatory response to cardiopulmonary bypass and with reperfusion injury. Diuretic therapy should be started as soon as possible, provided adequate hemodynamic pressures and pump flows can be maintained. Frequently it is necessary to utilize hemofiltration to remove excess fluid, and this should be initiated as soon as it becomes clear that the response to diuretic is inadequate to achieve fluid balance. Cannulae position and security should be carefully monitored as the patient diureses, as the cannulas can shift as the swelling diminishes. Routine re-positioning should always be done as patient condition permits; even minimal movement, such as tilting rather than turning the patient, can help to mobilize fluid and maintain skin integrity. It is unlikely that the patient will successfully wean off of ECMO until the overall fluid balance is approximately even.

Complications

Bleeding

Bleeding is the most frequent and serious complication of ECMO. The interactions of the blood elements with the cardiopulmonary bypass and ECMO circuits as well as endothelial damage due to surgical trauma make the management of hemorrhagic complications challenging. In cardiac ECMO patients, the risk of severe hemorrhage is highest in the immediate post-operative phase, when patients are likely to suffer from a multifactorial coagulopathy caused by dilution of clotting factors while on cardiopulmonary bypass, hypothermia, hypoxia, and acidosis.

Severe bleeding requires prompt replacement with the appropriate blood products (platelets, fresh frozen plasma, and/or cryoprecipitate), and may also require lowering of ACT parameters and administration of antifibrinolytic medications. Blood products are administered to maintain parameters established by the ECMO physician; typical transfusion thresholds in the post-operative cardiac patient are as follows:

- packed RBC to maintain a hematocrit of 35-45%
- platelets to maintain a platelet count of >100,000
- FFP to maintain fibrinogen >150

Additional blood products (cryoprecipitate, factor VII) may be required in the post-operative patient with difficult to control bleeding, keeping in mind that excessive correction of the ECMO patient's coagulopathy can lead to clot formation in the circuit. For this reason, platelets and cryoprecipitate should be administered post-oxygenator or directly into the patient's IV access in order to minimize this potential problem.

Rapid infusion of blood products must be closely monitored; the CVP, RAP, and LAP should be followed to prevent overdistention of the heart during administration. Ionized calcium and potassium should be monitored closely (especially in the setting of large volume PRBC transfusions) and maintained in the normal range. The patient's temperature should be maintained in the normal range to promote normal coagulation function, unless the care team has requested initiation of mild hypothermia (34-35°C) for neuroprotection after cardiac arrest.

Hemostatic agents such as aminocaproic acid are considered for persistent bleeding if bleeding persists despite ACT adjustment and appropriate blood product repletion. Aminocaproic acid acts by inhibiting plasminogen activators, interfering with fibrinolysis and allowing for more stable clot formation. Generally, a loading dose of 100 mg/kg is infused over 60 minutes in D5W, followed by a maintenance dose of 33.3 mg/kg/hour (the dose is adjusted to 15 -20 mg/kg/hour for renal failure.) The circuit must be closely observed for evidence of clot formation; discontinuation of the heparin infusion is not recommended during the administration of aminocaproic acid as this may increase the risk of clot formation within the circuit. The goal is to control the patient's bleeding while still maintaining the viability of the ECMO circuit. Aminocaproic acid infusions can also be used to control bleeding in the setting of planned surgical procedures undertaken while on ECMO.

Recombinant Activated factor VIIa (rFVIIa) is another hemostatic agent that some centers have reported using with success to control excessive bleeding while on ECMO. It forms a complex with tissue factor (TF) to activate factor X, which then induces thrombin formation from prothrombin. This results in the formation of a stable fibrin plug that is resistant to premature lysis. Since the effectiveness of the drug requires combining with TF and platelet accumulation at the site, it is thought that the best response occurs in the setting of surgical bleeding. The duration of rFVIIa hemostasis is dose-dependent; blood loss has been shown to decrease dramatically after 1 to 2 doses.[18] The potential for excessive clot formation in the circuit or thromboembolic events affecting the patient remain a concern, so it is generally reserved for severe, uncontrolled bleeding.

Surgical bleeding may require chest exploration. Large amounts of blood and clot in a body cavity act as potent stimulus for fibrinolysis, resulting in a vicious cycle of continuous bleeding. Repeated chest exploration may be necessary. Aggressive stripping of the chest tubes is necessary to reduce the chance of tamponade. The ECMO specialist needs to be aware that topical hemostatic agents, such as absorbable hemostat and thrombin spray with packing, may be placed directly into the chest cavity after surgical exploration. Packing these agents around the heart can contribute to tamponade, which can occur even with the mediastinum open. An increase in filling pressures and heart rate, followed by loss of venous return and a drop in venous saturation, indicates a need for re-exploration to rule out tamponade. Cardiac tamponade impedes the flow of venous return to the pump, sometimes abruptly. A quick method to determine if loss of venous return is due to tamponade versus hypovolemia is to turn the pump flow down 10-20 ml/min; Loss of venous return will continue to be an issue if tamponade is occurring. If the problem is decreased circulating volume, turning the pump flow down will allow for adequate venous return to the pump. Keep in mind that it may be difficult to differentiate between volume depletion and impending tamponade as both may, at least initially, respond to volume infusion.

Residual Cardiac Defects

A residual cardiac defect should be suspected if the post-operative patient fails to wean from ECMO, despite apparent return of cardiac function and recovery of other end organ injuries. A cardiac catheterization may be required to confirm this diagnosis, and if a residual defect is discovered further surgery may be required (19). Potential residual defects include an incompletely repaired or previously undiagnosed ventricular septal defect, new or previously undiagnosed aortopulmonary collaterals, and significant gradients across the pulmonary or systemic outflow tracts. Such patients may or may not need continued ECMO support after their re-operation.

Emergencies that require temporarily coming off ECMO

Rarely, an unexpected event such as air in the circuit requires temporary but sudden discontinuation of ECMO for a brief period of time. In the pulmonary ECMO patient, hand bagging or "emergency" ventilator settings often allow adequate support until ECMO can be resumed. In the post-operative cardiac patient with poor ventricular function, sudden discontinuation of ECMO support can result in cardiac arrest, with closed or open chest CPR required until ECMO support can be restored. Code medications should always be readily available at the bedside, and the ECMO specialist and bedside nurse should be aware of which members of the team are the immediate responders to an ECMO code situation and how they can be reached emergently.

Weaning from ECMO

In the post-operative cardiac patient, return of ventricular function capable of sustaining adequate cardiac output usually occurs within 48-72 hours after the initiation of ECMO; this recovery time course correlates with successful patient outcomes.[17] However, weaning must be individualized for each patient, and some patients may require a slower weaning process to successfully wean from ECMO. As flows are weaned, adequacy of cardiac output as assessed by venous saturation (or, in the patient with mixing, arterial-venous saturation difference), urine output, acid-base balance, and NIRS measurements will help to determine the readiness for decannulation. Of note, if a left atrial vent was placed, it must be removed to allow for successful weaning; adequate cardiac output cannot be achieved if one continues to remove blood from the left atrium. An echocardiogram at very low flows or with the circuit clamped can provide additional information regarding contractility and cardiac filling. Vasoactives may need to be added or increased in order to successfully separate from the ECMO circuit, keeping in mind that some vasoactives may increase afterload and result in more work for the ventricle. Thus it is essential to keep vasoactives in a dose range that adequately supports function without overworking the recovering ventricle. Prior to decannulation, the following should also be assessed:

- fluid balance (if needed, excessive fluid can be removed with hemofiltration)
- pulmonary vascular resistance (the patient may require nitric oxide to be added prior to decannulation if pulmonary hypertension is documented or the risk is high)
- lung function (ventilator settings should be adjusted to assure adequate oxygenation and ventilation)

If the patient is able to tolerate "idle" flows (10-15% of predicted cardiac output), this suggests a readiness for decannulation. Prior to clamping the circuit, goal hemodynamic and oxygenation parameters should be reviewed with the medical team. Adequate oxygen delivery for 60-120 minutes with the circuit clamped should be followed by separation from ECMO.

If there is very poor or no functional cardiac recovery after 3-5 days, the healthcare team should discuss options and possible outcomes with the family. These patients may be candidates for heart transplantation and/or a ventricular assist device. The decision regarding if and when to list a patient for transplantt should be made by a multidisciplinary team which includes cardiovascular surgery, cardiology, and critical care medicine; the family's wishes should be paramount in this process. Since the average time to receive a heart transplant is between four and six weeks, it is advantageous to list a patient once functional cardiac recovery seems unlikely. Patients with multiple genetic anomalies may or may not be appropriate candidates for ECMO post-operatively, and a discussion with the family and members of the medical team prior to surgery should include options of support that could be used, if needed, in the post-operative period.

Appendix: Outcomes in Cardiac ECMO

The following table summarizes the cumulative cardiac ECMO experience organized by age group and diagnosis (source: ELSO Registry, 2008)

		Total Runs	Avg Run Time (Hrs)	Longest Run Time (Hrs)	Sur-vived	% Survived
Congenital Heart Disease	Neonate	3,114	142	1,198	1,136	36%
	Infant	1,824	146	1260	769	42%
	Child	977	136	1133	421	43%
	Adult	92	127	733	30	33%
Cardiac Arrest	Neonate	44	113	517	10	23%
	Infant	45	122	533	18	40%
	Child	71	115	525	27	38%
	Adult	57	70	257	14	25%
Cardiogenic Shock	Neonate	37	165	621	14	38%
	Infant	25	150	1157	10	40%
	Child	51	124	428	20	39%
	Adult	133	112	900	56	42%
Cardiomyopathy	Neonate	92	214	867	57	62%
	Infant	103	225	1073	54	52%
	Child	300	201	1490	173	58%
	Adult	142	132	842	52	37%
Myocarditis	Neonate	41	264	868	20	49%
	Infant	51	222	1246	34	67%
	Child	143	191	1207	94	66%
	Adult	35	176	761	25	71%
Other	Neonate	280	194	1871	114	41%
	Infant	259	161	936	119	46%
	Child	413	153	1026	189	46%
	Adult	569	114	965	183	32%

References

1. Di Russo GB, Martin GR. Extracorporeal membrane oxygenation for cardiac disease: no longer a mistaken diagnosis. *Pediatric Cardiac Surgery Annual.* 2005; 8:34-40.

2. Ravishankar C, Dominguez TE, Kreutzer J, et al. Extracorporeal membrane oxygenation after Stage I reconstruction for hypoplastic left heart syndrome. *Pediatric Critical Care Medicine.* 2006;7:319-323.

3. Ungerleider RM, Shen I, Yeh T, et al. Routine mechanical ventricular assist following the Norwood procedure—improved neurologic outcome and excellent hospital survival. *Annals of Thoracic Surgery.* 2004;77:18-22.

4. Fenton KN, Webber SA, Danford DA, et al. Long-term survival after pediatric transplantation and postoperative ECMO support. *Annals of Thoracic Surgery.* 2003; 76:843-7.

5. Jonas RA. *Comprehensive Surgical Management of Congenital Heart Disease.* London, England: Hodder-Arnold; 2004.

6. Thiagarajan RR, Laussen PC, Rycus PT, et al. Extracorporeal membrane oxygenation to aid in cardiopulmonary resuscitation in infants and children. *Circulation.* 2007;116:1693-1700.

7. Fiser RT, Morris MC. Extracorporeal Cardiopulmonary resuscitatiin in refractory pediatric cardiac arrest. *Pediatric Clinics of North America.* 2008; 55:929-941.

8. Duncan BW, Ibrahim AE, Hraska V, et al. Use of rapid-deployment extracorporeal membrane oxygenation for the resuscitation of pediatric patients with heart disease after cardiac arrest. *Journal of Thoracic and Cardiovascular Surgery.* 1998;116:305-311.

9. Booth KL, Roth SJ, Thiagajaran RR. Extracorporeal membrane oxygenation support of the Fontan and bidirectional Glenn circulations. *Annals of Thoracic Surgery.* 2004;77:1341-8.

10. Pizarro C, Davis DA, Healy RM, et al. Is there a role for extracorporeal membrane support after stge I Norwood? *European Journal of Cardiothoracic Surgery.* 2001;19:294-301.

11. Aharon AS, Drinkwater DC, Churchwell KB, et al. Extracorporeal membrane oxygenation in children after repair of congenital cardiac lesions. *Annals of Thoracic Surgery.* 2001;72:2095-102.

12. Jaggers JJ, Forbess JM, Shah AS, et al. Extracorporeal membrane oxygenation for infant postcardiotomy support: significance of shunt management. *Annals of Thoracic Surgery.* 200;69:1476-83.

13. Diaz LK, Andropoulos DB. New Developments in cardiac anesthesia. *Anesthesiology Clinics of North America.* 2005;23:655-76.

14. Tortoriello TA, Stayer SA, Mott AR, et al. A noninvasive estimate of mixed venous oxygen saturation using near-infrared spectroscopy by cerebral oximetry in pediatric cardiac surgery patients. *Pediatric Anesthesia.* 2005;15:495-503.

15. McQuillien PS, Nishimoto MS, Bottrell CL et al. Regional and central venous oxygen saturation monitoring following pediatric cardiac surgery: concordance and association with clinical variables. *Pediatric Critical Care Medicine.* 2007;8:154-160.

16. Aiyagari RM, Rocchini AP, Remenapp RT, Graziano JN. Decompression of the left atrium during extracorporeal membrane oxygenation using a transeptal cannula incorporated into the circuit. *Critical Care Medicine.* 2006;34:2603-06.

17. Duncan BW, Hraska V, Jonas RA, et al. Mechanical circulatory support in children with cardiac disease. *Journal of Thoracic and Cardiovascular Surgery.* 1999;117:529-42.

18. Wittenstein B, Ng C, Ravn H, Goldman A. Recombinant factor VII for severe bleeding during extracorporeal membrane oxygenation following open heart surgery. *Pediatric Critical Care Medicine.* 2005;6:473-6.

19. Booth KL, Roth SJ, Perry SB, et al. Cardiac catheterization of patients supported by extracorporeal membrane oxygenation. *Journal of the American College of Cardiology. 2002;40:1681-6.*

Chapter 13 Questions

1. All of the following are contraindications to the use of ECMO in a patient with cardiac disease EXCEPT:
   a) end stage or inoperable disease
   b) single ventricle physiology
   c) extremes of size and weight
   d) significant neurological impairment
   e) directives to limit resuscitation

2. Which of the following can result in inadequate venous return to the ECMO circuit in the post-operative cardiac ECMO patient?
   a) cardiac tamponade
   b) hypovolemia
   c) dysrhytmia
   d) a and b
   e) a, b, and c

3. Interventions commonly undertaken to control bleeding in the post-operative cardiac patient on ECMO include all of the following EXCEPT:
   a) maintaining a platelet count over 100,000
   b) maintaining fibrinogen over 150
   c) use of aminocaproic acid
   d) chest exploration
   e) discontinuation of the heparin drip

Chapter 13 Answers

   1. b
   2. d
   3. e

14

Adult Extracorporeal Life Support

Elaine Cooley, RN BSN, RRT and Robert Bartlett, MD

Objectives

After completion of this chapter the participant should be able to:

- Understand criteria for going on ECLS
- Understand daily management routine
- Understand differences related to diagnoses
- Understand the management of difficult cases

Introduction

ECLS was first utilized in 1971 for support of an adult patient with respiratory failure. A randomized trial published in 1979 showed no benefit, and research on ECLS for adult respiratory failure stopped for a decade.[1] With refined techniques, some centers reported success in the 1990's and another randomized trial demonstrated the value of ECLS in 2007.

ECLS is used for acute severe respiratory failure (ARDS). This may be caused by primary injury (viral or bacterial pneumonia) or secondary failure (sepsis, shock lung trauma). The need for ECLS for adult cardiac support is also growing. Adult cardiac support may be required for acute cardiac failure due to myocarditis or infarction, or post surgical myocardial stun.

As of January 2008, the ELSO registry recorded over 2,500 adult patients supported by ECLS. Respiratory patients accounted for 56% of these patients, 32% cardiac and 11% ECPR. The adult ECLS respiratory patient averaged 247 pump hours per case. The longest recorded case was 2616 pump hours (~109 days).[2]

Adult Respiratory Cases

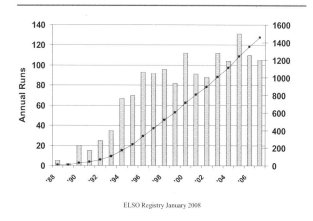

ELSO Registry January 2008

Figure 1: Annual Adult Respiratory ECLS Cases

Adult Diagnoses and Survival

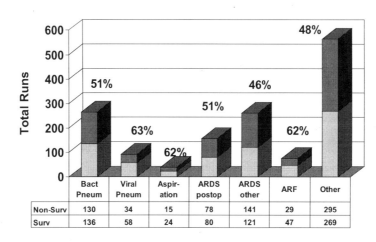

	Bact Pneum	Viral Pneum	Aspir-ation	ARDS postop	ARDS other	ARF	Other
Non-Surv	130	34	15	78	141	29	295
Surv	136	58	24	80	121	47	269

ELSO Registry January 2008

Figure 2: Outcomes

ECLS for Respiratory Failure

ARDS is characterized by refractory hypoxemia, persistent pulmonary inflammation, and increased vascular permeability.[3] Classification of ARDS includes primary lung injury (bacterial, viral or aspiration pneumonia, vasculitis, or other primary lung disease) or secondary lung injury (shock, trauma, sepsis, pancreatitis, etc).[3]

Acute Lung Injury (ALI) and ARDS include x-ray findings of bilateral patchy infiltrates, PF ratio <200, and poor lung compliance (<0.5cc/cm H_2O). These patients have capillary leakage, local or generalized edema and abnormal V/Q relationships.

Despite maximal medical therapy, ARDS mortality rates remain 30%-50%. This mortality is secondary to refractory pulmonary failure and multiorgan failure.

Patients with "severe" ALI or ARDS are classified as having a PF ration <100, A-aDO$_2$ >600mmHg, or transpulmonary shunt fraction >30% despite and after maximal medical treatment.[4] The use of ECLS is indicated in this group of patients. Acute respiratory failure can also be caused by status asthmaticus.

ECLS is used to keep these patients alive while the primary condition is treated.

Patient Selection

Case selection depends on both the patient condition and the capabilities of the team. Questions to be asked remain the same regardless if the patient is in your unit/hospital or at a referring hospital. There are 4 main concerns to identify:

- Is the underlying process reversible
- Do logistics allow you to provide ECLS to this patient
- Does the patient have a reasonable chance for survival
- Does the patient have any contraindications for ECLS

These are not always easy to answer. There may not be time to determine if the underlying process is reversible, or if the neuro status is adequate. The best interest of the patient and family wishes must be discussed before a decision is made.

Indications and contraindications vary widely between settings. The following Indications/Contraindications are recommended by ELSO.[5]

Indications: Acute severe lung failure with high mortality risk despite optimal conventional therapy. ECLS is considered at 50% mortality risk. ECLS is indicated in most circumstances at 80% mortality risk. Severity of illness and mortality risk is measured as precisely as possible using measurements for the appropriate age group and organ failure.

Respiratory Failure:

1. Hypoxic respiratory failure due to any cause (primary or secondary respiratory failure).
   a. 50% mortality risk, consider ECLS: PaO_2/FiO_2 <150 on FiO_2 >90% and/or Murray score 2-3
   b. 80% mortality risk, definite ECLS: PaO_2/FiO_2 < 80 on FiO_2 >90% and Murray score 3-4

2. CO_2 retention (asthma, permissive hypercapnea) $PaCO_2$ >80

Contraindications: Relative Contraindications – most contraindications are relative, balancing the risks of the procedure (including the risk of using valuable resources which could be used for others) vs. the potential benefits.

Respiratory Failure:

1. Mechanical ventilation at high settings (FiO_2> 90%, P-plat >30) for 7 days or more
2. Major pharmacologic immunosuppresion (absolute neutrophil count <400/ml3)
3. Age: no specific age contraindication but consider increasing risk with increasing age
4. Weight: over 100 kg (or some centers use a BMI of ~40)

Specific Patient Considerations:

1. Non fatal co-morbidities maybe a relative contraindication based on the individual case (i.e. diabetes and renal transplant and retinopathy and PVOD complicated by severe pneumonia)
2. Bridging to lung transplant: generally bridging to lung transplant is impractical because of limited donors.
3. Preexisting conditions which affect the quality of life (CNS status, end stage malignancy, risk of systemic bleeding with anticoagulation).
4. Futility: patients who are too sick, have been on conventional therapy too long, or have a fatal diagnosis
5. Contagious diseases which could be a risk to the treatment team may be considered a contraindication (HIV, Hepatitis C).

Pre ECLS Management

Many referral patients will improve with a standardized management protocol without the need for ECLS.

The University of Michigan ARDS Protocol is:

Mechanical Ventilation
- Pressure Controlled ventilation (limiting inspiratory pressure to 30 cm H_2O)
- Best Peep based on SvO_2
- Titrate FIO_2 for SaO_2 >90% & SvO_2 >70%
- Inverse I:E

Monitoring
- Continuous SaO_2
- Continuous SvO_2
- Arterial Line
- PA catheter
- Ventilator tidal volume pressure and minute ventilation

Treatments
- Prone positioning (12-18 hrs/day)
- Normal hematocrit (transfuse with PRBC's to Hct of 40-45)
- Diuresis to dry weight (Furosemide drip or CVVH)
- Chemical sedation or paralysis if needed
- Full enteral or parenteral nutrition
- Early tracheostomy
- Control fever
- Corticosteroids in patients with no pulmonary improvement after 7 days

If patient does not respond to this protocol (Pf ratio under 200) then ECLS is indicated

Circuit & Equipment Requirements

The basics include a pump (roller or centrifugal), membrane oxygenator, and monitoring devices (pressure, saturation, ABG's, clot formation, bubble detection, flow). Ports for withdrawing or infusing medications and blood products are necessary. Pumps must be selected and managed to prevent high negative inlet pressure which causes cavitation and hemolysis. Cavitation and hemolysis occurs when the inlet pressure exceeds ~ minus 200mmHg. The membrane lung must be made of solid (not porous) materials. In 2008 these devices in the U.S. are the Medtronic (spiral coil) and the Quadrox D from Maquet.

Respiratory patients greater than 40kg can go on ECLS with a clear primed circuit. Any sized patient can be placed on a clear primed circuit in an emergency, though the neonates do not respond as well to this method. Albumin (12.5 g) and CaCl (1g) are added to the prime. Once on ECLS a dose of a diuretic should be given to help excrete the additional crystalloid. It usually takes ~ 4 to5 units of PRBC's to return the Hct to the 40-45% level. Renal failure requiring renal replacement therapy occurs in ~ 40% of adult respiratory cases and ~50% of adult cardiac cases. (2) This requires a hemofilter to be placed into the ECLS circuit

Access for Respiratory ECLS

Venovenous cannulation is the preferred method for respiratory failure patients.

Cannula selection is very important to provide maximal support to the patient. It is advisable to have lines placed in the veins or arteries of vessels to be used for ECLS. These can be changed over a wire to ECLS cannulas. The largest cannula with the least resistance is needed to maximize your drainage potential. Percutaneous access is possible in 90% of adult patients. The technique for cannulating is discussed in another chapter.

Currently, two veins must be used for VV access. A Double Lumen Catheter (DLC) for adult patients is expected to be on the market in 2008. Venovenous mode can be performed utilizing AF (atrial-femoral) or FA (femoral-atrial) method. Most patients are managed with FA. Patients that are >50 kg do well with FA. Drainage occurs from the right femoral vein (RFV) and reinfusion through the right internal jugular vein (RIJV) to the atrium. Patients that have high intra abdominal pressures, are pregnant, or have any condition that impedes drainage from the RFV should use the AF mode. Drainage occurs from the RIJV (atrium) and reinfusion is through the RFV. Studies performed in the 1990's showed reduced recirculation in the FA mode.[6]

Management on VV ECLS

Management of the VV patient can be broken down into 5 categories.[7]
1. Flow and rest settings
2. Gas exchange
3. Anticoagulation
4. Monitoring
5. Other patient management

FLOW
Initially flow is increased to maximal, then set to maintain optimal oxygen delivery. Optimal support is seen when the ECLS flow maintains a SaO_2 >85% (accounting for some recirculation).

Ventilator settings: typical rest settings are pressure 25/10, rate 5 (i.e. ratio 2:1), FiO_2 .2-.3

GAS EXCHANGE

Sweep gas (typically 100% oxygen source) is used to regulate the $PaCO_2$ at a normal value.

In the absence of lung function, VV ECLS can supply all metabolic oxygen requirements, but the arterial saturation is usually 75-80%. This is ample oxyhemoglobin saturation for normal systemic oxygen delivery as long as the cardiac output and hemoglobin concentration are normal. However, arterial hypoxemia makes ICU staff uncomfortable. Education regarding oxygen delivery is important. Avoid the temptation to turn up the ventilator settings above rest settings during VV support.

ANITCOAGULATION

Heparin is the gold standard used for anticoagulant in ECLS. Other drugs such as Argatroban or Lepirudin have also been used (with concern for HIT) for anticoagulation.

Bleeding is the number one complication on ECLS. Measuring the ACT at the bedside is the most common method for monitoring and filtrating heparin effect. The activated clotting time can be reduced if needed for bleeding complications. Anticoagulation is a very complex topic and is reviewed in greater detail in another chapter.

MONITORING

Monitoring the patient on VV ECLS is best done with SaO_2 (patient) and SVO_2 (circuit) monitors. These monitoring devices allow you to analyze for recirculation, lung improvement or worsening respiratory status. A PA catheter is extremely useful for monitoring of the VV patient to monitor filling pressure, cardiac output, and pulmonary vascular resistance.

OTHER PATIENT MANAGEMENT

Patients on VV ECLS that have severe respiratory failure may require other interventions to help maintain adequate support. Patients are managed with minimal sedation. If VV oxygen delivery is not adequate to meet oxygen demands, patient oxygen consumption can be lowered with paralysis and systemic coolant. Tracheostomy decreases the need for sedation and facilitates weaning from the ventilator after ECLS. Use of paralytics is reserved for those patients who can not be maintained with a SaO_2 of >70%. Long term use of paralytics can cause significant muscle fatigue/wasting and can contribute to an extended recovery post ECLS. There are centers who keep their ECMO patients alert and awake throughout their ECMO run. Limiting sedation so that the patient is comfortable but can answer questions (with adequate support indicators) is an appropriate goal.

Resting the lungs is the most important goal while on ECMO. Maintaining the FiO_2 at 50% or less and limiting the inspiratory pressure below 30cm H_2O helps to minimize further damage to the lungs. Other rest and recruitment measures for the lungs include:

- Proning – 12-18 hrs/day
- Maintain ventilator rest settings
- Bronchoscopy /BAL as needed for diagnosis and clearing the airways
- Tracheostomy early after initiation of ECLS
- Diuresis – Lasix drip or CRRT as needed to achieve "dry weight."
- Aggressive management of any infectious/ surgical process that may be contributing to the situation.
- Appropriate nutrition – enteral feeds if tolerated, otherwise TPN

There is no hemodynamic support while on VV ECMO. The use of inotropes, vasodilators, blood volume replacement, etc. should be used to support the hemodynamic needs. Patients on VV who lose cardiac function require conventional CPR.

Daily management of these patients includes a CXR to evaluation lung inflation and cannula placement. CBC and platelets are measured daily. Other labs depend on the patient disease and condition. Coagulation is discussed in another chapter and will not be discussed here.

Routine daily care of the ECMO patient includes the same basic care for any ICU patient:

- Pain
- Skin Integrity
- Pulmonary Toilet – move side to side if you do not prone
- Mouth Care
- Eye Care
- Nutrition
- Neuro assessment

However, extra care must be used in prevention of bleeding. This includes:

- Gentle suctioning
- No percutaneous punctures
- Removal of any lines or tubes can lead to bleeding
- Gentle placement of NG/OG/Dophoff – use extra lubricant
- No subQ injections
- No placement of chest tubes (or any surgical procedure) without use of Bovie

Evaluation of Support

Determining adequacy of support for the adult VV patient can be a lesson in patience! Understanding oxygen delivery and consumption concepts are critical in managing these patients. In VV mode, infusate blood mixes with systemic venous blood return. At typical blood flow, the ratio of infusion blood to deoxygenated right atrial blood is usually around 3:1. If there is no native lung function, this results in arterial PCO_2 41, PO_2 40, Sat 80% and O_2 content of $17ccO_2/dL$ in the pulmonary artery. If there is no native lung function, this will be the composition of the gases in the arterial blood. It is important to realize that systemic arterial saturation around 80% is typical during VV support. As long as the hematocrit is over 40% and cardiac function is good, systemic oxygen delivery will be adequate at this level of hypoxemia.

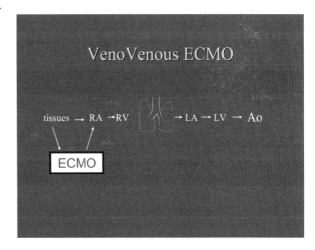

As the lungs get better you will see a step-up in the PA SvO_2 to SaO_2 reading.

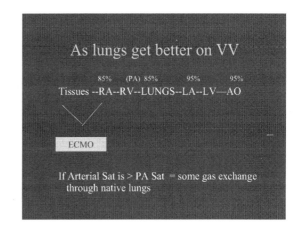

Trial and Decannulation

Preparation for trial off VV ECLS: Increase ventilator settings and be sure you have appropriate volume/medications on hand. Then discontinue the gas sweep to the oxygenator. If adequate gas exchange and hemodynamics are maintained by native lung function for 1-2 hours, cannulas can be removed. If lung function is borderline, cannulas can be left in place for 12-24 hours. Removal of percutaneously placed cannulas requires pressure held for 20-30 minutes. Patients with a percutaneously placed femoral venous cannula should have a Doppler Scan of the leg veins 2-3 days post-decannulation.

Patients found to have deep vein thrombosis (DVT) are managed with an inferior vena cava (IVC) filter.

Cardiac Support

Patients in cardiac failure require VA ECLS. In the ELSO registry, the average time on ECLS was 123 hours. Survival overall was 32%. The subgroup with myocarditis had 70% survival.[2] Adult cardiac support may be required in an ECPR setting for an acute myocardial infarction (MI), pulmonary embolus (PE), or cardiovascular collapse. It may be used as a bridge to ventricular assist device (VAD) support, or for post-op inability to come off cardiopulmonary bypass (CPB).

Emergent Referral

Emergent ECLS is referred to as ECPR (Extracorporeal-Cardiopulmonary Resuscitation) and may be required for those patients in extremis that experience sudden complete cardiovascular collapse.

The ability to respond with ECLS in a short period of time (5-15 minutes) will depend on how your program is set up. A rapid deployable system must be utilized. Some centers keep a pre-primed circuit at all times, others utilize a centrifugal pump and microporous oxygenator that can be prepared within 5 minutes. All supplies should be in one area that can be quickly moved to wherever the patient is located. The blood bank must be notified immediately for the need of emergency blood. The use of ECPR for patients in active cardiac arrest varies between institutions. ECLS is usually used in a witnessed arrest of 5 minutes or less with monitoring demonstrating adequate perfusion (strong pulse, pH>7.2). Survival for adult ECPR is 26% in the ELSO registry.

VA Access

Venous access can be either the RIJV or RFV. Arterial access can be through the right common carotid artery (RCCA), but the FA is preferred. If

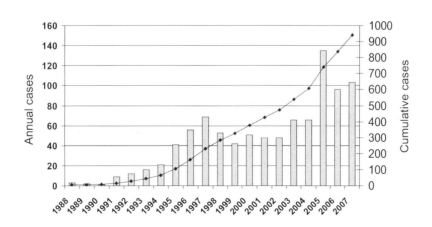

Cardiac Cases By Year
16 years old and over

ELSO Registry January 2008

Figure 3: Adult Cardiac Cases

the FA is used, a distal reperfusion cannula can be placed in the post tibial artery (PTA).

Patients that are cannulated through the groin and also have a component of respiratory failure may experience a phenomenon of perfusion mismatch, also sometimes identified as North-South Syndrome. Patients with North-South syndrome present with low upper body extremity saturations, while the lower extremity saturations are normal. The native cardiac output has improved and LV output is blocking the perfusion of oxygenated blood from the return cannula in the RFA.

Treatment is placement of a perfusion cannula in the RIJV to allow oxygenated blood to be infused into the RA. This is called VA-V ECLS. Monitoring a patient cannulated VA through the groin is best achieved by utilizing the saturation probe on the right hand. You can read more about this physiology in the chapter on ECLS physiology.

As with the pediatric population, some adults are placed on ECLS for inability to wean from CPB or immediately post-op. Typically the CPB cannulas are used and the chest is left open and covered with a plastic drape. Sedation requirements for cannulating VA are the same as with VV. Once the patient is stable on ECMO, sedation/narcotics should be turned off to assess neurologic status. Sedation can be restarted to keep the patient comfortable.

Management

The same basic principles applied to the VV patient apply to the VA patient. The main difference is that inotropes are not required and the arterial pressure is nonpulsatile.

Sedation should be at a level where the patient is comfortable but awake. Patients with an open chest require frequent assessment for pain and sedation. Patients on VA ECMO that have normal lung function may be more comfortable extubated. This allows for normal breathing and decreases the risk of a nosocomial infection/pneumonia. If the ventilator is used, keep it at rest settings. Typically VA patients that are being supported for primary cardiac failure do not require proning, or not able to be proned secondary to open chest.

Cardiac ECLS by Diagnosis
16 years old and over

	Runs	*% Survived*
Congenital Defect	85	32
Cardiac Arrest	52	21
Cardiogenic Shock	122	44
Myocardiopathy	133	33
Myocarditis	33	70
Other	515	32

ELSO Registry January 2008

Figure 4: Adult Cardiac Outcomes

Assessment of Support

In VA ECMO infusate blood mixes with blood in the aorta. The ratio of infusion to native aortic blood flow is typically 8:1. If native lung function is normal (O_2 content 21ccO_2/dL) and the FiO_2 is 0.21, this results in PCO_2 40, PO_2 200, saturation 100%, PO_2 100, saturation 98%, content 20ccO_2/dL. NOTE: the forgoing is true if infusion blood going into the femoral artery and flow is retrograde. The mixing will occur somewhere in the mid aorta. The higher the flow rate, the higher the level of mixing. During severe respiratory failure, at typical VA flow rate (80% of cardiac output), this can result in desaturated blood from the left ventricle perfusing the aortic arch and coronaries and fully saturated infusion blood perfusing the lower 2/3 of the body (North-South syndrome- see above).

Arterial oxygenation monitoring depends on the location of blood reinfused and location of the arterial line. Patients on VA utilizing the RCCA should be monitored from the left radial artery. Patients on VA-V bypass are best monitored by the arterial line in the right radial artery. Placement of saturation probes follows the same logic. Knowing the physiology of your patient and where the reinfusion of oxygenated blood goes is vital in making an accurate assessment of support.

Trial and Decannulation

Trialing off VA ECMO is more complex than on VV. Some institutions start a second heparin drip to the patient ~ 15-20 minutes prior to the start of the trial. Others may wean flow but not completely clamp off bypass. Some ECLS programs set a time frame for VA trials. Decisions must be made to either go back on ECLS or decannulate within that time frame. VA trials can be stressful for the patient and the circuit. Flashing the cannulas every 10-15 minutes can alter the patients' hemodynamics and potentially increase the risk of introduction of emboli.

Make sure you have the necessary pressors/ introps and volume available. Ventilator settings do not usually play as significant a role for the cardiac patient. The main focus is maintenance of blood pressure and perfusion. If blood pressure can be maintained on a modicum of pressor support while supporting adequate perfusion, then the patient can be decannulated. If cannulated percutaneously, the cannulas are pulled and pressure applied. If they were placed by cut-down, the site will be re-opened and the vessels either repaired or ligated (depending on location). Chest cannula can be removed at the bedside or if your policy requires, taken out in the operating room.

Troublesome Diagnosis and Treatments *(5)*

Management of air leaks:
- Small pneumothorax – (estimated 20% or less with no hemodynamic compromise and no enlargement over time) is best managed by waiting for absorption with no specific treatment.
- Symptomatic pneumothorax – (> 20%, enlarging, or causing hemodynamic compromise) should be treated by external drainage, using a small tube with appropriate preparation.
- Massive air leak or bronchopleural fistula (BPF) – defined as less than half of the inspired volume coming out as expired volume – can be managed by ECLS, in fact it is sometimes a specific indication for ECLS. As in any BPF, the first objective is to evacuate the pleural space so that the lung contacts the chest wall, leading to adhesions with closure of the visceral pleura. During ECLS this can almost always be managed by a single chest tube placed on high continuous suction (20-50 cm/H_2O), then limiting inspiratory pressure and volume. In some cases, it may be necessary to manage the airway by continuous positive airway pressure at 10, 5, or even 0 cm/H_2O for hours or days. When the air leak has sealed, airway pressure is gradually added until conventional rest settings are reached. Recruitment of the totally atelectatic lung may take one or more days.

BPF with a massive air leak directly from a bronchus or the trachea (after lung resection or trauma for example) should be managed initially as outline above, but direct endoscopic or thoracotomy closure is often required.

Pulmonary Embolism

Many patients with primary or secondary ARDS will have small (segmental) pulmonary emboli on contrast CT or angiography. Such emboli do not require any specific treatment aside from the heparinization, which accompanies ECLS. When **major or massive pulmonary embolism** is the cause of respiratory/cardiac failure, venoarterial ECLS can provide very successful management if cannulation and extracorporeal support can be instituted before brain injury occurs. Patients with major PE treated with ECLS have a 65% survival rate. (8)

After VA access and successful ECLS is established, document the extent of pulmonary embolism by appropriate imaging studies. Massive pulmonary emboli will usually resolve or move into segmental branches within 48-72 hours of ECLS support. The patient can be weaned from ECLS then from ventilation and managed with pulmonary embolism prophylaxis. Almost all such patients are managed with placement of an IVC filter. If heart/lung function has not recovered within two days, or if there is a secondary reason to get the patient off ECLS (GI bleeding for example), the patient should undergo pulmonary thrombectomy with cardiopulmonary bypass support. When thrombectomy is done it is usually necessary to continue ECLS for days until lung function is normal. A study of PE patients over a 14 year time span revealed a 62% survival for this group at one center.(8)

Lung Biopsy

The cause of severe respiratory failure may be unknown when the patient is started on ECLS. Although lung biopsy is the next step in diagnosis, it is potentially dangerous in patients on ECLS with anticoagulation. If pulmonary function rapidly improves during ECLS (the first few days) lung biopsy may be delayed until the patient is off anticoagulation. However, if pulmonary function is not improving and the primary diagnosis is not known, lung biopsy can and should be done within the first week on ECLS. Lung biopsy is best done by thoracotomy (or thoracoscopy) rather than transbronchially because of the risk of major hemorrhage into the airway with transbronchial biopsy. As with any thoracotomy during ECLS, it is best to leave the chest open, covered by an adhesive plastic drape, with definitive closure after ECLS. (5)

Rare conditions

ECLS has been used for rare causes of pulmonary failure with variable success. When considering ECLS for a specific diagnosis for the first time in any given center it may be helpful to consult the ELSO registry for the worldwide experience with that condition. Examples are:
- Vasculitis
- Autoimmune lung disease
- Bronchiolitis Obliterans
- Goodpasture syndrome
- Rare bacterial, fungal, or viral infections
- Bridge to and from lung transplant

Conclusion

The use of ECLS in the adult respiratory and cardiac population is growing. As more centers gain experience in the management of the adult ECLS patients, the overall survival may improve. With experience, one center had an average 5-year survival rate of 78% for adult respiratory failure. While adult ECLS is labor intensive and fraught with challenges, there is no better reward than seeing your patient return with their family at your next ECMO picnic!

References

1. Bartlett, RH. Historical Perspectives, Extracorporeal Membrane Oxygenation ECMO). American Academy of Pediatrics 2005.
2. Adult ECMO Registry of the Extracorporeal Life Support Organization (ELSO). Ann Arbor, Michigan. January 2008.
3. Brown, K., Haft, J., Bartlett, RH. Acute Lung Injury and Acute Respiratory Distress Syndrome: Extracorporeal Life Support and Liquid Ventilation for Severe Acute Respiratory Distress Syndrome in Adults. Respiratory Critical Care Medicine 2006; 27; 416-425.
4. Hemmila, M., Rowe, S., Boules, T., Miskulin, J., McGillicuddy, J., Schuerer, D., Haft, J., Swaniker, F., Arbabi, S., Hirschl, R., Bartlett, RH. Extracorporeal Life Support for Severe Respiratory Distress Syndrome in Adults. Annals of Surgery 2004, October; 240 595-607.
5. Extracorporeal Life Support Organization (ELSO). Ann Arbor, Michigan. Protocol/Guidelines for Adult Respiratory Failure 2008.
6. Rich,P., Awad, S., Crotti,S., Hirschl,R., Bartlett,R., Schreiner,R. Cardiopulmonary Support and Physiology: A prospective comparison of atrio-femoral and femoro-atrial flow in adult venovenous extracorporeal life support. J Thorac Cardiovas Surg 1998; 116:628-632.
7. Extracorporeal Life Support Organization (ELSO). Ann Arbor, Michigan. General Protocol/Guidelines for all ECLS Cases. 2008.
8. Maggio, P., Hemmila, M., Haft,J., Bartlett, RH. Journal of Trauma March 2007; 62;3 570-576.

Chapter 14 Questions

1. ARDS is characterized by:
   a). Refractory hypoxemia
   b). Persistent pulmonary inflammation
   c). Increased vascular permeability
   d). All of the above

2. When is ECLS indicated in most circumstances?
   a). When mortality risk is 50%
   b). When mortality risk is 40%
   c). When mortality risk is 80%
   d). When mortality risk is 60%

3. What is a relative contraindication for ECLS?
   a). Pt. on high ventilatory support for 3 days.
   b). Pt. on high ventilatory support for 6 days
   c). Pt. on high ventilatory support for 10 days
   d). There are no contraindications for ECLS

4. Patients greater than 40 Kg can go on ECLS with a clear prime circuit.
   a). True
   b). False

5. Patients on VV ECLS are better supported with less recirculation if they are cannulated and flow in which direction?
   a). Atrial-Femoral (AF)
   b). Femoral-Atrial (FA)

6. What is an acceptable arterial saturation for a patient on VV ECLS?
   a). Must be at least 95%
   b). Must be at least 90%
   c). Must be at least 85%
   d). Greater than 80% ok if Hct. is greater than 40.

7. If your VV patient has a PA saturation of 85% and the arterial saturation is 85%, what does this tell you?
   a). The pt. is not well supported
   b). The monitor is not working properly
   c). The patient must need more Hemoblobin
   d). The patients' lungs are not exchanging oxygen

8. What is the greatest risk to the patient when you cannulate the groin vessels for VA ECMO?
   a). Not enough ECMO flow available
   b). Loss of pulses in the affected foot
   c). Inability to turn patient
   d). A & C

9. Your patient has a small pneumothorax. What should you do?
   a). Have a surgeon place a chest tube immediately
   b). Increase the FIO_2 on the ventilator
   c). No specific treatment – wait for adsorption
   d). All of the above

10. You have placed your patient on with a clear prime circuit. What should you be thinking about?
    a). Give a diuretic
    b). Increase Hct. to 40-45%
    c). Start a hemofilter immediately
    d). A & B

Chapter 14 Answers

1. d
2. c
3. c
4. a
5. b
6. d
7. d
8. b
9. c
10. d

15

Medical and Surgical Management of the Congenital Diaphragmatic Hernia Patient on ECMO

Wolfgang Stehr, M.D., David Powell, M.D., and Billie Short, M.D.

Objectives

After completion of this chapter, the participant should be able to:

- Discuss an overview of the pre-ECMO treatment of the CDH patient
- Outline care of the CDH patient after being placed on ECMO
- Describe complications in the CDH patient that may occur on ECMO
- Describe management of surgical repair on ECMO

Introduction

The use of extracorporeal membrane oxygenation (ECMO) has revolutionized the care of infants born with a congenital diaphragmatic hernia (CDH). Despite significant scientific efforts there is still disagreement and lack of understanding of preoperative ventilation strategies, as well as clear knowledge as to which patients are likely to benefit from ECMO and what the correct timing of hernia repair is for the infant treated with ECMO. Historically, due to its high mortality, repair of CDH was a true surgical emergency. In the 1970's, ECMO was first utilized as a rescue therapy following repair of CDH when conventional methods failed.[1] In the 1980s, advancements in neonatal intensive care and a better understanding of the pathophysiology of pulmonary hypertension associated with CDH led to a strategy involving preoperative stabilization and delayed surgical intervention.[2] Retrospective reviews demonstrate an improvement of survival in infants treated with ECMO from 56% to 71%.[3-5] This chapter will outline the advances in the care

of the congenital diaphragmatic hernia patient pre-ECMO and discuss the approach used for treatment with ECMO.

CDH occurs in one in every 2500 live births. The most frequent posterolateral Bochdalek hernia results from a failure of closure of the pleuroperitoneal membrane segregating the chest from the abdomen during the eighth week of gestation. The resultant unilateral hernia is associated with a variable amount of bilateral pulmonary hypoplasia and pulmonary hypertension. The overall surface area of the alveoli and the vascular bed in infants with CDH is reduced. These smaller vessels are more prone to developing resistance such that even subtle insults can lead to profound increases in pulmonary vascular resistance.[36] Figure 1 shows the typical left sided CDH x-ray. The selective activation of

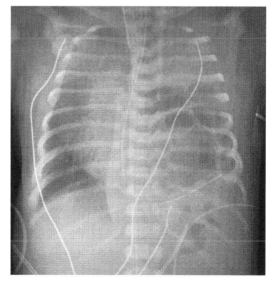

Figure 1. X-ray findings seen a typical left diaphragmatic hernia patient. Note that the nasogastric tube is in the left chest.

thromboxane synthetase pathways precipitated by CDH may in part contribute to pulmonary hypertension.[35] ECMO may allow for a rest period in which homeostasis of prostanoids can be achieved and lead more importantly to resolution of pulmonary hypertension.

Indications for ECMO

For an infant with a pre- or postnatal diagnosis of CDH, no criteria are absolutely predictive of outcome in general nor of the success of conventional therapy. Infants who undergo CDH repair without requiring ECMO support have a near one hundred percent survival rate.[23] Analysis of the Extracorporeal Life Support Organization (ELSO) database failed to identify reliable predictors of mortality in CDH patients requiring ECMO. There was a trend toward improved survival in patients who tolerated medical management for greater than 18 hours, had a longer gestational periode, a birth weight greater than 3.5 kg and a pre-ECMO pH greater than 7.4 or a P_aCO_2 less than 49.[34]

The most often-sited indication for ECMO in CDH patients is a "failure of conventional medical management." Traditional medical management strategies consist of mechanical ventilatory and vasopressor hemodynamic support and sedation in an effort to control pulmonary hypertension by hyperventilation and maintaining post-ductal oxygen saturations greater than 90%.[7] Achieving these goals required high respiratory rates and high peak inspiratory pressures resulting in pulmonary barotrauma. The lung injury resulting from this approach was clearly responsible for much of the historic morbidity of CDH infants. New intensive care strategies and technologies emphasize lower inspiratory pressures, permissive hypercapnia and spontaneous respirations in an attempt to minimize barotrauma.[8-10] High frequency oscillatory ventilation (HFOV) has been used as rescue therapy for children failing conventional ventilator management in the preoperative management of CDH.

Inhaled nitric oxide (NO) therapy has been successful in managing pulmonary hypertension in CDH patients. NO is a potent vasodilator derived from endothelial cells. In this setting, NO exerts its effects on the pulmonary vasculature and is rapidly metabolized before reaching the systemic circulation.[11,12] Unfortunately, in a randomized trial, the national inhaled nitric oxide study group (NINOS) did not find any benefit for CDH patients treated with NO in terms of need for ECMO or mortality.[13] In addition to the pulmonary hypoplasia and hypertension noted, some studies have documented lung immaturity in the patients with CDH. Attempts to improve function of the immature lungs by means of surfactant administration has been associated with improvement in lung compliance, pulmonary vascular resistance and gas exchange in a fetal lamb model of CDH,[14] however surfactant therapy shows no benefit in CDH patients in terms of survival, need for ECMO or development of chronic lung disease.[15] Classic objective criteria for institution of ECMO therapy include alveolar-arterial oxygen gradient of greater than 600 mmHg for 4 hours, oxygenation index greater than 40, $P_aO_2 < 40$ mmHg, or pH < 7.15 for 2 hours.

Exclusion Criteria

Available cannula sizes limit ECMO therapy to CDH infants weighing at least two kilograms. The required systemic anticoagulation for ECMO bypass, and the associated increased risk of intracranial hemorrhage (ICH) in premature infants limits eligible patients to a gestational age greater than 34 weeks.[7,16] Similarly, due to concerns for rebleeding, a child who has already suffered an ICH greater than grade II is generally excluded from ECMO. Infants with evidence of ongoing bleeding and coagulopathy are rarely considered for ECMO therapy. Neonates with concomitant lethal anomalies are not considered for ECMO. The initial investigation of all children with CDH should include an echocardiogram to evaluate for anatomic cardiac defects since CDH is frequently associated with other anomalies including congenital heart disease.

Technical Considerations

Compared to venovenous (VV) ECMO, venoarterial (VA) ECMO offers the added advantage of circulatory support and is less subject to mediastinal shift noted in patients with CDH. Recent studies, however, have shown that VV ECMO may be as efficient in supporting CDH patients as VA ECMO. [17-21] Although renal complications and inotrope use are less common with VA ECMO, VV ECMO is associated with fewer cerebral infarcts and seizures and the maintenance of pulsatile oxygenated blood flow through the lungs inducing production of endogenous nitric oxide,resulted in improved coronary blood flow and avoidance of increased left ventricular afterload. [17-21]

ECMO access is usually performed via a transverse or oblique incision in the right neck. For VA ECMO CDH patients are preferentially cannulated via the right internal jugular vein and right common carotid artery, for VV ECMO via the right internal jugular vein. Placement of central venous access through the right neck is therefore contraindicated in CDH patients. For VA ECMO, the tip of the venous cannula is placed at the level of the right atrium and the tip of the arterial cannula at the junction of the innominate artery and the ascending aorta. Proper cannulae position is confirmed by chest radiograph (Figure 3) or echocardiography. Optimal positioning of the catheters can be difficult in patients with CDH because herniated abdominal viscera in the

thorax tend to the shift the mediastinum. If there are concerns about catheter position &/or VRM alarms after going on ECMO, a echocardiogram should be done. Because of the sift of the heart, venous catheters that look I position on x-ray can be either against the wall or through the foramen ovale into the left atrium.

Diaphragm Repair

With the recognition that associated pulmonary hypertension and hypoplasia are the major contributors to mortality, rather than the presence of abdominal viscera in the chest (Figure 2), the timing of diaphragmatic hernia repair has shifted from emergent to delayed. ECMO support allows for time to achieve pulmonary vascular bed stabilization with subsequent surgical repair. [22,23] The optimal timing for repair (prior to ECMO, while on ECMO, or after completion of ECMO) remains controversial. Patients who require ECMO after emergent repair have a marked reduction in their survival rates. [24] One approach for those infants who require ECMO is to perform the CDH repair after stabilization of

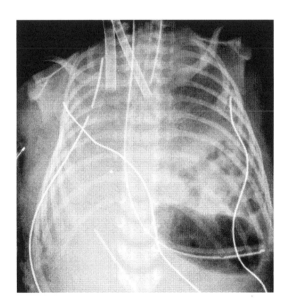

Figure 2. The typical picture of a patient with congenital diaphragmatic hernia on venoarterial ECMO. The ECMO cannulae are shifted to the right, indicating the shift of the heart into the right chest.

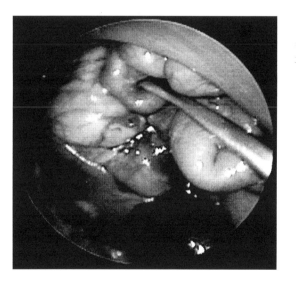

Figure 3: Surgical view of the bowel and liver in the chest of a congenital diaphragmatic hernia patient.

pulmonary hypertension and immediately prior to decannulation. ECMO can then continue postoperatively if undergoing the repair leads to deterioration of the patient's condition. Repair while on ECMO is associated with an increase in bleeding complications and high mortality.[25,26] Hemorrhagic complications can be decreased from 58 to 21% by postponing repair until pulmonary hypertension has improved enough to allow weaning off ECMO and a period of observation on conventional ventilation.[27] This strategy has led to optimizing survival rates in CDH patients requiring ECMO to 78%.[2,6,16,22] The CDH patient who can not wean from ECMO prior to repair likely has severe irreversible pulmonary hypoplasia. Discussion about salvage CDH repair on ECMO should include acknowledgement of the poor prognosis.

Management on ECMO – What the ECMO Specialist Should Know

Compared with other neonatal ECMO patients, the presence of a CDH requires recognition that abdominal contents is in the chest. Distended stomach or intestine in the thorax can cause mediastinal and vena caval shift, resulting in decreased venous return and venous return monitor (VRM) alarming may occur. If this bowel gas cannot be reduced by a sump nasogastric tube, the infant may need further sedation to reduce gastric/bowel gas entrapment. Neonatal ECMO patients in our center are not paralyzed unless absolutely necessary to reduce air entrapment and maintain venous flow.

Patients undergoing CDH repair prior to or while on ECMO support are at risk for major postoperative bleeding.

- *Management of patients placed on ECMO after surgical repair of the CDH –*
  - o Because of the bleeding risk, ACTs and coagulation management should focus on preventing bleeding. In our institution this is achieved by maintaining ACTs of 160-170 seconds (Hemochron), platelets >150,000mm³, and fibrinogen >150mg%.

  - o ECMO blood flow rates are being maintained at least at 120mL/kg/min during this coagulation management phase.
  - o When the chest x-ray improves and the ECMO physician determines that the patient can be weaned, the ECMO flows are weaned hourly as tolerated to idle. We limit the idling time to 4 hours to prevent increased bleeding since the ACTs during this time are between 190-200 seconds. ACTs are increased when flow is <150mL/min to reduce fibrin formation in the circuit.
  - o After successful idling period the patient should be taken off ECMO
  - o For patients who do not idle successfully, a trial "off" ECMO can be performed by clamping the venous and arterial lines above the opened bridge. The main risk associated with this procedure is clot formation in the ECMO cannula resulting in a potential thrombus of the cannula or superior vena cava. Therefore the catheters should be "flashed" (see below) every 5 minutes to prevent this and as soon as the patient has been "off" ECMO for >30 minutes, a heparin infusion should be started on the patient side. Flashing the catheters consist of opening the arterial and venous clamps, closing the bridge and allowing fresh blood to enter the catheters. This should only be done for a few seconds, but repeated every 5 minutes.
  - o If the patient is not stable after the "off" trial, the ECMO blood flow should be turned back to 120 mL/kg/min and the patient allowed to stabilize. ACTs should be reduced as above. These described "off" trials can be performed daily to determine when the patient is ready to be decannulated.
  - o At our institution, after the patient has been on ECMO for 21 days without improvement, we recommend terminating the ECMO therapy. This is discussed with the parents during the consenting

process on the day the patient is placed on ECMO.

- Management of patients placed on ECMO pre-surgery
  - o ACTs may be maintained as you would for any non-surgical ECMO patient.
  - o Higher levels of sedation may be required to prevent air entrapping in the stomach or bowel and hereby compromising venous return.
  - o Most centers will perform CDH repair after a successful idling period after the patient is successfully "off" ECMO.

- Management of patients on ECMO during CDH repair.
  - o Surgery on ECMO does not usually result in acute bleeding complications, but bleeding will start in the surgical areas after 6-12hrs, so management of ACTs and coagulation is important.
- ACTs in our institution are kept at 150-160 seconds (Hemochron) during surgery and for 4-6 hours post surgery. They are then increased to 160-180 seconds after this time period
- Amicar is usually started 60 minutes prior to surgery with a initial bolus followed by a continuous drip.
- Platelets are maintained ≥150-200,000 during the surgery and at least 24 hours post surgery and fibrinogen is kept >150.
- ECMO flows are kept ≥120ml/kg/hr until it is decided to attempt to wean.
- Patients are weaned off by 24-48 hours post surgery. Most require a 24 hour period of stabilization and then are weaned rapidly by weaning flows by 50mL/min per hour.

- Complications during ECMO
  - o Bleeding is the biggest complication for the CDH patient repaired either pre or on ECMO
  - o Venous return problems are common and require management of the gas entrapment in the stomach/bowel. Re-

member that volume is the number one cause of VRM alarms for most patients, but catheter placement in the beginning of the run can be a common cause in the CDH patient and bowel gas entrapment is the next most common in the CDH patient.
  - o Long-runs require meticulous management of ACT/coagulation, and lung recruitment. We change our circuits out if marked increases in fibrin/clots are noted and/or if we are at 10 days of ECMO (concern for raceway integrity).
    - An average CDH run in our institution is 10 days – one should not operate on a patient on ECMO with a 10 day circuit that has fibrin/clots. It is safer to change it out and wait until the patient is stable, since this increases the risk of having complications from the circuit due to low ACTs. The use of Amicar may help if the circuit can't be changed out.
    - If you have to change the circuit out, pre-treating the circuit with steroids is advised to decrease the activation of complement and other vaso-active mediators that result in worsening lung function.

CDH Outcome

While ECMO has contributed to improved survival in infants with CDH it is not without complications. Careful monitoring for potential hemorrhagic, neurologic and infectious complications are required and can necessitate discontinuing ECMO and death.

The overall incidence of bleeding in patients with CDH treated with ECMO is as high as 43% and may lead to death in up to 4.8%. Sites of hemorrhage include the surgical site, if the repair is undertaken before or during ECMO, ICH (the most common cause of hemorrhage-related mortality), pulmonary, gastrointestinal, urinary and umbilical.[27] The use of antifibrinolytic therapies significantly reduces bleeding at the surgical site, as well as red blood cell transfusions.[25]

The true survival rate for patients with CDH is difficult to predict due to the unknown number of fetuses that don't survive to delivery and patients who are too ill to survive transport. The multiple institution Congenital Diaphragmatic Hernia Study Group has attempted to determine the effect of ECMO on CDH survival.[29] The overall survival for CDH patients requiring ECMO is approximately 68%. A survival rate of 38.5 % was seen in patients who without ECMO would have a predicted mortality of greater than 80%. Right heart failure, hypoplastic lungs, sepsis, and intracranial hemorrhage have been identified as causes of long-term mortality. [20, 33]

Amongst surviving CDH patients, at least one-fifth to two-thirds will display neurodevelopmental problems.[30] CDH patients may be more susceptible to neurologic injury than other infants requiring ECMO.[30] Other long term morbidity includes chronic lung disease, gastroesophageal reflux and malnutrition.[31,32] Gastroesophageal reflux is a major problem in the CDH patient. Long-Term concerns for severe esophagitis need to be a concern passed on to the primary physician so proper treatment and followup can be arranged.

Summary

ECMO therapy has clearly saved the lives of many infants born with CDH. As the neonatal care of infants with CDH evolves, less invasive and morbid therapies will likely decrease the need for ECMO. Until then, ECMO continues to allow successful navigation of the critical period of pulmonary hypertension.

References

1. Bartlett RH, Gazzaniga AB, Huxtable RF, et al: Extracorporeal circulation (ECMO) in neonatal respiratory failure. J Thorac Cardiovasc Surg 74:826-833, 1977

2. Freckner B, Ehren H, Granholm T, *et al*: Improved results in patients who have congenital diaphragmatic hernia using preoperative stabilization, extracorporeal membrane oxygenation, and delayed surgery. J Pediatr Surg 32:1185-1189, 1997

3. vd Staak FHJM, Geven W, Oeseburg B, *et al*: Improving survival for patients with high-risk congenital diaphragmatic hernia by using extracorporeal membrane oxygenation. J Pediatr Surg 30:1463-1467, 1995

4. Heiss K, Manning P, Oldham KT, *et al*: Reversal of mortality for congenital diaphragmatic hernia with ECMO. Ann Surg 209:225-230, 1988

5. Sawyer SF, Falterman KW, Goldsmith JP, *et al*: Improving survival in the treatment of congenital diaphragmatic hernia. Ann Thorac Surg 41:75-78, 1986

6. Wung JT, James LS, Kilchevsky E, et al: Management of infants with severe respiratory failure and persistence of the fetal circulation, without hyperventilation. Pediatr 76:488-494, 1985

7. Kim ES, Stolar CJ: ECMO in the Newborn. Am J of Perinatol 17:345-356, 2000

8. Okuyama H, Kubota A, Oue T, *et al*: Inhaled nitric oxide with early surgery improves the outcome of antenatally diagnosed congenital diaphragmatic hernia. J Pediatr Surg 37:1188-1190, 2002

9. Bagolan P, Casaccia G, Crescenzi A, *et al*: Impact of current treatment protocol on outcome of high-risk congenital diaphragmatic hernia. J Pediatr Surg 39:313-318, 2004

10. Fournier L, Cloutier R, Major D, *et al*: Barotrauma in congenital diaphragmatic hernia. The killer? Can J Anesth 36:A67, 1991

11. Finer N, Etches P, Kamstra B, *et al*: Inhaled nitric oxide in infants referred for extracorporeal membrane oxygenation. J Pediatr 124:302-308, 1994

12. Roberts JD, Polaner DM, Lang P, *et al*: Inhaled nitric oxide in persistent pulmonary hypertension of the newborn. Lancet 340:818-819, 1992

13. The National Inhaled Nitric Oxide Study Group: Inhaled nitric oxide and hypoxic respiratory failure in patients with congenital diaphragmatic hernia. Pediatr 99:838-845, 1997

14. Wilcox DT, Glick PL, Karamanoukian H, *et al*: Pathophysiology of congenital diaphragmatic hernia, V: effect of exogenous surfactant therapy on gas exchange and lung mechanics in the lamb congenital diaphragmatic hernia model. J Pediatr 124:289-293, 1994

15. Van Meurs K. Congenital Diaphragmatic Hernia Study Group Is surfactant therapy beneficial in the treatment of the term newborn infant with congenital diaphragmatic hernia? J Pediatr 145:312-316, 2004

16. Lally KP: Extracorporeal Membrane Oxygenation in Patients with Congenital Diaphragmatic Hernia. Semin Pediatr Surg 5:249-255, 1996

17. Heiss KF, Clark RH, Cornish JD, *et al*: Preferential use of venovenous extracorporeal membrane oxygenation for congenital diaphragmatic hernia. J Pediatr Surg 30:416-419, 1995

18. Kugelman A, Gangiano E, Pincros J, *et al*: Venovenous versus venoarterial extracorporeal membrane oxygenation in congenital diaphragmatic hernia. J Pediatr Surg 38:1131-1136, 2003

19. Anderson HL III, Snedecor SM, Otsu T, *et al*: Multicenter trial of conventional venoarterial access versus venovenous double-lumen catheter access in newborn infants undergoing extracorporeal membrane oxygenation. J Pediatr Surg 28:530-535, 1993

20. Guner YS, Khemani RG, Qureshi FG, , *et al*: Outcome analysis of neonates with congenital-diaphragmatic hernia treated with venovenous vs venoarterial extracorporeal membrane oxygenation. . J Pediatr Surg 44, 1691–1701, 2009.

21. Dimmitt RA, Moss RL, Rhine WD, *et al*: Venoarterial versus venovenous extracorporeal membrane oxygenation in congenital diaphragmatic hernia: The Extracorporeal Life Support Organization Registry, 1990-1999. J Pediatr Surg 36:1199-1204, 2001

22. Bryner BS, West BT, HIrschl RB, *et al*: Congenital diaphragmatic hernia requiring extra-

corporeal membrane oxygenation: does timing of repair matter? J Pediatr Surg 44:1165–1172, 2009

23. Sigalet DL, Tierney A, Adolph V, *et al*: Timing of congenital diaphragmatic hernia requiring extracorporeal membrane oxygenation support. J Pediatr Surg 30:1183-1187, 1995

24. Sakai H, Tamura M, Hsokawa Y, *et al*: Effect of surgical repair on respiratory mechanics in CDH. J Pediatr Surg 111:432-438, 1987

25. vd Staak FHJ, de Haan AFJ, Geven WB, *et al*: Surgical repair of congenital diaphragmatic hernia during extracorporeal membrane oxygenation: hemorrhagic complications and the effect of tranexamic acid. J Pediatr Surg 32:594-599, 1997

26. Sell LS, Cullen ML, Whitlesy GC, *et al*: Hemorrhagic complications during extracorporeal membrane oxygenation: prevention and treatment. J Pediatr Surg 21:1087-1091, 1986

27. Vazquez WD, Cheu HW: Hemorrhagic complications and repair of congenital diaphragmatic hernias: does timing of the repair make a difference? Data from the Extrcorporeal Life Support Organization. J Pediatr Surg 29:1002-1006, 1994

28. Nagaraj HS, Mitchell KA, Fallat ME, *et al*: Surgical complications and procedures in neonates on extracorporeal membrane oxygenation. J Pediatr Surg 27:1106-1110, 1992

29. The Congenital Diaphragmatic Hernia Study Group: Does extracorporeal membrane oxygenation improve survival in neonates with congenital diaphragmatic hernia? J Pediatr Surg 34:720-725, 1999

30. Stolar CJ, Crisafi MA, Driscoll YT: Neurocognitive outcome for neonates treated with extracorporeal membrane oxygenation: Are infants with congenital diaphragmatic hernia different? J Pediatr Surg 30:366-371, 1995

31. D'Agostino J, Berbaum J, Gerdes M, *et al*: Outcomes for infants with congenital diaphragmatic hernia requiring extracorporeal membrane oxygenation: The first year. J Pediatr 30:10-15, 1995

32. Nagaya M, Akatsuka H, Kato J, *et al*: Gastroesophageal reflux disease occurring after repair of congenital diaphragmatic hernia. J Pediatr Surg 29:1447-1451, 1994

33. Davis PJ, Firmin RK, Manktelow B, *et al*: Long-term outcome following extracorporeal membrane oxygenation for congenital diaphragmatic hernia: the UK experience. J Pediatr 144:309-315, 2004

34. Newman KD, Anderson KA, Van Meurs K, *et al*: Extracorporeal Membrane Oxygenation and Congenital Diaphragmatic Hernia: Should Any Infant Be Excluded? J Pediatr Surg 25:1048-1053, 1990

35. Stolar CJ, Dillon PW, Stalcup SA: Extracorporeal Membrane Oxygenation and Congenital Diaphragmatic Hernia: Modification of the Pulmonary Vasoactive Profile. J Pediatr Surg 20:681-683, 1985

36. Geggel RL, Murphy JD, Langleben D, *et al*: Congenital Diaphragmatic Hernia: Arterial Structural Changes and Persisten Pulmonary Hypertension after Surgical Repair. J Pediatr Surg 107:457-463, 1987

37. Heerema AE, Rabban JT, Sydorak RM, *et al*: Lung pathology in patients with congenital diaphragmatic hernia treated with fetal surgical intervention, including tracheal occlusion. Pediatr Dev Pathol 6:536-546, 2003

Chapter 15 Questions

1. The CDH patient placed on ECMO pre-surgery may have all following problems on ECMO except:
   a) Increased risk for bleeding
   b) Average run time of 10 days
   c) Require increased sedation secondary to bowel gas entrainment and reduced venous return
   d) Venous return problems early in the run can be secondary to catheter placement due to the shifting of the mediastinum.

2. If surgery is done on ECMO, bleeding complications will occur within the first 1-2 hours
   a) True
   b) False

3. Your patient has idled successfully and the surgeons want to go to the OR, but your circuit now has multiple areas of clot/fibrin formation. It is best to go ahead with the surgery and get the patient off ECMO instead of changing the circuit prior to ECMO.
   a) True
   b) False

4. If you have to change the circuit, it is best to pre-treat with steroids to decrease the effect of activation of complement and other vasoactive mediators on pulmonary function.
   a) True
   b) False

Chapter 15 Answers

   1. a
   2. b
   3. b
   4. a

16

Extracorporeal Life Support during Cardiac Arrest (ECPR)

Heidi J. Dalton MD, FCCM and Sharad Menon MD

Objectives

After completion of this chapter, the participant should be able to:
- Discuss the indications for ECPR
- Discuss the contraindications for ECPR
- Outline the team members needed to provide ECPR
- Discuss the outcome of the ECPR patient population

Introduction

A primary goal of cardiopulmonary resuscitation is to achieve neurologically intact survival. While some recent reports find that 2/3 of patients can be successfully resuscitated to return of spontaneous circulation (ROSC) following in-hospital cardiac arrest, intact neurologic survival remains poor for many patients. Those patients who have prolonged (>30 minutes) episodes of conventional cardiopulmonary resuscitation (CPR) prior to ROSC have dismal outcomes.[1-4] A recent review of the National Registry of Cardiopulmonary Resuscitation database revealed a rate of survival to discharge of 27% for pediatric in-hospital cardiac arrest, with 65% of survivors having a "good" neurologic outcome, although outcome was assessed by chart review for discharge status and not long-term evaluation.[6] Other studies have shown similar results with a high rate (63–70%) of ROSC after CPR, but with lower survival to discharge rates (10–27%).[6-8]

The success of extracorporeal support in providing cardiopulmonary support for a variety of patients has led to use of extracorporeal life support (ECLS) or extracorporeal membrane oxygenation (ECMO) as a resuscitation adjunct for patients failing conventional resuscitation. ECLS and ECMO will be used interchangeably in this text. The use of ECLS in circumstances of cardiac arrest has come to be termed "ECPR", for extracorporeal life support during CPR. While ECPR was originally described in patients following repair of congenital heart defects who suffered a sudden arrest, it has now been used in a variety of circumstances for patients both with and without primary heart disease. Multiple centers have reported successful use of ECPR in adults and children. However, because of the cost, the complexity of the technique, and the resources required, ECPR is not offered in all centers as a rescue for pediatric patients with refractory cardiac arrest. The increasing importance of such programs, however, is highlighted by recommendations such as that of the American Heart Association, which states, "…to consider extracorporeal CPR for in-hospital cardiac arrest refractory to initial resuscitation attempts if the condition leading to cardiac arrest is reversible or amenable to heart transplantation, if excellent conventional CPR has been performed after no more than several minutes of no-flow cardiac arrest, and if the institution is able to rapidly perform extracorporeal membrane oxygenation."[9] One large pediatric study has shown that good outcome can be achieved when extracorporeal CPR is started after 30 to 90 minutes of refractory standard CPR for in-hospital cardiac arrests.[5]

Table 1 shows the summary of published literature regarding pediatric extracorporeal cardiopulmonary resuscitation. Most of the patients in these series were cardiac patients with survival to discharge rates of 8% to as high as 80%. Duration of CPR prior to ECLS ranged from 4 to 127 minutes.[9]

If you decide to do ECPR

The key to successful deployment of ECLS during resuscitation is appropriate equipment, personnel and teamwork. Planning ahead for an ECPR event starts with identification of WHO is an appropriate patient and, equally important, who is NOT. As an example, some centers will only perform ECPR in the Cardiac ICU environment, some anywhere within the ICU, some anywhere in the hospital, and some centers will also consider patients who arrive in the ED in arrest as appropriate candidates. To prevent confusion, it is best to have a defined protocol that outlines which patients ECPR will be considered appropriate for and to make sure that those clinicians who care for patients (ED, cath lab, ICU, floor patients, etc) are aware of these criteria. While there are no universally agreed upon criteria for who is NOT a candidate for ECPR, there are patients that the medical care team (and family as appropriate) do not feel appropriate for ECPR consideration. If possible, these patients should be formally identified to nursing staff and care personnel to prevent confusion in the event of arrest.

Despite protocols and planning, however, it is likely that events will arise that will make it difficult to always know which patients ECPR should be initiated for. Thus, the ultimate responsibility of calling for ECPR should be designated to one person—usually an ICU physician or surgeon (either attending or fellow) who is present at the resuscitation and is part of the ECPR team. Whatever mechanism is designed to initiate ECPR, calling for it early in the resuscitation is best. It is much easier to CANCEL an ECPR implementation it is to initiate it during a prolonged resuscitation.

The team typically consists of cardiothoracic and/or general surgeons, ECLS specialist/perfusionist, intensive care specialist and nursing staff familiar with initiation and management of a patient on ECLS. Each member of the team should understand their particular role. Maintaining efficiency by use of mock "ECPR" codes or "water drills" for these often rare events is useful. Identifying personnel who are responsible for entering orders, getting blood, running for supplies, "crowd control", family updates, and communication are as vital roles to the team as the personnel who actually place the cannulas and

Table 1. Modified from: Fiser RT, Morris MC. Extracorporeal Cardiopulmonary Resuscitation in Refractory Pediatric Cardiac Arrest. Pediatr Clin N Am 55(2008) 929-41.

Author	Patient Population	No. of patients successfully cannulated	Number of survivors to discharge	Duration of CPR in Minutes: median (range) or Mean±SD
Aharon, et al	Post-cardiotomy	10	8 (80%)	42 (5-110)
Alscufi, et al	ICU	80	27 (34%)	Favorable outcome: 46 (14-95) Unfavorable outcome: 41 (19-110)
Dalton, et al (ref 8)	Cardia	11	6 (55%)	42 (42-110)
Cengiz, et al	ELSO registry	161	64 (40%)	Not reported
Del Nido, et al (ref 7)	Post-cardiotomy	11	6 (55%)	65 ± 9
De Mos, et al	ICU	5	2 (40%)	All: 31-77 Survivors: 35-48
Duncan, et al	Cardiac	11	7 (64%)	55 (20-103)
Hamrick, et al	<1Yr old post-cardiotomy	12	1 (8%)	Not reported
Parra, et al	Cardiac	4	4 (100%)	16 (12-20)
Posner, et al	ER	2	1 (50%)	50-90
MacLaren, et al	Septic shock	18	10 (55%)	Not reported
Morris, et al (ref 19)	ICU	64	21 (33%)	Survivors: 50 (5-105) Non-survivors: 46 (15-90)
Shah, et al	Cardiac	27	9 (33%)	Not reported
Theurani, et al	Cardiac	15	11 (73%	54 (4-127)

start the circuit. The cardiopulmonary resuscitation is continued by a physician who is FOCUSED on ensuring that proper CPR is continued—failure to give adequate perfusion with CPR will be associated with poor ECPR outcomes. Recent reports of the inadequacy of compressions and poor CPR techniques by resuscitating personnel as well as other reports of improved conventional CPR outcomes with optimal compressions and CPR techniques (but without need for ECPR), highlight how important the process of CPR is, whether ECPR is required or not. While CPR is in progress, the ECPR circuit is primed and readied for connection to the patient. Some centers maintain a pre-primed, sterile circuit which is used for ECPR and some centers use a compact circuit which is setup but primed only when ECPR is required. New pumps and oxygenator systems allow for priming times of only a few minutes, as compared to the traditional roller head/ silicone lung systems which required much longer priming times. Pre-primed circuits have been stored for up to 30 days without noted infection or other complications when put in use.

To truly have an ECPR system, all required personnel should be available in-house 24/7. However, if this is not possible, a system that gets required surgical and initiation personnel to the bedside in a matter of minutes is needed. While good survival has been obtained with prolonged resuscitation prior to ECPR, a shorter duration of pulseless activity is always desirable.

Another important aspect of a successful ECPR team is to have a well-designed means for cannulation. Cannulas are placed in the cervical, femoral, or thoracic sites as patient situation and size dictates. Because of the varied size of pediatric patients as compared to adults, obtaining timely vascular access resulting in adequate pump flow can be challenging. In addition to appropriate surgical personnel, needed equipment such as a cannula cart complete with varying sizes of catheters for all sizes of patients, a tray or instrument set for insertion, drapes, appropriate connectors and other items need to be immediately available at the bedside. One other caution is in the circumstance where transthoracic cannulation is undertaken. As many surgeons are used to having trained scrub nurse personnel assist with opening chests and placing cannulas in the OR, ensuring that these processes also flow well in an emergent situation outside the OR environment should be practiced to prevent frustration and fraying tempers when an actual event occurs.

As patients undergoing ECPR have either little or no intrinsic cardiac output, patients are cannulated with a venoarterial approach except for unusual circumstances. Once cannulation is complete, radiography or echocardiography is performed to assess cannulation placement. Echocardiography offers the advantage that cardiac function can also be assessed. In cases of severe left ventricular dysfunction, consideration is given to placement of a left atrial catheter via blade septectomy or a transthoracic left atrial cannula placement to decompress the left side of the heart. Failure to decompress the left heart in instances where the aortic valve poorly opens can lead to pulmonary venous hypertension and massive pulmonary hemorrhage. This will then turn a primary cardiac failure patient into a pulmonary and cardiac failure patient, making recovery even more difficult.

Post Cannulation Care

Although there are no pediatric studies that demonstrate the effectiveness of hypothermia post-arrest in improving outcome, the current trend is to maintain the patient's core body temperature between 33-35°C for 24-48 hrs. A randomized trial of hypothermia versus normothermia after cardiac arrest is in progress and results are eagerly awaited. Unfortunately, this trial will not be completed for several years so conventional wisdom will have to guide patient care decisions in the meantime. One issue, on which clinicians agree even now however, is that preventing fever following arrest is optimal and this goal can be easily obtained with ECLS temperature control. Other goals following cannulation are to maintain normal blood pressure for age by adjusting flow on pump while being on minimal vasoactive support. The patients are placed on "resting" ventilatory support with a low rate (<10 breath/ min), high PEEP to maintain some lung inflation (8–15 cmH2O) and low inspired oxygen concentration (<0.4). Sweep flow and FiO_2 delivery adjustment are used for normalizing blood gas parameters. Anticoagulation with unfractionated heparin while on ECMO is titrated to maintain activated clotting times between 180 and 220 seconds.

A few practical points regarding patient care are to pay close attention to normalization of organ function and acid-base balance once ECLS has begun. Several reports have outlined the fact that failure to normalize lactate levels and acidosis within 24 hours and to reverse renal and hepatic insufficiency are all associated with poor outcome. Some have suggested that failure to normalize these parameters may result from a sense of security that being on ECLS brings, without realizing that the support provided is inadequate and taking measures to improve it. In hypothermic patients, following clinical exam for adequacy of support is difficult, as these patients are often peripherally vasoconstricted and skin color is poor. Following lactate levels, acidosis, mixed venous saturations, urine output, brain oximetry, and other adjunct measures of tissue perfusion are all helpful during ECLS support. Of paramount importance following arrest is the need to assess neurologic function as much as possible. This may best be accomplished by clinical exam, eliminating sedation or neuromuscular blockade until neurologic activity such as patient movement can be assessed. Other measures such as EEG monitoring, CT scan, and evoked potentials are other ways to monitor brain function non-invasively. Although NIRS monitoring is currently used in many centers, the true reliability of these monitors in assessing brain blood flow and long term neurologic outcome is unknown.

Single-ventricle patients pose special considerations for post-ECLS support. The optimal oxygenation status is unknown, although most clinicians maintain patients on room air and allow saturations in the 80's similar to what would be observed in the "natural" state if ECLS was not in place. These patients frequently require increased blood flow to support both pulmonary and systemic circulations, especially if they have a Blalock-Taussig shunt. Single ventricle patients may also require additional cannulas to obtain adequate venous drainage, especially if the patient has a completed Fontan procedure where the IVC/pulmonary and RA circulations may be separate.

Failure of cardiac function to return within 72 hours of cannulation has been associated with poor outcome. While function may not have returned to a level to allow separation from the ECLS circuit, a continuous improvement in cardiac and other organ function should be observed after successful ECPR. For patients who are post-cardiotomy, cardiac catheterization should be strongly considered if cardiac function does not return quickly to identify any residual lesions which can be repaired either surgically or with cath lab interventions. "Myocardial stunning", which is the term given for asystole or minimal contractility noted following initiation of ECLS, is often seen in the first hours following initiation of VA ECMO for ECPR. While the exact etiology of this is unknown, it may relate to changes in cellular calcium concentration (thus maintaining normal ionized calcium levels is important) or from the sudden increase in the left ventricular afterload and decreased left ventricular preload that occurs with VA ECMO. While this condition seems to be self-limited in many patients, others respond to cardiac pacing, vasoactive manipulations including afterload reduction with milrinone or nitroprusside, and some require emergent left atrial decompression to prevent pulmonary venous congestion and pulmonary hemorrhage. Maintaining the intracardiac filling pressures at low-normal levels to augment epicardial blood flow is also an important component of cardiac recovery.

Although renal insufficiency or failure requiring renal replacement therapy or filtration to maintain fluid balance is frequent in ECPR patients, it should be remembered that renal failure and use of dialysis is associated with worse outcome. The lack of pulsatility during VA ECLS support may be one factor in the development of renal insufficiency, although again, no specific etiology other than a proposed period of poor perfusion to the renal system has been identified as the ultimate cause of renal disease during ECLS.

Other patient management issues (feeding, sedation, medications, etc.) should follow routine ECLS care algorithms.

Advantages and Disadvantages

By providing cardiac and pulmonary rest and adequate tissue perfusion while on ECMO, ECPR provides a period of stability for resolution of the underlying pathologic problems which led to the refractory cardiac arrest in the first place..

By regulating temperature in the mild hypothermic to normothermic range through the ECMO circuit and thereby avoiding hyperpyrexia in the immediate post resuscitation period, acute exacerbation of neurologic injuries associated with fever can potentially be avoided.

Outcome

Review of the ELSO Database finds that a total of 1781 patients have been placed on ECPR, of whom 634 (36%) were discharged or transferred alive from the ICU (Table 2).[12]

In a recently published meta-analysis of ECPR, 288 patients were identified with 40% surviving to hospital discharge. Venoarterial ECMO was used in 99% of patients and 63% were cannulated through an open chest. Median length of duration of ECMO was 4.3 days. The overall occurrence of complications was high (59%). The most commonly occurring complications were neurological (27%), renal (25%), sepsis (17%), bleeding (7%) and multisystem organ failure (9%).[13]

Another review from the National Registry of CPR found 199 pediatric patients placed on ECMO during arrest with an overall survival of 44%. In 59 survivors who had neurologic outcome recorded, 95% had favorable outcomes based on Pediatric Cerebral Performance Scores. By multivariate analysis, pre-arrest renal insufficiency, metabolic or electrolyte abnormality at the time of arrest, and use of sodium bicarbonate or tromethamine were associated with decreased survival. Underlying cardiac illness was associated with an increased survival to discharge.[14]

In another study from a single institution over a six year period, 32 children underwent ECPR out of a total of 329 in-hospital cardiac arrests. Eighty-two percent of the patients had an underlying cardiac disease. Overall 73% of the patients survived to hospital discharge and 75% of survivors had no change in their PCPC and POPC (gross neurological outcome) scores from baseline to discharge. Of patients who received chest compressions >60 minutes, 40% survived without gross neurological injury.[15]

In another report, 80 children undergoing ECPR with various underlying pathologies, including 39 postoperative patients from a single institution, the survival rate was noted to be 34% with a mean duration of CPR of 40 minutes. Most importantly, the duration of CPR prior to ECMO initiation did not correlate with survival and good neurological outcome was obtained even in patients undergoing prolonged CPR.[16]

Another study analyzing the ELSO database over a period of 13 years noted 682 patients undergoing ECPR with a 38% survival to discharge. Risk factors for death included pre-ECMO pH<7.2, non cardiac pathology, CPR while being on ECMO,

Table 2.

	Total Patients	Survived ECLS	Survived to DC/ Transfer
Neonatal	492	309 (63%)	184 (37%)
Pediatric	908	473 (52%)	348 (38%)
Adult	381	138 36%)	102 (27%)
Total	1781	920 (52%)	634 (36%)

ECLS Registry Report, International Summary July, 2009

renal, neurological, and pulmonary hemorrhage complications.[17]

One fact regarding ECPR outcome that requires further investigation is that cardiac patients are often reported to have improved outcome when compared to non-cardiac patients. Whether this represents disparity in access to ECPR between cardiac and non-cardiac patients (as many cardiac ICUs have ECPR systems which are not always available to other patients, and may have cannulating personnel who are familiar with cannulating in arrest situations and using multiple access sites) or underlying physiologic factors which make non-cardiac patients less amenable to survival is unknown at the current time. An addendum to the ELSO registry that has been designed to capture specific data on cardiac arrest patients may help give more detailed information regarding factors which help predict what patients and what features are associated with good and bad outcomes in the future.[18, 19]

A recent study which sought to identify risk factors for acute neurological injury in children undergoing ECPR, found 22% of patients had acute neurological injury, which was defined as occurrence of brain death, brain infarction, or intracranial hemorrhage identified by ultrasound or computerized tomography imaging. Brain death occurred in 11% of patients, cerebral infarction in 7%, and intracranial hemorrhage in 7%. The in-hospital mortality rate in patients with acute neurological injury was 89%.[20]

Summary

ECPR has been successfully used to rescue many patients with refractory cardiac arrest with good short-term neurological outcomes. For ECPR to be most successful, it must be deployed rapidly while the patient is undergoing excellent CPR. Early activation of the ECPR team could possibly shorten CPR duration and might improve survival and outcome. More research needs to be done to refine the populations and circumstances which offer the best outcome with ECPR, evaluate the cost/benefit ratios, and establish the long-term neurodevelopmental outcomes in survivors. Variability in patient care techniques from center to center, equipment used, and protocols followed also make it difficult to extrapolate one center's experience to another. To even attempt to standardize how ECPR is performed, needed information as to the optimal means of providing support should be obtained through collabortive efforts.

References

1. Schindler MB, Bohn D, Cox PN, McCrindle BW, Jarvis A, Edmonds J, Barker G. Outcome of out-of-hospital cardiac or respiratory arrest in children. N Engl J Med. 1996 Nov 14;335(20):1473-9.
2. Zaritsky A, Nadkarni V, Getson P, Kuehl K. CPR in children. Ann Emerg Med. 1987 Oct;16(10):1107-11
3. Innes PA, Summers CA, Boyd IM, Molyneux EM. Audit of paediatric cardiopulmonary resuscitation. Arch Dis Child. 1993 Apr;68(4):487-91.
4. Lopez-Herce J, Garcia C, Dominguez P, et al. Characteristics and outcome of cardiorespiratory arrest in children. Resuscitation. 2004;63:311–320
5. Morris MC, Wernovsky G, Nadkarni VM Survival outcomes after extracorporeal cardiopulmonary resuscitation instituted during active chest compressions following refractory in-hospital pediatric cardiac arrest. Pediatr Crit Care Med. 2004 Sep;5(5):440-6.
6. Nadkarni VM, Larkin GL, Peberdy MA, Carey SM, Kaye W, Mancini ME, Nichol G, Lane-Truitt T, Potts J, Ornato JP, Berg RA; National Registry of Cardiopulmonary Resuscitation Investigators. First documented rhythm and clinical outcome from in-hospital cardiac arrest among children and adults. JAMA. 2006 Jan 4;295(1):50-7.
7. del Nido PJ, Dalton HJ, Thompson AE, Siewers RD. Extracorporeal membrane oxygenator rescue in children during cardiac arrest after cardiac surgery. Circulation. 1992 Nov;86(5 Suppl):II300-4.
8. Dalton HJ, Siewers RD, FuhrmanBP, Del Nido P, Thompson AE, Shaver MG, Dowhy M. Extracorporeal membrane oxygenation for cardiac rescue in children with severe myocardial dysfunction. Crit Care Med 1993; 21: 1020-8.

9. Fiser RT, Morris MC. Extracorporeal Cardiopulmonary Resuscitation in Refractory Pediatric Cardiac Arrest. Pediatr Clin N Am 55(2008) 929-41

10. Lopez-Herce J, Garcia C, Dominguez P, et al. Characteristics and outcome of cardio-respiratory arrest in children. Resuscitation. 2004;63:311–320

11. Fiser RT, Morris MC. Extracorporeal Cardiopulmonary Resuscitation in Refractory Pediatric Cardiac Arrest. Pediatr Clin N Am 55(2008) 929-41

12. ECMO Registry of the Extracorporeal Life Support Organization, Ann Arbor MI, July 2009.

13. Tajik M, Cardarelli M Extracorporeal membrane oxygenation after cardiac arrest in children: what do we know? Eur J Cardiothorac Surg 2008; 33: 409-417

14. Raymond TT, Cunnyngham CB, Thompson MT, Thomas JA, Dalton HJ, Nadkarni VM; for the American Heart Association National Registry of CPR Investigators. Outcomes among neonates, infants, and children after extracorporeal cardiopulmonary resuscitation for refractory in-hospital pediatric cardiac arrest: A report from the National Registry of CardioPulmonary Resuscitation. Pediatr Crit Care Med. 2009 Nov 17. [Epub ahead of print]

15. Prodhan P, Fiser RT, Dyamenahalli U, Gossett J, Imamura M, Jaquiss RDB, Bhutta A. Outcomes after extracorporeal cardiopulmonary resuscitation (ECPR) following refractory pediatric cardiac arrest in the intensive care unit. Resuscitation Vol 80, Issue 10, October 2009, Pages 1124- 1129

16. Alsoufi B, Al-Radi OO, Gruenwald C, Lean L, Williams WG, McCrindle B W, Caldarone CA, Van Arsdell GS Extracorporeal life support following cardiac surgery in children: analysis in a single institution Eur J Cardiothorac Surg (2009), doi:10.1016/jejcts.2009.02.015

17. Thiagarajan RR, Laussen PC, Rycus PT, Bartlett RH, Bratton SL. Extracorporeal Membrane Oxygenation to aid cardiopulmonary resuscitation in infants and children. Circulation.2007;116:1693-1700.

18. Del Nido PJ, Dalton HJ, Thompson AE, Siewers RD. Extracorporeal membrane oxygenator rescue in children during cardiac arrest after cardiac surgery. Circulation. 1992 Nov;86(5 Suppl):II300-4.

19. Morris MC, Wernovsky G, Nadkarni VM Survival outcomes after extracorporeal cardiopulmonary resuscitation instituted during active chest compressions following refractory in-hospital pediatric cardiac arrest. Pediatr Crit Care Med. 2004 Sep;5(5):440-6.

20. Barrett CS, Bratton SL, Salvin JW, Laussen PC, Rycus PT, Thiagrajan RR Neurological injury after extracorporeal membrane oxygenation use to aid pediatric cardiopulmonary resuscitation Pediatr Crit Care Med 2009;10:445-451

Chapter 16 Questions

1. What mode of ECMO is predominantly used for patient undergoing ECPR for refractory cardiac arrest?
   a) VV
   b) VVDL
   c) VA
   d) VA+V

2. Survival rate amongst children requiring prolonged conventional CPR (greater than 30 min) has not been attained
   a) True
   b) False

3. AHA's recommendation for initiating ECPR for in-hospital refractory cardiac arrest includes:
   a) condition leading to cardiac arrest is reversible or amenable to transplant
   b) patient has received excellent CPR with no more than several minutes of no flow cardiac arrest
   c) patient can be rapidly placed on ECMO
   d) All of the above

4. Patient on VA ECMO with severe left ventricular dysfunction are at increased risk for development of severe pulmonary venous hypertension, pulmonary edema and hemorrhage. Immediate measures to resolve the pulmonary venous hypertension would include:
   a) Increasing the ventilator oxygen level
   b) Lowering the pump flow rate and allowing more blood to enter the pulmonary circuit
   c) Providing a left atrial vent either directly via mediastinal cannulation or doing a blade atrial septectomy in the cardiac catheterization lab.
   d) To ignore the problem as the patient is fully supported on VA ECMO

5. Attention to CPR while preparing for ECPR initiation is unimportant, as the patient will soon be supported well with perfusion supplied by the ECLS circuit .
   a) True
   b) False

6. The prognosis is best for which of the following patients undergoing ECPR for refractory cardiac arrest:
   a) patients with underlying respiratory disease
   b) patients with underlying cardiac disease
   c) patient in septic shock
   d) patient with multiple trauma

7. In a recently published study reviewing the National Registry of CPR, noted all of the factors to be associated with decreased survival for patients undergoing E-CPR ,except:
   a) pre-arrest renal insufficiency
   b) metabolic or electrolyte abnormalities
   c) underlying cardiac illness
   d) use of bicarbonate or tromethamine

Chapter 16 Answers

1. c
2. b
3. d
4. c
5. b
6. b
7. c

17

Hemofiltration and Hemodialysis on ECMO

Daphne C. Hardison, RN, BSN and Geoffrey Fleming, MD

Objectives

After completion of this chapter, the participant should be able to:

- Define hemofiltration vs. hemodialysis and outline criteria for use
- Outline equipment needed
- Pros and cons of Setup Options
- Clinical management goals.

Background

Acute renal failure (ARF) is the rapid deterioration of renal function that may be associated with adequate urine output (non-oliguric) or with diminished to absent urine output (oliguric). ARF has been categorized by the location of dysfunction within the renal system and includes: pre-renal, post-renal and intrinsic ARF. Although these categorizations give a simple anatomic reference when considering causes of ARF, these categories have significant overlap and are inadequate for precise nomenclature. A strict definition for ARF is lacking but accepted diagnostic criteria include an increase in serum levels of creatinine (SCr), glomerular filtration rate (GFR) or blood urea nitrogen (BUN).[1-3] Current consensus guidelines utilize a change in SCr normalized to the patient's own baseline rather than an absolute threshold level for all patients. One such consensus criteria for ARF, the RIFLE criteria, utilizes either serum creatinine or urine output to estimate glomerular filtration rate in order to categorize ARF into Risk of renal injury, Injury to the kidney, Failure of kidney function, Loss of kidney function, and End-stage kidney disease[4] . This adult scoring system was modified for pediatric use by normalizing creatinine to body surface area as an estimation of glomerular filtration rate, the pRIFLE criteria.

Acute renal failure (ARF) in the pediatric intensive care unit occurs commonly, with a wide variation in the reported incidence, ranging from 4.5 % to 85 % depending upon the criteria used for the definition of ARF. [5-11] The majority of ARF cases are secondary to hypotension leading to poor renal perfusion and systemic inflammatory response syndrome (SIRS) of severe sepsis, with only 7% of ARF mediated by primary renal disease. In a recent study of pediatric patients with secondary ARF, 42% demonstrated renal dysfunction on admission to the intensive care unit, of which 55% had persistent ARF beyond the initial 48 hours[5]. ARF occurs more commonly in the subpopulation of critically ill patients on extracorporeal membrane oxygenation (ECMO), with an incidence of 12% to 69%.[12-15] A recent ECLS Registry report demonstrates 3-25% of patients reported to the database required either hemodialysis or hemofiltration on ECMO.[16]

The development of ARF during critical illness is associated with an increased mortality, and may be 8-fold higher as compared to patients without ARF.[9-11] Additionally, renal failure composes 4-13% of organ failure associated with the multiple organ dysfunction syndrome, with associated mortality rates of 0.6 -100%.[17] The increased mortality risk associated with ARF is also true for the population on ECMO, and in multivariate analysis has been shown to be an independent risk factor for mortality.[12-15, 18-24] Hence, renal failure is common in the ECMO population and is an associated independent risk factor for mortality.

Significant fluid overload has also been associated with an increased mortality risk in critically ill patients. In retrospective analysis, multiple authors have found fluid overload (>10-15%) to be independently associated with mortality.[25-29] Additionally, patients with multi-organ failure who were able to achieve dry weight during renal replacement therapy had higher survival than those who did not.[29] Fluid overload has been associated with a longer duration of ECMO, with reports of return to dry or ideal body weight prior to successful decannulation.[30-31] Inability to return to dry weight during the ECMO course is also an independent risk factor for mortality with acute renal failure.[24]

Introduction

Continuous renal therapies of today had origins that began in the 1980's, with the earliest descriptions using pump assisted continuous arterio-venous hemofiltration (CAVH). Dr. Robert Bartlett led the way in utilizing this therapy in the management of patients on ECMO and was among the early authors in literature[32-34]. These pump assisted therapies required arterial cannulation which increased the morbidity of the therapy. Dr. Canaud described continuous venovenous hemofiltration (CVVH) for adults in 1988 (29) and Dr. Yorgin described the therapy applied to children in 1990.[31] The success of venovenous circulation using a pump for continuous ultrafiltration helped reduce the morbidity of the therapy. Over the years the therapy has fundamentally been delivered in the same fashion but with some modifications and refinements of technique.

ECMO frequently triggers an acute inflammatory reaction associated with diffuse endothelial dysfunction and capillary leak syndrome. Renal dysfunction may occur as a result of this inflammatory response or may be due to instability prior to ECMO cannulation. In addressing renal dysfunction, diuretics are often employed to manage fluid overload with variable success. When the use of diuretic fails to improve fluid balance, the patient may need to undergo renal replacement therapy (RRT). Fluid balance becomes important as return to dry weight has been associated with time to decannulation on ECMO.[35-36] Additionally, fluid overload > 10% has been associated with mortality in the pediatric literature.[25] Multiple studies have shown that earlier and more aggressive CVVH improves mortality in the post-operative cardiac patient.[37-38]

Hemofiltration versus hemodialysis

The choice of modality depends upon the local practices of those managing renal replacement therapy, however a combination of hemofiltration and hemodialysis is common. Renal replacement therapy employs only two physiologies for solute and fluid movement, with both methods requiring sequestration of blood on one side of a semi-permeable membrane. Dialysis employs a diffusive clearance while hemofiltration or ultrafiltration employs convective clearance. Hemodialysis involves the diffusion of solutes down a concentration gradient from areas of high to low concentration. Dialysate is passed across the membrane counter current to blood flow allowing equilibration of plasma and dialysate solute concentrations to occur. This process may remove or add solute to the plasma water space depending upon the composition of dialysate compared to the plasma. Water will also move along a gradient in effect "following" the solute. Diffusive clearance is very effective at removal of small solute, including serum ions and urea, with subsequent fluid removal as a consequence. In addition, other solutes such as antibiotics, narcotics and other medications will cross the membrane. Diffusion gradients change dependent upon blood flow rates, dialysate flow rates, and starting concentration gradients. Continuous therapy employing countercurrent dialysate for solute clearance is considered continuous venovenous hemodialysis (CVVHD)

Hemofiltration uses a pressure gradient for fluid movement instead of solute concentration gradients. A positive hydrostatic pressure drives water across the membrane from the blood side to the filter side and solutes are essentially dragged through the membrane with the water. This process removes isotonic plasma water and is considered slow continuous ultrafiltration (SCUF). Due to the possibility of large shifts of volume during convective therapies a filter replacement fluid (FRF) is often utilized to replace fluid lost by convection. Fluid given is removed in equal quantities for isovolemic hemofiltration, yet the plasma composition will eventually resemble the FRF allowing for solute management. There are multiple names for the types of hemofiltration performed including SLEF (slow extended hemofiltration), SCUF (slow continuous ultrafiltration), CVVH (continuous venovenous hemofiltration), and CVVHDF (continuous venovenous hemodiafiltration).

Regardless of the modality employed, the goal of renal replacement therapy is to precisely control serum electrolytes, clear toxins, and provide fluid removal for the patient with renal failure.

Equipment

There are multiple manufacturers of dialysis machines and filters including Minntech (Minnesota USA), Gambro (Stockholm Sweeden), Fresenius Medial Care (Homburg Germany), Baxter International Inc (Illinois USA), B-Braun (Melsungen Germany), and Nx Stage (Massachusetts USA). The primary workhorse of the therapy is the hemodiafilter across which diffusion and/or convection occurs. The most popular membranes in use today are polyacrylontirile (AN69) and polysulfone; however polyamide, polycarbonate and polymethlymethacrylate are available. Newer synthetic materials have improved biocompatibility and reduced complement

activation which are felt to limit immunoreactivity to the membrane. Membranes are predominantly hollow fiber in structure, in which blood flows through a series of small tubes held together in a bundle, allowing for a low resistance in a high surface area membrane. Additional equipment required may include high flow stopcocks, infusion pumps, or scales. Placing the filter in-line with the ECMO circuit we will call "passive" CRRT and attaching a CRRT machine with a hemodiafilter to the ECMO circuit we will call "active" CRRT, although the reader should realize these are arbitrary designations.

During passive CRRT hemodiafilters are placed in-line from the high pressure arterial side returning to the low pressure venous side utilizing a high flow stopcock and ¼"X1/16" tubing. The hemodiafilter may be placed either pre-oxygenator to venous limb, or post roller pump and pre oxygenator to venous limb.(Figure 1) A flow of approximately 100 to 200 ml/min can be achieved through this shunt, which produces ultrafiltrate at a rapid rate due to the relatively high transmembrane pressure gradients. To transition the therapy from SCUF to

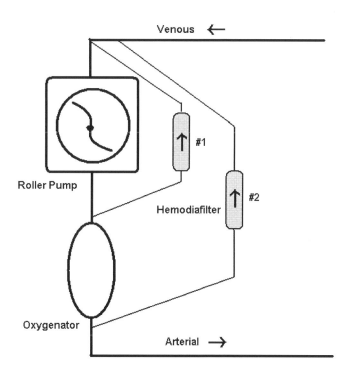

Figure 1. Schematic diagram of ECMO circuit with hemodiafilters in-line with connections from the arterial limb to the venous limb. #1 demonstrates post pump, pre-oxygenator access and #2 demonstrates post oxygenator access with both returning to the venous limb.

CVVH, FRF may be infused into the patient utilizing standard infusion pumps. The rate of ultrafiltrate flow may be regulated utilizing an infusion pump which draws from the hemodiafilter and empties into a reservoir. To convert the therapy to CVVHD, dialysate is infused through the appropriate port in the hemodiafilter using infusion pumps countercurrent to blood flow. In both convective and diffusive therapies it is important to accurately monitor fluid infusion and retrieval. To this end multiple measuring devices have been used from urinometers to scales to weighing fluids.

Active CRRT is accomplished by connecting CRRT machines to the circuit. The inlet or arterial limb of the CRRT machine is usually connected to the low pressure (venous) limb of the ECMO circuit with the return outlet or venous limb from the machine connected to the venous limb of the ECMO circuit, possibly at the bladder. (Figure 2) Although this may also be achieved by accessing the high pressure (arterial limb) of the ECMO circuit, internal alarms in the CRRT machine may become a problem as they were designed to monitor low pressure venous access and return. These alarms usually include "low pressure alarm", "access disconnection", or "return pressure high". Most machines come with the limits internally set but can be manipulated to confer compatibility to the ECMO circuit. A "return pressure high" alarm would lead the specialist to consider either moving the return port to a lower pressure side of the ECMO circuit or to troubleshoot the site of re-infusion. There should not be a return pressure high alarm alert on the venous, pre-raceway side unless there is a clot or occlusion at the site. Access disconnection is the most common occurrence and in an ECMO system running with high pressures this can be a continual problem alarm. One solution is to turn the stopcock by ¼ of a turn to give the machine the chance to read an actual pressure, other options would include moving the access to a more negative or less high pressure site, such as the venous side pre-raceway. However, remember that hemolysis is a concern with highly turbulent flow in a small aperture, as may occur with a partially closed stopcock.

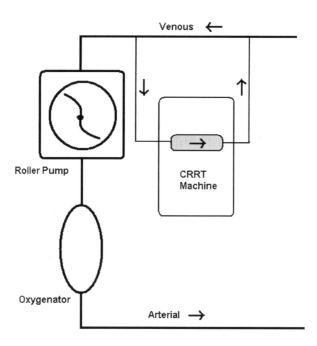

Figure 2. Schematic diagram of ECMO circuit with CRRT machine connected to the venous limb. Both the inlet (arterial) and outlet (venous) lines from the CRRT machine are connected to the venous limb of the ECMO circuit.

Pros and Cons of Setup Options

Passive hemofiltration can be placed within the ECMO circuit with minimal cost, ease of set up, and utilization of less blood volume than a complete CRRT machine circuit. This system acts as a shunt that will require increased ECMO flows to achieve adequate patient flow. The smaller patients typically only need a blood flow of 30 ml/minute across the hemodiafilter for adequate therapy. Due to high blood flow on ECMO, the flow across the filter may result in clearance that can be rapid and excessive for smaller patients. Using ultrasonic flow probes to measure actual blood flow to patient and to the hemodiafilter may assist in monitoring the flow through this shunt relative to total flow. Electrolytes should be monitored frequently especially in the case of SCUF as rapid ion shifts are possible. Utilization of infusion pumps for fluid control during passive hemofiltration /hemodialysis may lead to large volume shifts due to potential inaccuracies of the pumps. This may be magnified in the smaller patient with a lower blood volume relative to larger blood flows across the filter. Infusion pumps have frequently been found to be inaccurate in the ECMO setting and can put children at risk for excessive fluid loss and ultrafiltration.[39]

The use of an active pump-driven system results in more accurate control of blood flow and fluid removal, however may be more technically involved due to machine alarms on the CRRT. Additionally, there is the cost of the machine and the required circuit to include. The blood flows are set and maintained by the pump system to allow for either standard convective or diffusive models of hemofiltration. This can allow for higher rates of solute clearance with decreased risks for hypovolemia and electrolyte shifts. For small infants, the minimal ultrafiltration rate of 10 mL/hr may be problematic when using the Prisma ® system, but surmountable by creative fluid accounting methods.

No data exist to support recommendation of active CRRT over passive CRRT on ECMO. Hence each center will need to review available equipment, safety monitoring and previous experience to decide between passive and active CRRT on ECMO.

Coagulation Management Differences

There is no significant change to anticoagulation management during CRRT on ECMO whether using a passive or active system. Heparin clearance during renal failure is markedly reduced, and the addition of a hemodiafilter to the circuit may increase heparin clearance. Hence usual monitoring practices, the activated clotting time in many centers, need to be followed closely for needed heparin adjustments to maintain adequate anticoagulation.

Management Goals

Establishment of fluid and electrolyte balance goals is essential in the care of the ECMO patient when using a CRRT therapy. Frequent assessment of intake and output status is necessary to stay within goal parameters. This is especially challenging in the patient population requiring frequent blood product administration. It is easy to have excessive fluid removal resulting in exacerbation of the renal dysfunction. Goals for renal support need to be reviewed by members of the team including physicians, bedside nursing and ECMO team members.

Other Indications for Hemofiltration and Hemodiafiltration

Hemodialysis can be used in tandem with ECMO to treat urea cycle disorders, specifically hyperammonemia.[40] In this setting a standard hemodialysis machine which requires higher blood flow rates than CRRT may be connected to the circuit to provide rapid clearance of ammonia. The connection is similar to CRRT, however the duration of therapy will be limited and driven by ammonia levels. Other extracorporeal therapies may be employed during ECMO, including plasmapheresis for sepsis, and leukophoresis in pertussis.[41] These therapies are delivered using a pump-driven active system and are connected to the circuit as in active CRRT.

Conclusion

Fluid and electrolyte imbalances are common in the ECMO patient population frequently related to the severity of their disease process. Current data support early use of renal support, which limits fluid overload, and may confer survival benefits.[42-46] There are multiple strategies for the technical application of CVVH and CVVHD with no demonstrable benefit of active over passive CRRT.

References

1. Montagnino B, Currier H. The Child with Genitourinary Dysfunction. In: Hockenberry M, Wilson D, Winkelstein M, editors. Wong's Essentials of Pediatric Nursing. 7th ed. Elsevier Mosby. *2005 p. 1001-1003.*
2. Singri N, Ahya SN, Levin ML. Acute Renal Failure. *JAMA* 2003;289:747-751.
3. Albright RC Jr . Acute renal failure: a practical update. *Mayo Clin Proc* 2001;76:67-74.
4. Bellomo R, Ronco C, Kellum JA, Mehta RL, Palevsky P, ADQI Workgroup. Acute renal failure-definition, outcome measures, animal models, fluid therapy and information technology needs: the Second International Consensus Conference of the Acute Dialysis Quality Initiative (ADQI) Group. *Crit Care Med* 2004;8(4):R204-12
5. Akcan-Arikan A, Zappitelli M, Loftis LL, Washburn KK, Jefferson LS, Goldstein SL. Modified RIFLE criteria in critically ill children with acute kidney injury. *Kidney Int 2007;71:1028-35*
6. Karlowicz MG, Adelman RD, Nonoliguric and oliguric acute renal failure in asphyxiated term neonates. *Pediatri Nephrol 1995;9(6):718-22.*
7. Moghal NE, Brocklebank TJ, Meadow SR. A review of acute renal failure in children: Incidence, etiology, and outcome. *Clin Nephrol 1998;49 (2):91-95.*
8. Williams DM, Sreedhar SS, Mickel JJ, Chan JCM. Acute kidney failure: A Pediatric experience over 20 years. *Arch Pediatr Adolesc Med 2002;156:893-900.*
9. Bunchman, TE, McBryde KD, Mottes TE, Gardener JJ, Maxvold NJ, Brophy PD. Pediatric acute renal failure: Outcome by modality and disease. *Pediar Nephrol 2001;16:1067-1071.*
10. Hui-Stickle S, Brewer ED, Goldstein SL. Pediatric ARF epidemiology at a tertiary care center from 1999-2001. *Am J Kid Dis 2005;45(1):96-101.*
11. Baily D, Phan V, Litalien C, Ducruet T, Merouani A, Lacroix J, et al. Risk factors of acute renal failure in critically ill children: A prospective descriptive epidemiological study. *Pediatr Crit Care Med 2007;8(1):29-35.*
12. Sell LL, Cullen ML, Whittlesey GC, Lerner GR, Klein MD. Experience with renal failure during extracorporeal membrane oxygenation: treatment with continuous hemofiltration. *J Pediatr Surg 1987;22(7):600-2.*
13. Adolph V, Heaton J, Steiner R, Bonis S, Flaterman K, Arensman R. Extracorporeal membrane oxygenation for non-neonatal respiratory failure. *J Pediatr Surg 1991;26(3):326-7.*
14. Raithel SC, Penningon G, Boegner E, Fiore A, Weber TR. Extracorporeal membrane oxygenation in children after cardiac surgery. *Circulation 1992;86 (SuppII):II305-II310.*
15. Weber TR, Kountzman B. Extracorporeal membrane oxygenation for non-neonatal pulmonary and multi-organ failure. *J Pediatr Surg 1998;33:1605-1609.*
16. *ELSO International Registry Report, July 2008 (Ann Arbor, MI)*
17. Typpo K, Mariscalco M. Multiple Organ Dysfunction Syndrome. In: Wheeler DS, Wong HR, Shanley TP, editors. Pediatric Critical Care Medicine. Basic Science and Clinical Evidence. 1st ed. London: Springer Verlanger: *2007. p 1445-56.*
18. Bartlett RH, Andrews AF, Toomasian JM, Haiduc NJ, Gazzaniga AB. Extracorporeal membrane oxygenation for newborn respiratory failure: forty-five cases. *Surgery* 1982;92(2):425-33.
19. Kirkpatrick BV, Krummel TM, Mueller DG, Ormazabal MA, Greenfeld LJ, Salzberg AM. Use of extracorporeal membrane oxygenation for respiratory failure in term infants. *Pediatrics* 1983;72(6):872-876.
20. Weber TR, Connors RH, Tracy RF, Bailey PV, Stephens C, Keenan W. Prognostic determinants in extracorporeal membrane oxygenation for respiratory failure in newborns. *Ann Thorac Surg* 1990;50(5):720-723.

21. Duncan BW, Hraska V, Jonas RA, Wessel DL, Del Nido PJ, Laussen PC, Mayer JE, Lapierre RA, Wilson JM. Mechanical circulatory support in children with cardiac disease. *J Thorac Cardiovasc Surg* 1999;117(3):529-542.

22. Kist-van Holthe tot Echten JE, Goedvolk CA, Doornaar MBME, van der Vorst MMJ, Bosman-Vermeeren JM, Brand R et al. Acute renal insufficiency and renal replacement therapy after pediatric cardiopulmory bypass surgery. *Pediatr Cardiol* 2001;22:321-326.

23. Morris MC, Ittenbach RF, Godinez RI, Portnoy JD, Tabbutt S, Hanna BD, et al. Risk factors for mortality in 137 pediatric cardiac intensive care unit patients managed with extracorporeal membrane oxygenation. *Crit Care Med* 2004;32(4):1061-1069.

24. Swaniker S, Kolla S, Moler F, Custer J, Grams R, Bartlett RH et al. Extracorporeal life support outcome for 128 pediatric patients with respiratory failure. *J Pediatric Surg* 2000;35(2):197-202

25. Goldstein SL, Currier H, Graf JM, Cosio CC, Brewer ED, Sachdeva R. Outcome in children receiving continuous venovenous hemofiltration. *Pediatrics* 2001;107:1309-1312.

26. Michael M, Kuehnle I, Goldstein SL. Fluid overload and acture renal failure in pediatric stem cell transplant patients. *Pediatr Nephrol* 2004;19:91-95.

27. Gillespie RS, Seidel K, Symons JM. Effect of fluid overload and dose of replacement fluid on survival in hemofiltration. *Pediatr Nephrol* 2004;19:1394-1399.

28. Foland JA, Fortenberry JD, Warshaw BL, Pettignano R, Merritt RK, Heard ML et al. Fluid overload before continuous hemofiltration and survival in critically ill children: A retrospective analysis. *Crit Care Med* 2004;32:1771-1776.

29. Goldstein SL, Somers MJG, Baum MA, Symons JM, Brophy PD, Blowey D et al. Pediatric patients with multi-organ dysfunction syndrome receiving continuous renal replacement therapy. *Kidney International* 2005;67:653-658.

30. Canaud B, Garred LJ, Christol JP, Aubas S, Beraud JJ, Mion C. Pump assisted continuous venovenous hemofiltration for treating acute uremia.. *Kidney Int* 1988;24(supp):S154-S156.

31. Yorgin PD, Krensky AM, Tune BM. Continuous venovenous hemofiltration. In: Paul WE, ed. *Pediatric Nephrology*. 1990;4:640-2.

32. Bartlett RH, Bosch J, Geronemus R, Pagnini E, Ronco C, Swartz R. Continuous arteriovenous hemofiltration for acute renal failure. *ASAIO Trans* 1988;34:67-77.

33. Mault JR, Dechert RE, Lees P, Swartz, Port JK, Bartlett RH. Continuous arteriovenous filtration: an effective treatment for surgical acute renal failure. *Surgery* 1987;101:478-84.

34. Heiss KF, Pettite B, Hirschl RB, Cilley RE, Chapman R, Bartlett RH. Renal insufficiency and volume overload in neonatal ECMO managed by continous ultrafiltration. *ASAIO Trans* 1987;33:557-560.

35. Kelly R, Phillips D, Foglia R, et al. Pulmonary Edema and Fluid Mobilization as Determinants of the Duration of ECMO Support. *Journal of Pediatric Surgery* 1991;26(9):1016-1022.

36. Anderson H, Coran A, Bartlett R, et al. Extracellular Fluid and Total Body Water Changes in Neonates Undergoing Extracorporeal Membrane Oxygenation. *Journal of Pediatric Surgery* 1992;27(8):1003-1008.

37. Swaniker S, Kolla S, Moler F, Custer J, Grams R, Bartlett RH et al. Extracorporeal life support outcome for 128 pediatric patients with respiratory failure. *J Pediatric Surg* 2000;35(2):197-202.

38. Golej J, Boigner H, Burda G, Hermon M, Kitzmueller E, Trittenwein G. Peritoneal dialysis for continuing renal support after cardiac ECMO and hemofiltration. *Wien Klin Wochenschr* 2002;114:733-738.

39. Jenkins R, Harrison H, Chen B, Arnold D, Funk J. Accuracy of intravenous infusion pumps in continuous renal replacement therapies. *ASAIO* 1992;38:808-810.

40. Summar M, Pietsch J, Deshpande J, Schulman G. Effective hemodialysis and hemofiltration driven by an extracorporeal membrane oxygenation pump in infants with hyperammonemia. *J Pediatr* 1996;128:2379-382.

41. Grzeszczak M, Churchwell K, Edward K, Pietsch J. Leukopheresis therapy for severe infantile pertussis with myocardial and pulmonary failure. *Ped Crit Care Med* 2006;7(6):580-582.

42. Meyer RJ, Brophy PD, Bunchman TE, et al.. Survival and renal function in pediatric patients following extracorporeal life support with hemofiltration. *Pediatr Crit Care Med* 2001;2:238-242.

43. Maqsood M, Ming Y, Robin M, Ramana R, et al. Early hemofiltration improves survival in post cardiotomy patients with renal failure. *Eur J Cardiothorac Surg* 2004;26:1027-1031.

44. Bent P, Han T, Buxton B, et al. Early and intensive continuous hemofiltration for severe renal failure after cardiac surgery. *Ann Thorac Surg* 2001;71:832-837.

Chapter 17 Questions

1. Fluid removed during hemofiltration or SCUF
    a) Occurs due to concentration gradients.
    b) Occurs due to pressure gradients.
    c) Contains no ions (sodium e.g.)
    d) Is called dialysate.

2. Troubleshooting alarms on CRRT machines during ECMO:
    a) Requires an understanding of the site of attachment to the ECMO circuit.
    b) May require adjustment of alarm limits on the CRRT machine.
    c) Requires close attention for safety purposes
    d) all of the above

3. Heparin dosages may need to be altered when CVVH is added into the system because.
    a) The hemodiafilter absorbs all heparin
    b) Dilution due to the extra blood volume contained in the hemodiafilter
    c) Heparin clearance is significantly affected by renal failure.
    d) It is necessary to give platelets at initiation of CRRT on ECMO.

Chapter 17 Answers

1. b
2. d
3. c

18

Plasmapheresis for the ECMO Patient

Jeffrey B. Sussmane, MD and Edward Wong, MD

Objectives

After completion of this chapter, the participant should be able to:

- Understand the physiologic basis of Apheresis
- Describe the different modalities of Apheresis
- Describe the most common indications for Plasmapheresis
- Understand the principles of Operation
- Understand the set up and initiation of Plasmapheresis for the ECMO Patient
- Describe the responsibilities of the Pheresis specialist
- Understand the physiologic considerations during Plasmapheresis
- Calculate the fluid balance of the patient
- Review the complications of Plasmapheresis

Introduction

Huang Di, the "Yellow Emperor" of China, in the middle of the third millennium BCE, first introduced the concept of balancing circulating "forces" within the body to promote health and treat disease.[1] Galen popularized the concept of forces within the body, the "four humours", in the Roman Empire. Managing circulating humours was done routinely in an attempt to improve or restore health.[2] The Greek verb "aphaeresis" meaning "to take away, withdraw or separate" continues to be a central concept and application in Western Medicine. The term Plasmapheresis is used interchangeably for a variety of clinical applications. It may refer to the removal, exchange, modification, or filtration of circulating blood components, with or without the returning of a blood component. Therapeutic Plasma Exchange (TPE) is the most frequent Plasma "pheresis" modality performed. TPE utilizes either a centrifuge or filter to separate or remove the plasma components and replace a plasma component concurrently. The goal is to remove, replace, or deplete unique circulating substances that are responsible for the disease process.

The process of removing cellular components (Cytapheresis) includes; Red Cell Pheresis or Erythrocytapheresis, which is the removal of red blood cells (RBCs). Therapeutic Leukodepletion is employed for the removal of large numbers of circulating white blood cells (WBCs: lymphoblasts, myeloblasts, granulocytes or monocytes), thereby decreasing aggregates that interfere with blood flow during the acute presentation of Leukemia. Leukapheresis often refers to Peripheral Stem Cell Collection, which is performed to remove specific CD34+ progenitor cells, from peripheral blood for storage and reinfusion during the process of Stem Cell Transplantation.

The application of TPE includes infection, inflammatory, autoimmune, oncologic, metabolic, neurologic, or renal diseases.[3] The American Society of Apheresis (ASFA) has recently published a review of the indications for TPE and the likelihood of response.[3,5] In the past 10 years, many hospitals have developed apheresis programs due to the growing success and increased therapeutic use of this procedure.[4,5] The technique has also gained widespread acceptance in Europe.[6] TPE is generally a supportive therapy used in conjunction with ongoing care, and has been shown to increase the chance of recovery and survival in critically ill children and adults.[5-20]

Selected Indications for Plasmapheresis

Disease	ASFA Category	Disease	ASFA Category
ABO Incompatible Hematopoetic Progenitor Cell Transplantation	II	Heart Transplant Rejection	III
ABO Incompatible Solid Organ Transplantation	II (kidney, heart [infants]) III (liver)	Hemolytic Uremic Syndrome; Thrombotic Microangiopathy; and Transplant Associated Microangiopathy	III (aHUS, TMA, TAM) IV (Pediatric, diarrheal)
Acute Disseminated Encephalomyelitis	III	Hyperleukocytosis	I (Leukostasis)
Acute Liver Failure	III	Hypertriglyceridemic Pancreatitis	III
Acute Inflammatory Demyelinating Polyneuropathy (Guillain-Barré Syndrome)	I	Idiopathic Thrombocytopenic Purpura	IV
ANCA-Associated Rapidly Progressive Glomerulonephritis (Wegener's Granulomatosis)	II	Malaria	II (severe)
Anti-Glomerular Basement Membrane Disease (Goodpasture's Syndrome)	I	Multiple Sclerosis	II (Acute CNS inflammatory demyelinating disease)
Autoimmune Hemolytic Anemia (Warm Autoimmune Hemolytic Anemia; Cold Agglutinin Disease)	III WAIHA III CAD	Myasthenia Gravis	I
Catastrophic Antiphospholipid Syndrome	III	Overdose and Poisoning	II (mushroom poisoning) III (other compounds)
Chronic Inflammatory Demyelinating Polyradiculoneuropathy	I	Paraneoplastic Neurologic Syndromes	III
Cyroglobulinemia	I	Sepsis	III
Focal Segmental Glomerulosclerosis	III (primary) II (recurrent)	Thrombotic Thrombocytopenic Purpura	I

Principles of Therapeutic Plasma Exchange (TPE) Operation

TPE, for the patient on ECMO, is performed in an Intensive Care Unit by individuals who are ECMO certified or under the direct supervision of an ECMO specialist. The direct supervision of a qualified ECMO physician is also necessary. The patient's weight, sex, height, hematocrit, and procedure specific information are programmed into the machine software and the machine is wheeled next to the ECMO circuit. A unique TPE circuit is loaded into a centrifugal machine for each therapy. The appropriate prescribed fluids are connected to the TPE and the circuit is primed automatically by the specific software program chosen for each therapy. A filtration system may alternatively be used. Replacement fluids, anticoagulant, and priming solutions are dependant on size of patient and chosen before the therapy based on the child's condition. The access to systemic circulation is drawn directly from the ECMO circuit, without interruption or alteration of the ECMO flow. Once the TPE circuit is connected to the ECMO circuit, blood is pumped into the machine with an anticoagulant that is automatically calculated and added as the blood enters the centrifuge. In some centers, the systemic anticoagulation provided by the heparin in the ECMO circuit suffices and no further anticoagulant is needed. A fully heparinized ECMO circuit may negate the need for additional anticoagulation. Heparinized or otherwise coated ECMO circuits may affect the anticoagulation necessary for the TPE circuit. The need for additional or alternative anticoagulation should be evaluated for each patient and each therapy.

In those centers using a centrifugal based plasma separation technique, the centrifuge separates the blood into layers primarily based on density. Red cells are the densest and collect against the centrifuge wall first, or farthest outside on the centrifuge plate, followed by white cells, platelets, and plasma. Centrifugal TPE utilizes optical sensors to detect each layer interface to minimize contamination of each cell and fluid layer. The desired components are automatically removed to collection bags and the remaining blood components, along with appropriate replacement fluids, are returned to the patient.

Rotary peristaltic pumps automatically control the amount of blood pumped from the patient, the amount of the component sent to the collection bag, the specific amount of anticoagulant, and (when programmed) the appropriate constitution of reinfused fluids. Warmers can be added to the circuit to warm replacement fluid to prevent hypothermia caused by infusion of room temperature or cold fluids. This is generally unnecessary with a functioning heat exchanger during ECMO, as these fluids are entered pre-heat exchanger. Most apheresis machines also have the capability of selecting the percentage of fluids for automatic reinfusion. This is done in direct proportion to the percentage of fluid removed; thus decreasing the possibility of the patient developing hypovolemia or hypervolemia. Multiple audiovisual alarms alert the operator to potential problems.

TPE may also be performed using a filtration technique. An anticoagulated extracorporeal circuit passes the blood through a filter. Separation of the plasma is achieved and reinfusion of the cellular components then occurs. This technique performs well for specific plasma filtration scenarios but is reliant upon the filter pore size.[10-16]

Specific Apheresis Considerations for the ECMO Circuit

Apheresis is indicated when a there is an acute clinical need to separate blood components. Therapeutic Apheresis, including: total plasma exchange, red blood cell exchange, Leukopheresis, and peripheral blood stem cell collection can be easily performed by the Apheresis specialist during ECMO. A stopcock is placed on the venous line, pre-bladder for the access of the withdrawal specimen. The returning line is placed downstream on the venous line, again pre-raceway. As all Apheresis Specialists managing the ECMO pump should be Certified ECLS Specialists, this procedure can be performed with relative ease, eliminating venous access (catheter) problems and alteration of total ECMO flow. The parallel Apheresis circuit does not affect ECMO circuit flows. Once therapy is stabilized the ECMO flows will remain unchanged. The initial "total" ECMO circuit compliance may transiently change, during the initiation of Apheresis. If the ECMO venous drainage is unrecognized as borderline or marginal, the venous pressure alarm may sound ("chirp"), suggesting an acute decrease in venous return. The servo regulation of the pump may also suddenly reduce ECMO flow. This may require an additional volume bolus during initiation of Apheresis. The Apheresis protocol and software from the manufacturer should be followed for continued maintenance of the separation therapy. Unique conditions may require the manual programming of the device, or overriding specific parameters. The scope and nature of every unique scenario is beyond the scope of this manual and when this occurs it may be best to acquire additional expertise from the manufacturer or a more experienced center before beginning the therapy.

Responsibilities
- Verify procedure with Apheresis / ECMO specialist, physician and family
- Assist in explaining indication, procedure, and risks to family.
- Record patient height, weight, hematocrit, and indication.
- Send baseline pre-procedure labs- CBC, ICa^+ and electrolytes (notify Physician of results).
- Labs for specific procedures (notify Physician of results).
  - TSM (red cell exchange)
  - CD34+, disease markers and HIV (need consent), for peripheral blood stem cell harvest
  - Specific Disease markers and HIV (need consent)
  - Anti-inflammatory panels
- Extra labs for multiple procedures (notify Physician of results).
  - Mg (is this total or ionized?) & PO_4 & ICa^+
  - PT/PTT
  - FDP, Fibrinogen
  - IgG
- Standby emergency replacement fluid (PRBC's, Albumin, FFP, NS).
- Connect apheresis access line (using sterile and airless technique) to venous pigtail close to patient (pre-bladder).

- Connect apheresis return line (using sterile and airless technique) to any of the venous pigtails downstream from access line and pre-raceway
- Halfway through procedure, or if symptomatic for hypocalcemia, send ICa^+ (Notify Physician of results).
- Monitor ACT's; If decision to utilize citrate to chelate calcium to prevent clotting in the Pheresis circuit is made, adjustments in heparin may be necessary.
- If patient deteriorates stop apheresis immediately, notify Physician STAT and follow ECLS protocol.
- When procedure is completed disconnect apheresis access and return line (using sterile and airless technique) and flush pigtails with 1 cc NS and place port cap on site.
- Post-procedure send
  - ICa^+, Mg^+, Electrolytes and PT/PTT (notify Physician of results)
  - Anti-inflammatory panel (optional? What labs? It won't come back fast enough to affect clinical care)
  - IgG

Specific humoral considerations of Therapeutic Apheresis

Therapeutic Plasma Exchange - TPE is a systemic immunomodulatory therapy. It removes specified plasma volumes and returns predetermined replacement fluids, most commonly plasma and or albumin. The manipulation of removing, diluting, and returning foreign plasma components initiates an immune response which can be seen in the elevation of all major circulating immune complexes 1-3 hours post treatment. There is also serum elevation of complement, including C3a, C4a, C5a and an increase in the total number of circulating granulocytes and macrophages within the first two treatments. Lymphocytes increase in treatment three and the T helper/suppressor ratio increase in treatment four. TPE involves cycling 100% of the patient's total blood volume thereby removing putative pathologic material in the patient's plasma.

The efficacy of treatment may be measured by a reduction in concentration of pathologic and toxic substances such as pro-inflammatory cytokines.[21,22] The aggressive use of IgG concomitant with TPE has been widely reported for pre-transplant patients and for blood group incompatibilities incurred with transplantation and rejection.[23-25] This should also be considered for all extended therapies, due to the significant reduction of circulating Immunoglobulins during repeated procedures especially those using albumin as replacement. Circulating inflammatory mediators are widely recognized as contributing to the morbidity and mortality of certain clinical conditions. This is the predominant pathophysiologic condition during sepsis and the application of Plasmapheresis has been directly shown to improve outcome and reduction of the "humoral" imbalance.[27,28,29] The direct filtration of these mediators has not been possible until the recent improvement in the biocompatibility of membranes.. Although no longer available a Polymixin-B-immobilized fiber has been shown to significantly decrease circulating levels of endotoxin after TPE[31] but no study has shown a benefit to these absorptive therapies. An immunoadsorption column with Protein A covalently bound to a microprocessed silicone filter, (Prosorba®, has been widely utilized to prevent graft vs. host reactions in organ recipients and the reduction of immunologic blood group incompatibilities in kidney transplant patients.[30] However, this column has been recently discontinued and it is unclear if it will become available in the future.

Cardiorespiratory, Metabolic and Hematalogic Considerations

The clinical application of TPE begins with the age of the patient and the determination of the intravascular volume. Additional venous access is not necessary during ECMO. The type of priming fluid for the circuit is dependent on the patient's age. The older typical centrifuge circuits require 350 ml for priming and have a circuit volume of approximately 150 ml. The 18 kg child will have approximately a 12% dilution from the circuit and this may be primed with blood to minimize the dilutional effects of priming. These packed red blood cells will prevent further dilution of the hematocrit and anemia and for certain children, as well as possible hypovolemia.[32-35] Smaller children are at greater risk while larger children (> 20 kg) may tolerate priming with colloid or crystalloid. The choice of replacement fluids also varies depending on the diagnosis, indication, and/or institutional preference. The decision to utilize fresh frozen plasma or fractionated human albumin as priming and replacement fluid should be made clinically, based on the immunologic, protein, pulmonary, and cardiovascular condition of the child. Crystalloid solutions (normal saline) and colloid solutions (albumin or fresh frozen plasma) may be utilized alone or in combination. The risk of transfusion and physiologic complications increases with the use of foreign protein, but children with unstable or suboptimal physiology often benefit from the use of a combination of fresh frozen plasma and fractioned human albumin.[36,39] Fresh frozen plasma is the replacement of choice if coagulation factors are depleted; however, administration requires immunologic compatibility and carries an increased risk of exposure to foreign protein. There are newer circuits primed with less than 100 ml and circulating less than 50 ml. These circuits may allow crystalloid priming for children greater than 8 kg.

TPE treatments are usually from one to three hours in duration. They may be ordered once a day or every other day, for a period of 3-14 days. The number of treatments is dependent upon patient response and can usually be established after the completion of the first two treatments. Improved lab values and clinical status will become apparent for the rapid responder within the first 24 hours. Repeated therapies for conditions that are slowly responding should be cycled every 4 to 7 treatments with a day or two without TPE. This will minimize the depletion of endogenous healthy circulating cofactors. Replacement of many cofactors may be carried out utilizing fresh frozen plasma and should be utilized for extended therapies. Specific cofactors may need to be measured and replaced as needed. Many centers routinely measure IgG levels and replace accordingly. Careful monitoring of inflammatory mediators, coagulation profiles, protein and Immunoglobulins will trace improvement and depletion of cofactors.

It is important to calculate the plasma volume to exchange. One blood volume plasma exchange will replace 63% of the circulating blood volume or toxin. A two blood volume plasma exchange will remove 86%. Single volume exchanges are typically performed, better tolerated, and successful when repeated after a day or two time delay. TPE can be performed on an either daily or every other day profile depending on the indication.. The typical total course for sepsis is four to ten treatments. Many centers will increase this to fourteen treatments for sepsis, although supporting data is not available. The unpublished data from Miami Children's Hospital (MCH) typically will provide 5 to 7 treatments that successfully treat the rapid responders. We will institute a 2 day holiday before proceeding with additional treatments for slow responders, as all plasma and protein bound substances are readily removed during TPE and need to be reconstituted. The initial TPE calculation commonly recommends that a one and one half (1 ½) blood volume exchange is appropriate. Although many centers continue to perform single volume exchanges for consecutive treatment we perform 1 ½ volume exchanges throughout the TPE therapy for the sicker patients. It should be noted that the plasma volume calculated includes the plasma volume of the patient and the plasma volume of the extracorporeal ECMO circuit.

Cardiorespiratory Considerations

Sudden decreases in preload, acute changes in peripheral vascular resistance, and alteration of right ventricular compliance may occur from both the exposure to the extracorporeal circuit and volume shifting. The initiation of any extracorporeal circuit must take into consideration the underlying right and left ventricular lusitropic and inotropic condition, as well as the peripheral vascular resistance. Ventilated ECMO patients who are marginally preload dependent may suffer a decrease in pulmonary blood flow and left ventricular pressure. Larger patients generally respond to flow adjustments and volume replacement with solutions containing protein and rarely require inotropic support. Warming of the replacement fluids can help prevent complications such as hypothermia and "sickling" in susceptible patients. There is no evidence of a primary change

in pulmonary compliance or of alteration in gas exchange, but there may be a sudden change in peripheral vascular resistance from exposure to foreign surfaces usually amenable to volume infusion. There may be an improvement in left ventricular function[36] after therapy with the reduction of circulating mediators, seen more commonly in gram negative sepsis.[27,37]

Metabolic Considerations

The most frequently encountered electrolyte disturbances and complications result from abnormalities in ionized calcium, when citrate is used as an additional anticoagulant. Hypocalcemia is most frequently seen in patients with severe liver dysfunction, those receiving fresh frozen plasma, or during procedures with a high citrate to whole blood ratio.[37,38] Children should also be observed for complications of hypokalemia as a result of citrate toxicity. Depletion of plasma proteins, especially coagulation factors, and immunologic factors may occur if repeated procedures are required. Prevention and management of hypocalcemia includes administration of supplemental calcium (gluconate or chloride). Monitoring of pH, base excess, and metabolic alkalosis should be performed.

Hematologic Considerations

High blood flow rates may create hemolysis if the circuit is twisted or kinked. Significant hemolysis may precipitate DIC or mimic a transfusion reaction. Hemolysis may be detected by monitoring the plasma color or obtaining plasma hemoglobin levels. Monitoring of hemoglobin, hematocrit, platelets and coagulation factors such as PT/PTT, fibrinogen, and FDP are also essential for evaluation of hematologic status. There may be a shifting of the ACTs as well. A decrease in circulating immunoglobulins or coagulation cofactors may be addressed by the infusion of fresh frozen plasma, IVIG, fibrinogen concentrates, or cryoprecipitate.

Circuit Priming

The fluid status of the patient needs to be carefully evaluated. The goal is usually to leave the patient in a fluid balance range of no more than 75-125% of calculated baseline. The Cobe Spectra® machine default volume level is 100% baseline (no net increase or decrease). Crystalloid prime is often used for children larger than 45 kg. Colloid prime is recommended for children 20 to 45 kg. Blood prime may be ordered by the physician for any child. Children less than 20 kg often require one unit of crossmatch compatible, CMV negative, irradiated, leukodepleted blood to prime the apheresis circuit. The methods of blood priming will be dependent on the physician's clinical decision. Blood priming with reconstituted blood (FFP with RBCs.) This should be considered when the extracorporeal volume is large relative to the patient, such as a neonate, and when the hematocrit is desired to be normal or high. This is not a method for keeping the hematocrit normal or high or to maintain some coagulation factor level]. If you want to increase the hematocrit, on an anemic or volume overloaded or volume intolerant patient PRBC's are the component of choice for priming. Plasmapheresis is usually calculated to be volume neutral and does not require packed RBCs. You can divert the waste and/or not do a rinseback to decrease volume. However, it is safer to program the apheresis instrument to keep the patient volume neutral, negative or positive.] Clinically stable children often tolerate either solution.

A Cobe ® Spectra circuit requires 345 ml to prime. The circulating internal volume is 150 ml and the rinse-back volume is 195 ml. If rinse-back is given when the procedure is programmed to leave the patient at 100% balance, then the patient will be 195 cc positive at the end of the procedure. One should not rinse-back at the end of a procedure unless there is a need to increase the patient's volume or to return RBCs. The recorded values can be subtracted from final run values to measure total volume given.

Calculation: Fluid balance = (replacement rate + AC rate) x 100) plasma flow rate

When blood priming with reconstituted whole blood to a desired hematocrit, the formula is:

Volume of RBC post dilution =
(Hct RBC from banked blood bag) x (vol. RBC bag)

(Desired Hct for prime)

The volume of diluent to add to PRBC bag = (Total vol. RBC after dilution) - (Initial vol. PRBC bag). The volume of RBCs after dilution = Volume of diluent -volume of initial PRBCs.

The diluent may be a combination of FFP, 5% Albumin or Normal Saline. Reconstituted whole blood is obtained with PRBCs and FFP.

Example:
RBC Hct = 70%
RBC volume = 220 ml
Desired Hct for prime = 30%
Volume of RBC unit after dilution =
$\frac{(0.70) \times (220 \text{ ml})}{(0.30)} = 513 \text{ ml}$

Volume of diluent = 513 ml - 220 ml = 293 ml

Add 293 ml of fluid to the original unit of PRBC's to achieve a desired Hct of 30 %

When blood priming with packed red blood cells or reconstituted whole blood, the machine should be programmed with the Hct of the PRBC or whole blood unit. When the blood reaches the return saline manifold, the procedure and record the "volume-processed" values recorded for anticoagulant (AC), inlet, plasma. This volume may be replaced if applicable. Plasma processed from prime is added to the target values as this will correct the run so the desired patient blood product is removed.

Anticoagulation Issues

Anticoagulation is initiated to minimize clotting of the blood as it travels through the circuit. The most frequently used anticoagulant is citrate. The most common form used is ACD-A. Most ACD-A is processed from the circuit when exposed to the calcium in the circuit collection. Each 100 ml of ACD-A contains 2.2 g sodium citrate hydrous, 730 mg citric acid anhydrous, and 2.45 g dextrose anhydrous. The infusion rate for AC is dependent on the total blood volume and type of replacement fluid (ml of AC/min/liter of total blood volume). The

Spectra control program will minimize the citrate reactions by adjusting this flow rate. The clinical condition may alternatively require the use of heparin. However, some centers will use the heparin from the ECMO circuit to anticoagulate the TPE circuit. Heparin binds antithrombin III and blocks clotting factor activity of VII, IX, X, XI, XII. The use of heparin requires the monitoring of clotting times. A convenient bedside determination of in vivo clotting is the measurement of an Activated Clotting Time (ACT). An accepted range for ACT's utilizing the I-stat® technique is 130-150 seconds, unless the ECMO patient requires increased anticoagulation. An ACT of 130 seconds may be within the "normal" range for blood clotting but the heparin should be infused directly into the circuit to perform regional anticoagulation of the circuit and minimize systemic anticoagulation and its associated complications.

Patient Care of ECMO TPE Patient

Full explanation and understanding is essential prior to the insertion of the venous access device as well as the actual apheresis procedure. Providing the patient and family with written materials about the purpose and benefits of the TPE procedure and allowing time to answer any questions or concerns before beginning the procedure promotes a better environment. Informed consent for the line placement, blood products and procedure is standard.

Orders include type of procedure, replacement fluid, volume to be processed, and ending fluid balance should all be checked and verified. The patient's height, weight, and gender are important for programming the machine. The baseline labs include a CBC, ionized calcium (ICA+), electrolytes, Mg (ionized or total?), PO_4, PT, PTT (for multiple runs, this is usually not needed because the patient is heparinized-you have to obtain a heparin absorbed sample to adequately assess the PT and PTT). Vital signs include EKG, temperature, B/P, and O_2 saturation. A detailed medication history is required. Continuous cardiac and O_2 saturation monitoring of all ECMO patients must occur during the procedure. Blood pressure and heart rate are recorded at least every 15 minutes. Some patients require pre-medication with Solu-Medrol ®, or Benadryl ®. Sedation and pain medication should be monitored

during this plasma dilution and replacement. During the treatment the patient must be monitored for signs of hypocalcemia, hypotension, hypothermia, or any signs of possible additional transfusion reactions. The ionized calcium is repeated at least one hour or midway into the procedure if citrate is infused. After the procedure, ICa^+, CBC, Mg^+, and PO_4^{-2} are measured. If the patient requires multiple treatments, protein, IgG, coagulation factors, and PT/PTT are measured. A hepabsorbed specimen may also be required to remove the heparin effect while evaluating other clotting factors and tendencies. Plasma/protein bound medications may also be removed during apheresis. A clinical assessment of the patient should be performed at the start of every procedure and includes vital signs, neurological status, and the examination of the extracorporeal circuit. The date and time of initiation of treatment must be recorded. The effluent color or texture of fluids, and any mechanical problems during treatment are recorded. Documentation should also include fluid replacement used, any change in patient status during treatment and any intervention, date and time of end of treatment, and the patient tolerance to treatment. Pretreatment labs and labs drawn during the treatment should also be recorded. Family understanding and participation should also be documented.

Complications

The Apheresis Program at Miami Children's Hospital began in 1994 and has provided care to over 230 patients with almost 1000 procedures in the first 12 years. Clinical events that required intervention occurred in 47% of our treatments, with one fatality. Decreased blood pressure was noted in 5.6%, increased blood pressure 3.5 %, hypocalcemia in 11%. Non-interventional events (nausea, vomiting, increased heart rate, tingling) occurred in 6.2% of patients. (Unpublished results, J Sussmane, MCH). Other complications of vascular access included hematoma at the site of catheter insertion, pneumo/hemothorax, retroperitoneal bleed, infection, thrombosis, and air embolism.

Hypocalcemia is the most frequent complication. The contributing factor is citrate anticoagulant in the PRBC bag, in the ACD-A (if used) and if FFP is used. The patient may complain of tingling/numbness of lips, fingers, or toes; at times, they may also feel lightheaded or dizzy. Although symptomatic monitoring may not be possible in sedated or paralyzed patients. In cases of severe hypocalcemia, the patient can develop dysrhythmias. The calcium in the blood binds to citrate causing gradual depletion of the circulating ionized calcium. Electrolytes are monitored before, during, and after each procedure with special emphasis on magnesium, ionized calcium, and potassium levels. For procedures more than an hour in length, the calcium levels must be monitored every hour until the end of the procedure. Calcium gluconate or calcium chloride drips can be infused throughout lengthy treatments. As an emergent response to arrhythmias, it is recommended to stop the procedure and administer IV calcium chloride. If the calcium level is within normal limits, the procedure can be resumed with ongoing calcium monitoring. The management of hypocalcemia includes slowing down the inlet flow (20 cc/min), sending a stat ionized calcium and giving calcium replacements such as calcium chloride 10% (20-25 mg/kg/dose) and calcium gluconate 100-500 mg/kg/d continuous drip in 4 divided doses.

Coagulation abnormalities are commonly twofold. First is a depletion of coagulation factors as they are removed during TPE. This can be compounded by the fact that albumin, or any replacement fluid, that does not contain coagulation factors will add a dilutional effect to the plasma. Recovery of coagulation factors is characterized by a rapid four hour increase and a slower rise in circulating cofactors during the next 24 hours after a single exchange. When multiple treatments are performed over a short period (three or more treatments per week), the depletion in clotting factors is more pronounced and may require several days for spontaneous recovery.[37] By using fresh frozen plasma as a replacement fluid, the risks of iatrogenic hemodilution of circulating coagulation cofactors can be minimized. There is an increased risk of using human products that should always be considered.[38] One of the other considerations in the use of FFP is the need to maintain antithrombin III levels for heparin effectiveness.

Transfusion Reaction – Contributing factors include ABO mismatch (not following blood bank and hospital protocols) and multiple transfusions. Prevention includes administration of leukodepleted blood product and pre-medication of sensitive patients. Patients that receive multiple treatments or transfusions may have a better response if an antihistamine is administered before treatment. When a transfusion reaction occurs, the procedure is discontinued and transfusion reaction protocols are followed. Maintain perfusion by giving crystalloids and osmotic diuretics. Check urine for hemolysis.[46] Thrombocytopenia can result from loss of platelets in the discarded plasma, during dilution, or via filter thrombosis. There is a greater loss of platelets using the centrifugal method than by membrane plasma separation. Wood and Jacobs (1986) have also shown decreases in the hematocrit by 10% after each plasmapheresis treatment in the absence of any extracorporeal losses or hemolysis.

Hypothermia – Contributing factors are due to the circuit exposure, the use of cold/cool replacement fluids, and patient size. It is also due to the rapid loss of circulating volume that patients may experience chills or shivering. Preventive measures include using warmed replacement fluids. Slowing down the inlet flow may improve hypothermia. It may help to also warm to the infusing replacement fluid via circuit warmer.

Apheresis Specialist Training and Competencies

An outline of our recommendations and guidelines to certify individuals as Apheresis Specialists upon successful completion of the following three modules:

Module I - Didactic - The Apheresis Specialist Candidate will complete 32 hours of didactic lectures. These hours will include a formal lecture program. Upon completion of these hours, a written test will be given. A passing score of 85% must be achieved.

Module II - Water Labs - The Apheresis Specialist Candidate will complete 8 hours of supervised water lab training plus a final test of Emergency Drills. This does not include individual practice sessions which are required in order to pass the final test. These practice hours will vary according to the individual's skill level but will not be less than 4 hours.

Module III - Clinical Orientation -The Apheresis Specialist Candidate will complete a minimum of 36 hours of clinical orientation. Upon completion of these hours, the Nurse Manager and Extracorporeal Coordinator of the ECLS Team will review the skills checklists. If any skill requirements have not been met, further bedside orientation may be warranted.

Re-certification – Emergency water lab check-off four times annually. Didactic and/or practical continuing education in the form of lectures, workshops, or animal laboratory experience of not less than eight (8) hours per year.

Planned maintenance, calibration testing and Procedure for equipment failure

The performance of all medical equipment is tested according to relevant standards by the clinical engineering department. A planned maintenance program and calibration testing that assures accuracy of equipment is performed by the clinical engineering department in collaboration with the apheresis section toestablish longevity of the system. All calibration and maintenance testing is based on the recommendation of the manufacturer.

In the event of equipment failure, notification to the service dispatch promptly occurs. The repair response is required within 24-hours. Once repair is completed, notification to the clinical engineering department is issued and all service repairs documentation are sent to the clinical engineering department for safe keeping and tracking.

Apheresis Check List

Patients Name:_____   Date:_____
Reviewed by Medical Director or Designee Date: _____ Signature:_____
Account#:_____   Apheresis Specialist_____

Date/Notes	Done	Procedure
		• Pheresis Consult obtained. o Attending notified.

		• Appropriate staff notified.
		  o Fellow on call.
		  o Nurse Manager/CNS

		• Family provided with Apheresis brochure, indications, risks, procedure and understanding of participation is documented.

		• Pre-apheresis criteria met:
		  o Informed consent /blood transfusion consent obtained
		  o Appropriate labs reviewed & parameters met.
		  o CBC with diff. (platelets > 50,000, Hgb > 8, Hct > 24).
		  o PT, PTT (<13 - ≤ 35)
		  o Ionized calcium (≥ 1.0)
		  o If patient is less than 18 kg, do type & cross match & sent to blood bank (request Hct on bag).

		• Labs reviewed by Physician & Apheresis specialist (H/H, PT, PTT, ICa⁺) Corrective action taken before procedure

		• Patient is prepared for Apheresis treatment
		  o Physician / Apheresis specialist evaluates patient, (including height (cm), weight (kg), & temperature.
		  o History/physical/medication assessment done.
		  o Patient/Family teaching reinforced. Consent reviewed. Documented in medical record.
		  o Patient sedation reviewed for procedure.
		  o Machine primed & ready for use

		• Patient's pre-pheresis condition reviewed & documented. Pheresis started.

		• Reassessment/document (mid-procedure) by Physician and Specialist:
		  o sedation status
		  o neuro status
		  o vital signs
		  o treatment tolerance
		  o evidence of hypocalcemia:
		• Patients condition reviewed & documented post procedure including:
		  o sedation status
		  o neuro status
		  o vital signs
		  o tolerance of procedure
		
		• Two hours post completion, obtain CBC, & ionized CA⁺
		• Procedure & condition reviewed with family and documented in medical record.

		• Quality Clinical Indicators Documented
		• Case reviewed by medical director, Nurse Manager and Team.
		• Quality Process control continued

References

1. Ni Maoshing, The Yellow Emperor's Classic of Medicine, Shambhala Publications, Inc. 1995

2. Kambic HE, Nose Y. Historical perspective on plasmapheresis. Therapeutic Apheresis, 1997. 1:83-108.

3. Friday J, Kaplan A. Indications for therapeutic plasma exchange. Up-To-Date www.uptodateonline.com. Accessed January 13, 2005.

4. Madore F. Plasmapheresis: technical aspects and indications. Crit Care Clin. 2002; 8:375-392.

5. McMaster P., Shann F; The use of Extracorporeal Techniques to remove humoral factors in sepsis, Pediatr Crit Care med. 2003;30,4(1):2-7

6. Pisani E. Regulatory framework for plasmapheresis in the European Union: industry's viewpoint. Hematology & Cell Therapy, 1996, 38 Suppl 1:S35-38.

7. Clark WF, Rock GA, Buskard N, et.al. Therapeutic plasma exchange: An update from the Canadian Apheresis Group. Ann Int Med. 1999; 131:453-462.

8. Linenberger ML. Price TH. Use of cellular and plasma apheresis in the critically-ill patient: Part 1: technical and physiological considerations. J Int Care Med. 2005; 20:18-27.

9. Kellum JA, Venkataraman R. Blood purification in sepsis: an idea whose time has come. Crit Care Med. 2002; 30:1387–1388.

10. Busund R, Koukline V, Utrobin U, et al. E Plasmapheresis in severe sepsis and septic shock: a prospective, randomised, controlled trial. Int Care Med. 2002; 28:1434-1439.

11. Custis, George Washington Parke, Recollections of Washington (1860); " The Death of George Washington, 1799"

12. Malchesky PS. Sueoka A. Matsubara S. et al. Membrane plasma separation. 1983. Therapeutic Apheresis. 2000; 4:47-53.

13. Yeh JH, Chen WH, Chiu HC. Complications of double-filtration plasmapheresis. Transfusion. 2004; 44:1621-1625.

14. Unger JK, Haltern C, Dohmen B, et al. Maximal flow rates and sieving coefficients in different plasmafilters: effects of increased membrane surfaces and effective length under standard-ized in vitro conditions. J Clin Apheresis. 2002; 17:190-198.

15. Gurland HJ, Lysaght MJ, Samtleben W, et al. A comparison of centrifugal and membrane-based apheresis formats. Int J Artif Org. 1984; 7:35-38.

16. Madore F. Plasmapheresis. Technical aspects and indications. Crit Care Clinics. 2002; 18:375-392.

17. DePalo T, Giordano M, Bellantuono, et al. Therapeutic apheresis in children, Int J Artif Org. 2000; 23:834-839.

18. Rock G, Buskard NA. Therapeutic plasmapheresis. Curr Opin Hematol. 1996; 3:504-510.

19. Nenov VD, Marinov P, Sabeva J. Current applications of plasmapheresis in clinical toxicology. Nephrol Dial Transp. 2003; 18 Suppl 5:56-58.

20. Pond SM. Extracorporeal techniques in the treatment of poisoned patients. Med J Aust. 1991; 155:62-63.

21. Motohashi K, Yamane S. The effect of apheresis on adhesion molecules. Therapeutic Apheresis & Dialysis: Journal of the International Society for Apheresis, the Japanese Society for Apheresis, the Japanese Society for Dialysis Therapy. 2003; 7:425-430.

22. Gardlund B, Sjolin J, Nilsson A, et al. Plasma levels of cytokines in primary septic shock in humans: correlation with disease severity. J Inf Dis. 1995; 172:296–301.

23. Pisani BA, Mullen GM, Malinowska K, et.al, Plasmapheresis with intravenous immunoglobulin G is effective in patients with elevated panel reactive antibody prior to cardiac transplantation. J Heart Lung Transplant. 1999; 18:701-706.

24. Warren DS, Zachary AA, Sonnenday CJ,. et al. Successful renal transplantation across simultaneous ABO incompatible and positive crossmatch barriers. Am J Transp. 2004; 4:561-568.

25. Abraham KA, Brown C, Conlon PJ, et al. Plasmapheresis as rescue therapy in accelerated acute humoral rejection. J Clin Apheresis. 2003; 18:103-110.

26. Debray D, Furlan V, Baudoouin V, et. al, Therapy for acute rejection in pediatric organ transplant recipients. Pediatr Drugs. 2003; 5:81-93.

27. Stegmayr B. Plasmapheresis in severe sepsis or septic shock. Blood Purif. 1996; 14:94–101.

28. McMaster P, Shann F. The use of extracorporeal techniques to remove humoral factors in sepsis. Ped Crit Care Med. 2003; 4:2-7.

29. Busund R, Koukline V, Utrobin U, et al. E Plasmapheresis in severe sepsis and septic shock: a prospective, randomised, controlled trial. Int Care Med. 2002; 28:1434-1439.

30. Felson DT, LaValley MP, Baldassare Ar, et. at, The Prosorba column for the treatment of refractory rheumatoid arthritis: a randomized double-blind, sham-controlled trial. Arthritis Rheum. 1999; 42:2153-2159.

31. Aoki H, Kodama M, Tani T, et al. Treatment of sepsis by extracorporeal elimination of endotoxin using polymyxin B-immobilized fiber. Am J Surg. 1994; 167:412–417.

32. Gorlin JB. Therapeutic plasma exchange and cytapheresis in pediatric patients. Transfus Sci. 1999; 21:21-39.

33. Urbaniak SJ. Therapeutic plasma and cellular apheresis. Clinics in Haematology. 1984; 13:217-251.

34. Grima KM. Therapeutic apheresis in hematological and oncological diseases. J Clin Apheresis. 2000; 15:28-52.

35. Kliman A, Carbone PP, Gaydos LA, et al. Effects of intensive plasmapheresis on normal blood donors. Blood.1964; 23:647-656.

36. Pahl E, Crawford SE, Cohn RA, et al. Reversal of severe late left ventricular failure after pediatric heart transplantation and possible role of Plasmapheresis. Am J Cardiol. 2000; 85:735-739.

37. Berlot G, Tomasini A, Silvestri L, et al. Plasmapheresis in the critically-ill patient. Kidney International - Supplement. 1998; 66:S178-181.

38. Baldini GM, Silvestri MG. Quality assurance in hemapheresis: quality of fresh frozen plasma. Int J Artif Organs. 1993; 16 Suppl 5:226-228.

39. Strauss RG. Apheresis donor safety--changes in humoral and cellular immunity. J Clin Apheresis. 1984; 2:68-80.

Chapter 18 Questions

1) What does apheresis mean?
2) Name the three modalities of Apheresis.
3) Name three common indications for Plasmapheresis.
4) Where does the inflow portion of the Pheresis circuit become attached to the ECMO circuit?
5) Where does the outflow portion of the Pheresis circuit become attached to the ECMO circuit?
6) A "one volume" plasma exchange will exchange what percentage of the circulating blood volume?
7) A "two volume" plasma exchange will exchange what percentage of the circulating blood volume?
8) What is the most common complication of a Pheresis patient?

Chapter 18 Answers

1. "to take away, withdraw or separate"
2. Plasmapheresis, Erythrocytapheresis, Leukopheresis
3. Sepsis, Guillian Barre, Myasthenia
4. Inflow is attached before the bladder on the venous line
5. Outflow is attached after the inflow but before the raceway
6. 63%
7. 86%
8. Hypocalcemia

19

Cooling Neonates for Cerebral Protection on ECMO

Stephen Baumgart, MD

Objectives

After completion of this chapter, the participant should be able to:

- Discuss cooling criteria, candidates/non-candidates
- Outline the technique of whole body cooling while on ECMO
- Describe monitoring while cooling, esp. coagulation while on ECMO
- Describe outcome of patients treated with cooling while on ECMO

Introduction:

Therapeutic hypothermia has been introduced recently for treating a highly select population of near-term/term neonates with hypoxic-ischemic insults manifesting shortly after birth (<6 hours). Two recent studies[1, 2] suggest that cerebral cooling with either whole body cooling (to 33.5°C, 92°F core esophageal temperature, ie, moderate hypothermia), or selective head cooling (10°C, 50°F along with mild whole-body cooling to a core temperature of 34°C, 93°F) reduces the risk for death or moderate to severe neurological sequelae from >60% to <50% (Figure 1).[1] The (NICHD) Experts Panel Workshop held in May 2005 emphasized the need to use standardized protocols for hypothermia treatment and to provide continual follow-up until school age to develop and refine therapy for hypoxic-ischemic brain injury.[3]

Definitions for Hypothermia.

Gunn & Gunn have suggested the following classification for degrees of hypothermia: mild 1-3°C below normal (*ie* from 37°C down to about 34°C); moderate 4-6°C below normal down to 31°C; severe 8-10°C below normal down to 27°C; and profound ≥15-20°C below normal to as low as 15°C- sometimes performed with deep hypothermic circulatory arrest during surgical repair of complex congenital heart disease.[4]

- Mild hypothermia 36-34°C
- Moderate hypothermia 33-31°C
- Severe hypothermia 30-27°C
- Profound or deep hypothermia 26-15°C

Monitoring During Hypothermia.

Esophageal, abdominal skin, and axillary temperatures are monitored and recorded every 15 minutes for the first 4 hours of cooling, every hour for the next 8 hours, and every 4 hours during the remaining 72 hour period of hypothermia. Above all, hyperthermia >37.5°C axillary temperature is avoided, since fever in this setting contributes to brain injury.[5]

Infants otherwise receive routine clinical care, including the continuous monitoring of vital signs (mild sinus bradycardia 80-90 beats-per-minute, and a small decrease in blood pressure usually <10 mm Hg are commonly observed, and rarely require but are responsive to intervention with volume infusion and/or pressor therapy) and pulse-oximetry (usually normal). Additionally, frequent surveillance blood samples for in particular: blood counts and electrolyte disturbances: (hyper-, hypo-kalemia,

FIGURE 1. Neonatal Network (data adapted[1])

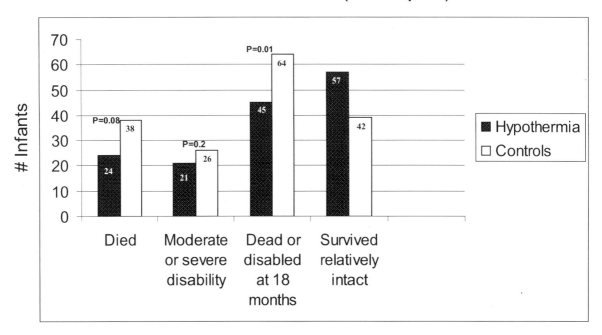

Figure 1. Results of the Neonatal Network Hypothermia Trial (Adapted from data by Shankaran S, Laptook AR, Ehrenkkranz RA, Tyson JE, McDonald SA, Donovan EF, Fanaroff AA, Poole WK, Wright LL, Higgins RD, Finer NN, Carlo WA, Duara S, Oh W, Cotton CM, Stevenson DK, Stoll BJ, Lemons JA, Guillet R, Jobe AH, for the NICHHD, Neonatal Research Network: Whole-body hypothermia for neonates with Hypoxic-ischemic encephalopathy. N Engl J Med 2005; 353:1574-84).[1] They reported 64/106 contol infants were dead or seriously disabled at 18-22 months of age and of these 38 had died, i.e. [64-38] left 26 seriously disabled survivors. From a study population of 106 control infants 68 survived; i.e. [68-26 disabled] leaves 42 survivors relatively intact. They also reported 45/102 hypothermic infants were dead or disabled at 18-22 months with 24 having died, leaving 21 seriously disabled subjects. From 102 treated infants 78 survived; i.e. [78-21] or 57 survived relatively intact. The authors additionally reported, however, that primary outcome data was available for 205 of the 208 infants enrolled. Of the three infants lost to follow-up, we presumed all survived and this may favorably bias these survival-intact estimates represented in this figure.

hyper-, hypo-natremia [SIADH], calcium and magnesium, hypo- hyper-glycemia), coagulopathy (PT/PTT, platelets and fibrinogen), and for major organ dysfunction (*eg*, liver enzymes, ALT/AST), which may all be altered during moderate hypothermia. Serial blood gas determinations are included to monitor and treat in particular pH, ventilatory, and acid-base disturbances. Blood gas data should be adjusted for temperature at 33.5°C and during re-warming. We perform these blood studies at 6, 12, 14, 36, 48, 60, 72, 96, and 120 hours after initiating hypothermia and during re-warming. Most ECMO centers additionally monitor ACT's during heparin infusion for bypass, and we recommend using the same protocol guidelines while cooling asphyxi-

ated babies on bypass with particular attention to maintaining plasma fibrinogen and platelets within normal ranges.

EEG Monitoring During Hypothermia.

We provide continuous EEG neuro-monitoring as part of our hypothermia protocol, although the EEG is not included in our clinical criteria for initiating hypothermia.[1] A full montage video-EEG (modified International 10-20 system for newborns) is recorded by computer for about 96 hours to include cooling and recovery periods. Using raw EEG data, amplitude-integrated EEG (aEEG) is also reviewed for characterization of background

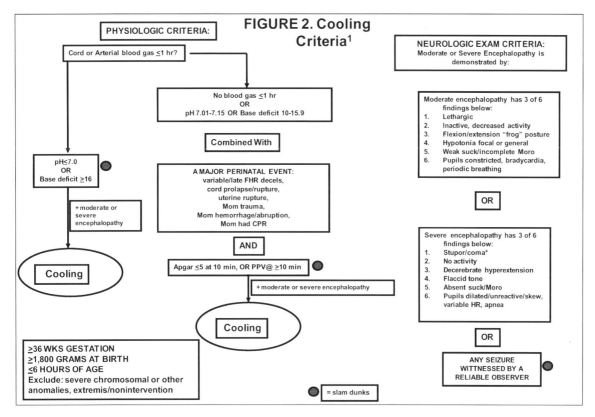

Figure 2. Summary diagram of criteria for initiating moderate whole body hypothermia for cerebral protection in moderate to severely asphyxiated neonates. (Adapted from Shankaran S, Laptook AR, Ehrenkkranz RA, Tyson JE, McDonald SA, Donovan EF, Fanaroff AA, Poole WK, Wright LL, Higgins RD, Finer NN, Carlo WA, Duara S, Oh W, Cotton CM, Stevenson DK, Stoll BJ, Lemons JA, Guillet R, Jobe AH, for the NICHHD, Neonatal Research Network: Whole-body hypothermia for neonates with Hypoxic-ischemic encephalopathy. N Engl J Med 2005; 353:1574-84).[1]

pattern and detection of seizures. Seizure detection is confirmed on raw EEG data and therapy provided (e.g., Phenobarbital).

Criteria for Infants Eligible for Cooling.[Figure 2]

To receive cooling therapy, infants must be more than or equal to **36 weeks completed** gestation, must arrive for treatment **within six hours of birth** and have experienced a hypoxic-ischemic (HI) insult. Moribund infants not receiving resuscitation and life support are obviously excluded. Premature neonates are also excluded since hypothermia in this population is associated with increased mortality.[6] Evidence of HI injury includes: requirement for resuscitation at delivery (in particular an Apgar score ≤5 requiring positive pressure ventilation at 10 minutes of life), arterial/venous/mixed umbilical vessel blood pH of ≤7.00, or having a significant base deficit of at least -16 mEq/L. Also qualifying for therapy are blood gas disturbances within the first hour of life with pH 7.01-7.15 and/or a base deficit between -10 to -15.9 mEq/L, along with an ominous perinatal history (fetal heart rate decelerations, umbilical cord prolapse or rupture, uterine rupture, severe maternal trauma preceding birth, and abruption of the placenta, or the expectant mother experienced any life-threatening event requiring CPR). Clinical signs of a moderate to severe encephalopathy must also be present (an infant who is lethargic, or completely stuporous, has diminished or completely absent activity and muscle tone, having weak or absent sucking and Moro reflexes, with fixed-constricted or unresponsive dilated pupils, having fixed flexion or extension posturing of extremities, or a seizure observed by an experienced clinician). Infants with such symptoms persisting for several days have about a 60 percent risk for death before hospital discharge, while a majority of survivors experience moderate to severe life-long neuro-developmental disabilities (cerebral palsy, deafness, blindness, mental retardation, and/or recurrent seizure disorder)(Figure 1).[1, 7]

Performing Hypothermia.

Infants meeting these criteria are placed supine at admission and before 6 hours of age[8] (wearing only a diaper) onto a water-filled cooling blanket, pre-cooled to 5°C (41°F- similar to a household refrigerator box temperature, eg 37°F). We use a Blanketrol II Hyper-Hypothermia System, Cincinnati Sub-Zero Inc., a device familiar to our ER and OR staff where it's used to reduce high fevers in young children. This same device was used in the Neonatal Network trial.[1] A warmed, flexible esophageal temperature probe is then positioned in the distal third of the esophagus (measured nares-to-auditory meatus-to-xyphoid process and minus 2 cm), and the water mattress cooling unit's thermostatic-controller is then immediately set to 33.5°C. Blanket water temperature rapidly cools the baby (30-40 minutes), then water temperature increases to about 34°C (93°F) to maintain the esophageal probe at 33.5°C.[1] A second, larger pediatric-size blanket is also attached parallel into the cooling system. Water circulates through both blankets with the larger blanket hung on an IV rack at bedside serving as a capacitor to diminish fluctuations in the esophageal temperature (to less than ±1.0 C).[9] Although we use a warmer bed platform as a convenient crib, the over-head warmer is not turned-on during the cooling period. Abdominal-wall skin temperature is also monitored with a surface probe, available with the warmer bed (in monitoring mode, warmer off). With esophageal temperature set to 33.5°C, we've observed that the majority of heat loss occurs via surface cooling.[10, 11]

After 72 hours at the set point of 33.5°C, the automatic controller on the cooling system is increased by 0.5°C per hour, and blanket re-warming occurs. After six hours, the esophageal probe and cooling blankets are removed, and the anterior abdominal wall skin temperature is then regulated using the radiant warmer's servomechanism set at 36.5°C (**warmer on**). Body temperature is monitored at a separate site (usually axillary) as a safety precaution to prevent hyperthermia >37.5°C.[12] The purpose for re-warming slowly is to avoid rapid shifts in critical electrolytes (calcium and potassium). Cardiac arrhythmias (ventricular tachycardia), fever, and seizures were observed more commonly with rewarming during the Network study[1], and in particular re-warming overshoot (fever >37.5°C either axillary or esophageal) is to be avoided by reducing the warming device servo-control in 0.5°C increments.[5]

Performing Hypothermia While on ECMO.

We've envisioned three scenarios combining whole body cooling therapy for asphyxia-related encephalopathy with ECLS on ECMO: [1] an infant is admitted who first meets criteria for cooling then while already hypothermic additionally meets criteria for ECMO and continues esophageal temperature maintenance at 33.5°C completing 72 hours at this temperature while on bypass, who is then rewarmed while on bypass to 36.5°C; [2] an infant is admitted who meets criteria for both cooling and ECMO concurrently, spending the first 72 hours at 33.5°C who is then rewarmed on bypass; and [3] an infant starts cooling after an event on bypass, and continues cooling while coming off of bypass and is subsequently rewarmed. We've only actually encountered the first two scenarios, and have eluded perinatal asphyxia while on ECMO. Resuscitation with ECMO with and without whole body cooling is under investigation by the Neonatal Network, and a multi-center randomized control trial is planned.

Four of our 44 hypothermia treated patients have required ECMO during cooling at esophageal temperature 33.5°C. The primary implement for maintaining systemic hypothermia was the ECMO apparatus' servo-regulated water-bath/blood warmer device with or without the concomitant use of the

FIGURE 3. ECMO Circuit with Temperature Probe

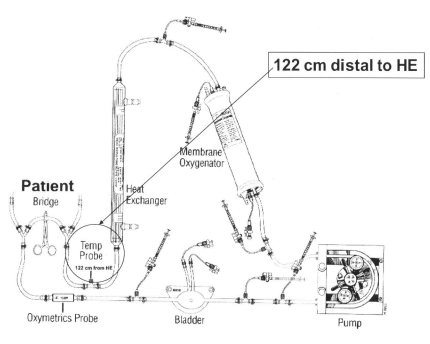

Figure 3. Schematic diagram of our ECMO circuit , Medtronics, Minneapolis, MN, demonstrating the location of the blood-path temperature monitoring probe 122 cm distal to the heat exchanger and proximate to the arterial cannula entering the baby's core circulation.

Blanketrol cooling unit. We've demonstrated two methods for cooling babies on ECMO.[13]

In three cases (**Method 1**), the primary implement for maintaining systemic hypothermia was the ECMO apparatus' servo-regulated water-bath/blood warmer (also a Cincinnati Sub-Zero device) set between 33.0-33.5°C. Blood path temperature was monitored proximate to the arterial cannula, and 122 cm distal to the heat-exchanger (HE).(Figure 3) This length of non-warmed tubing results in some environmental cooling of the blood path by about 1.5-2°C before reaching the infant. Infant core esophageal temperature was measured continuously using the Blanketrol II cooling unit in the **monitor only** mode. The temperature on the ECMO water bath (initially set at 33.5°C) was adjusted in ±0.2°C increments until the core esophageal probe temperature stabilized to read at or near a constant 33.5°C (Figure 4). Patient #3 had CDH, presented with HI injury at birth, and went directly onto ECMO

and cooling was initiated and maintained via this method. Blood path temperature was noted to be consistently lower than the target 33.5°C, leading to lower and variable esophageal temperatures (Figure 4). The patient subsequently withdrew from ECMO support due to a pulmonary hemorrhage after 4 hours on ECMO/cooling.

In the most recent case (**Method 2**), we set the Cincinnati Sub-Zero water bath on the ECMO cart to be constant at 35.0°C. In our circuit (Medtronics, Minneapolis, MN), the blood path temperature probe is 122 cm distal to the HE and reliably revealed blood temperature entering the baby at 33.5°C. We continued managing the baby on the cooling blanket as well, set to automatically control our target esophageal temperature to 33.5°C. During rewarming, both temperatures were increased by 0.5°C/hr until the baby's esophageal temperature reached 36.5°C. Patient #4 was started on ECMO for worsening pulmonary hypertension after 24

FIGURE 4. Patient #3 cooled via Method 1 (ECMO water bath, manually adjusted)

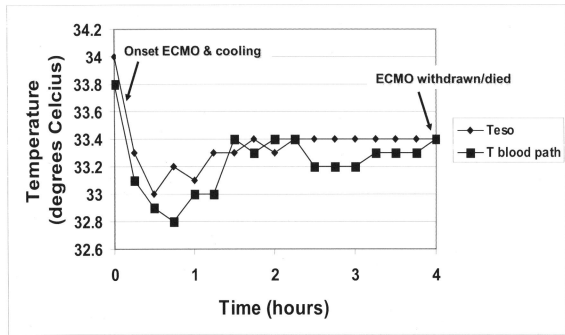

Figure 4. Cooling temperatures using only the ECMO circuit's heat exchanger water bath. The cooling blanket has been removed, and the esophageal temperature is monitored while the water bath temperature is manually "tweaked" in ±0.2°C increments by the ECMO specialist. Some variation in temperature is seen, probably from overdampening in the operater's response.

FIGURE 5. Patient #4 cooled via Method 2 (ECMO water bath + Blanketrol)

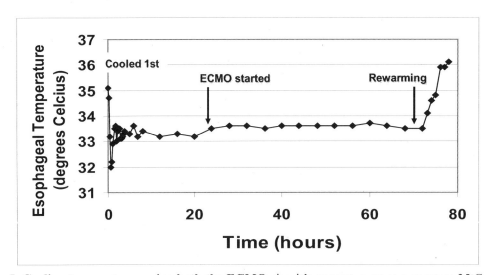

Figure 5. Cooling temperatures using both the ECMO circuit's apparatus set at a constant 35°C, and the cooling blanket servo-regulated to maintain esophageal temperature at 33.5°C. Varience in esophageal temperature is minimized at ≤1.5 %.[13]

hours of cooling and was maintained via this latter method. Of the four cases, this resulted in the least esophageal temperature variation (Figure 5).

Temperature variance for this method was only 1.5% including cooling induction (range 35.1-32.0°C).We suggest the latter method preferred for maintaining whole-body hypothermia when treating asphyxiated infants on ECMO.

Editorial

Giles J Peek MD FRCS

There is no doubt that hypothermia is a powerful weapon in the armamentarium against brain injury. ECMO provides unprecedented control over body temperature and makes it extremely easy to induce therapeutic hypothermia. This is well tolerated and theoretical fears regarding altered coagulation have not lead to problems in clinical practice. The duration of hypothermia is an interesting question, some authorities opining that the longer duration the better the effect, but 72 hours seems to be the accepted norm in 2009. In the UK we have been conducting a randomised controlled trial of therapeutic hypothermia in babies receiving ECMO (NEST,Neonatal ECMO Study of Temperature, IS-RCTN72635512) which has been recruiting since June 2006 and has enrolled 102 out of a total sample size of 118 patients (14/11/2009). The protocol can be downloaded from http://www.npeu.ox.ac.uk/nest. Hopefully by the time you are reading this chapter the results should be published. In terms of practical application of hypothermia, avoidance of rapid changes in temperature is important. I particularly enjoyed the authors elegant solution to this problem of using an additional water blanket hung on a drip stand as a thermal "compliance chamber" to smooth the temperature fluctuations. In our experience we have found urinary catheters with integral temperature probes an efficient method of monitoring patient temperature as esophageal probes can be easily displaced when the patient is moved.

References

1. Shankaran S, Laptook AR, Ehrenkkranz RA, Tyson JE, McDonald SA, Donovan EF, Fanaroff AA, Poole WK, Wright LL, Higgins RD, Finer NN, Carlo WA, Duara S, Oh W, Cotton CM, Stevenson DK, Stoll BJ, Lemons JA, Guillet R, Jobe AH, for the NICHHD, Neonatal Research Network: Whole-body hypothermia for neonates with Hypoxic-ischemic encephalopathy. N Engl J Med 2005; 353:1574-84.

2. Gluckman PD, Wyatt JS, Azzopardi D, Ballard R, Edwards DA, Ferriero DM, Polin RA, Robertson CM, Thoreson M, Whtelaw A, Gunn AJ, CoolCap study group: Selective head-cooling with mild systemic hypothermia after neonatal encephalopathy: Multi-center randomized trial. Lancet 2005, 395:365-70.

3. Higgins RD, et al.: "Hypothermia and Perinatal Asphyxia: Executive Summary of the National Institute of Child Health and Human Development Workshop. J Pediatr, 2006; 148:170-5.

4. Gunn AJ & Gunn TR: The 'pharmacology' of neuronal rescue with cerebral hypothermia. Early Human Development, 1998; 53:19–35.

5. Yager JY, Armstrong EA, Jaharus C, Saucier DM, Wirrell EC: Preventing Hyperthermia Decreases Brain Damage Following Neonatal Hypoxic-Ischemic Seizures. Brain Research, 2004; 1011:48-57.

6. Silverman WA, Fertig JW, Berger AP: The influence of the thermal environment upon the survival of the newly born premature infant, Pediatrics, 1958; 22:876-886.

7. Sarnat HB & Sarnat MS: Neonatal encephalopathy following fetal distress. Arch Neurol, 1976; 33:696-705.

8. Gunn AJ, Gunn TR, deHaan, Williams CE, Gluckman PD: Dramatic neuronal rescue with prolonged selective head cooling after ischemia in fetal lambs. J. Clin Invest, 1997; 99:248-256.

9. Shankaran S, Laptook A, Wright LL, Ehrenkranz A, Donovan EF, Fanaroff AA, Stark AR, Tyson JE, Poole K, Carlo WA, Lemons, JA, Oh W, Stoll, BJ, Papile LA, Bauer CR, Stevenson DK, Korones SB, McDonald S: Whole-Body Hypothermia for Neonatal Encephalopathy: Animal Observations as a Basis for a Random-

ized, Controlled Pilot Study in Term Infants. Pediatrics, 2002; 110:377-85.

10. Baumgart S, Massaro A, Chang T, Glass P, Tsuchida T and Short BL: Whole Body Cooling Therapy: Is It Really a Cooling Mattress? Abstract, Published: Society for Pediatric Research, Toronto, May 2007.

11. Stayer SA, Steven JM, Nicolson SC, Jobes DR, Stanley C, Baumgart S: The metabolic effects of surface cooling neonates prior to cardiac surgery. Anesthesia and Analgesia, 79:834-839, 1994.

12. Mayfield SR, Bhatia J, Nakamura KT, Rios GR, Bell EF. Temperature measurement in term and preterm neonates. J Pediatr 1984;104:271-275.

13. Baumgart S, Massaro A, Chang T, Glass P, Tsuchida T and Short BL: Therapeutic Hypothermia and ECMO. Accepted for presentation, 23rd Annual CNMC-ECMO Symposium, Feb 2007, Published: Society for Pediatric Research, Toronto, May 2007.

Chapter 19 Questions

1. The complications of moderate whole body hypothermia include which of the following:
   a) mild bradycardia
   b) cardiac stun
   c) suppression of clotting ability
   d) seizures, or cold induced brain coma

2. Moderate whole body cooling has been studied extensively at what temperature(s):
   a) 33.5±0.5°C esophageal
   b) 34.0°C deep rectal (5 cm beyond the anal verge)
   c) 36.5°C axillary
   d) all of the above

3. Which of the following are criteria for initiating whole body cooling?
   a) Gestation ≥36 completed weeks at birth
   b) post-natal age ≤6 hours
   c) Umbilical cord blood pH ≤7.00 or base deficit ≥16
   d) Any clinically observed seizure
   e) All of the above

Chapter 19 Answers

1. a. and c.
2. a. only
3. e.

Responsibilities of the ECMO Specialists and RN Staff

Lisa Williams, MHA, BSN, RNC-NIC and Billie Lou Short, MD

Objectives

After completion of this chapter, the participant should be able to:

- Define the role of the bedside RN, RT, and ECMO Specialist
- Outline the role for each individual in emergencies
- Outline the role of each individual for routine care

Introduction

ECMO is established and coordinated by many different disciplines in the various hospitals. Medical management of the ECMO patient is dependent on the case. In our organization newborn respiratory cases are managed by the Neonatologist on clinical service, neonatal heart patients are managed by the Critical Care ECMO attending, and pediatric respiratory cases are managed by the Critical Care ECMO attending. The bedside ECMO Specialist is either an RN or RT specially trained in ECMO and is responsible for managing the ECMO patient, under the direction of the ECMO physician. The ECMO Specialist and bedside nurse work together in the care of the patient, each with specific roles and responsibilities as outlined in the next sections. Care of the ECMO patient with cardiac disease is covered in a separate chapter.

Responsibilities of the ECMO Specialist and the Nursing Staff

Caring for the patient on ECMO is similar to the care of any critically ill patient requiring intense medical intervention. Additional care involves managing the ECMO circuit, which is the responsibility of the ECMO specialist. The specialist, bedside nurse, and ECMO physician need to work together as a team with other personnel. Issues that arise during the course of the ECMO therapy will need to be discussed between the nurse, specialist, and ECMO physician, to provide a complete and organized plan of care. Family involvement is another important component of planning care for the ECMO patient. The bedside nurse and specialist's responsibilities will vary from one ECMO center to another.

Patients receiving ECMO therapy have a variety of needs. Nursing care is vital to the stabilization and management of these patients. Pairing of these patients will depend on the policies of each institution, the experience of the ECMO specialist, and the acuity of the patient. Written guidelines outlining the staffing requirements for different levels of patients may be helpful in planning for staffing purposes.

In addition to routine cares, nursing actions will be focused primarily on observation of the patient's vital signs, detection of changes in clinical status, and prevention of complications. The ECMO patient is extremely vulnerable to multiple and catastrophic complications, and nursing care can be the most effective way to avoid some of these problems.

Patient Assessment – Dual Responsibilities:

A. Patient Procedures

Any procedure that requires moving the patient such as x-ray or evaluation of skin integrity, etc. requires the bedside RN and the ECMO Specialist to work together. The ECMO specialist is responsible for the ECMO catheters, assuring that they are not kinked or moved improperly during the procedure. If there is concern about movement of the patient, the ECMO physician should be called to the bedside to assist.

Patient movement to other areas of the hospital for tests and procedures (CT, cardiac catheterization) has become more commonplace. A policy or guideline written by key members off your ECMO team will help to guide staff who are not accustomed to moving ECMO patients. This policy/guideline should include the number and type of staff needed to move and their roles, necessary supplies and equipment, and a checklist to be used to assess readiness before moving. In general, a member of the ECMO team takes the lead role and is responsible for guarding the cannulas during transport as well as controlling the speed/flow of transport.

B. Neurologic Assessment

The most serious complications observed in ECMO patients have been central nervous system (CNS) related. CNS problems appear to be related to hypoxia, acidosis, hypercarbia, or other insults suffered prior to ECMO. Frequent neurologic checks should be performed, including: fullness of the fontanelle (as applicable), reflexes, movement, pupil size, level of consciousness, and presence of seizure activity. One of the first signs that a patient has had an intraventricular hemorrhage (IVH) is the cessation of spontaneous respirations, or dramatic changes in BP, blood pH and hematocrit. If this occurs, a neuro check should be performed immediately and the ECMO physician should be notified. Obtaining a hemoglobin and hematocrit (H/H) can assist in determining if a bleed has occurred. Keep in mind that a low pump PCO_2 and over sedation can also cause the patient to become apneic. Review the patient sedation record and obtain a pump gas before taking any further action.

C. Cardiovascular Assessment

Once on bypass, the ventilator settings will be dramatically reduced to minimize barotraumas, in most patients. The patient is critically ill; their condition is still labile. Patients should have minimal

handling and a quiet environment. Nursing and medical procedures should be coordinated, allowing the patient long periods of rest. Maintaining a neutral thermal environment (unless otherwise indicated) and offering comfort measures, such as bundling, will not only serve as a restraining measure but also as a comfort/sedative measure. By keeping the patient quiet and calm, their oxygen consumption will be decreased. Sedation should be given as ordered, in an effort to maintain oxygen consumption to a minimum without decreasing the patient's respiratory drive.

Nursing care of the ECMO patient involves frequent observation of the patient's vital signs (VS). VS should be obtained hourly, from the monitor, so that early detection of problems or complications can be dealt with in a timely fashion. "Hands-on" care, including VS, should be done every four hours in an effort to cluster care. Provision for a neutral thermal environment (NTE) is an important factor in decreasing metabolic oxygen requirements. Hypothermia will significantly increase oxygen consumption and can promote pulmonary vasoconstriction. These conditions promote hypoxia and acidosis which notably decrease surfactant production. Axillary temperatures should be done every 4 hours and PRN for temperature instability. Overhead warmer and/or the ECMO water baths can be adjusted to effect a change in the patient's temperature. The bedside nurse and specialist will work together to determine which method should be used, as to avoid warming or cooling the patient too quickly.

Patent ductus arteriosis (PDA) should be suspected in any neonatal ECMO patient with persistently poor perfusion, low urine output, acidemia, and/or low PO_2 despite increasing bypass flows. A systolic murmur may not always be audible if the ductus is opening and closing or if it is very large. Other symptoms may include an active precordium, bounding pulses, crackling rales, and tachycardia. These patients are usually treated with fluid restriction and diuretic therapy to decrease the intravascular volume.

Cardiac Stun is the partial or total absence of the ventricular component of the cardiac output. The cause of Cardiac Stun is not well understood. The patient will develop an aortic pulse pressure of

< 5mmHg and a PO_2 nearly equivalent to the Pump PO_2. The phenomenon is transient and usually lasts for 1 - 64 hours.

D. Respiratory Assessment

A thorough respiratory assessment should be performed on the ECMO patient every 4 hours. Through inspection, auscultation, and close clinical observation, the ECMO specialist and nurse can identify potential complications and evaluate the infant's response to treatment. A daily chest x-ray should be done on all ECMO patients. Observation of the quality of respirations and the skin color should be done before disturbing the patient. Respiratory effort is usually irregular in rate and shallow, primarily abdominal (infants) rather than thoracic breathing. During the initial days on ECMO, the patient's breath sounds will be difficult to auscultate, with minimal air entry noted. The reduction of the ventilator settings during the ECMO course causes a collapse of the lungs, usually producing a typical "white out" appearance on the chest x-ray. As the lungs and the patient's respiratory effort improve, so too will the breath sounds and x-ray. The nurse should observe the patient for signs and symptoms of atelectasis, i.e. unequal breath sounds, elevated PCO_2, acidosis, and hypoxia. Some of these symptoms will not be as evident, as the patient is on bypass. Vigilant pulmonary care including endotracheal tube (ETT) suctioning every 4 hours is needed to maintain patency of the ETT and clear secretions. Care should be exercised so that the suction catheter does not extend beyond the end of the ETT, causing trauma and potential pulmonary bleeding. Despite careful suctioning of these patients, sometimes bleeding will occur. The observation of blood (bright or dark red) in the ETT secretions requires attention. Increasing the PEEP or Peak Inspiratory Pressure (PIP) will help to control or stop the bleeding. Chest physiotherapy (CPT) may be done in some institutions to help mobilize secretions. "Sigh bagging" the patient for five (5) minutes after suctioning may help in the re-expansion of the atelectatic lungs.

Pediatric and adult patients with significant lung injury requiring prolonged ECMO runs may have collapsed lungs for a period of time. Sometimes, no breath sounds can be auscultated.

E. Fluid, Electrolytes and Nutrition

Record all intake and output accurately - include blood removed for all lab tests, blood gases and ACTs and all drainage from chest tubes, wounds, hemofiltration. Record urine output. Replace outputs as ordered by physician. Monitoring of the patient's hematocrit should be done every 12 hours and more frequently if bleeding is an issue.

Maintenance IV fluids, HAL, IL, and Heparin drips are administered into the ECMO circuit or the patient, depending upon institutional policy. Whole blood glucose should be monitored every 6-8 hours and PRN. The major causes of hyperglycemia in ECMO patients are stress and sepsis. ECMO patients who are septic or hypothermic may also become hypoglycemic. Hypothermia will cause the infant to rapidly decrease body stores of brown fat to increase heat production. This metabolic process produces heat but also requires oxygen and glucose to complete the process. NOTE: Maintenance IVs, vasoactives and sedative/narcotic drips are infused via the patient's central line in cardiac, pediatric, and adult ECMO patients unless there is limited IV access.

Abdominal girths should be measured every four hours. An increasing abdominal girth could indicate excessive air in the stomach/bowel, or bleeding into the abdomen. The nurse should check the placement and reposition the OG tube for optimal drainage of air and secretions. The abdominal distention can inhibit diaphragmatic breathing, which could result in hypoventilation, especially when the patient is on low bypass flows. If the patient has excessive OG drainage, the ECMO physician should notified, as it may indicate a need for replacements for an electrolyte loss. Gastrointestinal hemorrhage can occur while on bypass. If the OG drainage is coffee ground in appearance, the physician will order antacids (i.e., Cimetidine) as appropriate. If the drainage is frank blood or the amount is significant, iced saline lavages may be ordered. Accurate measurements of OG output should be maintained and the pH should be closely monitored.

Gut prophylaxis is ordered routinely in the pediatric and adult ICU patient. Commonly used medications for acid control in these patients are Protonix or Zantac.

F. Infection Control

Strict maintenance of aseptic technique and Universal Precautions is essential when caring for the patient on ECMO. The ECMO circuit usually has numerous ports which provide access for withdrawing or infusing fluids/blood. These ports as well as the patient lines serve as possible routes for infection. Frequent hand washing and the use of non-latex gloves is required of everyone who will be entering one of these sites. All IV lines and circuit ports must be prepped with an antimicrobial agent prior to entry. All access ports should have a blind cap or a syringe attached to them. Excessive use of alcohol to prep lines causes the polycarbonate plastic to crack. This will cause either blood loss from the circuit or air entry into the circuit. For this reason, this institution uses Betadine ONLY for prepping any ECMO line. Chlorhexidine preps are also used in other institutions.

G. Skin Integrity

Prior to the initiation of ECMO, patients have often required large amounts of crystalloid or colloid fluids in an effort to maintain blood pressure. At some point, the patient will experience "capillary leak" resulting in a generalized edema. This edema puts the ECMO patient at risk for skin breakdown due to a limited ability for movement. Use of an egg crate mattress, water mattress, or sheep skin will help in the prevention of skin breakdown. The nursing staff should also change the patient's position frequently. Care to prevent accidental decannulation is paramount when moving the ECMO patient; it requires the assistance of the ECMO specialist. A thorough inspection of the skin should be done every time the position is changed and any areas that appear reddened or broken should be noted and attended to. Lotion may be applied during routine baths. Gentle massage of the skin will help to improve circulation to the skin and promote reabsorption of excess extravascular fluid. The use of alcohol and adhesive tape remover should be minimized, as they have a drying effect on the skin. Change the patient's diapers frequently, especially if the patient is stooling, as this could cause skin breakdown to occur.

With the exception of periodic position changes, the ECMO patients have limited mobility for days. Efforts to avoid hyperextension of joints should be made, position the patient using blanket rolls to support the arms and legs. Passive range of motion should be performed at least once a shift as tolerated. Physical and occupational therapy consults may be appropriate for extended immobilizations, especially in older patients that are kept sedated and/or paralyzed.

H. Parent Interaction

Parents of patients on ECMO are generally overwhelmed by the severity of their child's illness and by the equipment and technology. It is important that the staff provide opportunities for the parents to ask questions. Offer explanations that provide information in an understandable manner. Remember, even parents with an understanding of medical terminology may find that what appears to be a simple statement to you may sound like a foreign language to them, especially in the early days of the ECMO course. Consistent messages from all members of the team decrease the chances of misunderstanding. The activities the parents may participate in are limited while on ECMO, but they could be allowed to assist with bathing and applying lotion to the skin, for instance. Encourage the parents to have contact with their child. They may choose to spend time at the bedside talking or reading to their child and lightly stroking the patient as tolerated. They may bring in pictures to place at the bedside or other items such as music boxes or small toys. Audio recordings from parents and family members may be helpful for older children. Institutions that have child life services may find that their involvement is helpful. Social work assessment is typically required for patients of this acuity.

ECMO Specialist Responsibilities

The ECMO specialist is a person who has been specially trained to care for long term modified heart-lung bypass circuits. The specialist's educational backgrounds vary from registered nurses, respiratory therapists, perfusionists, nurse practitioners, and physician assistants. Each institution mandates the qualifications they feel are necessary for individuals to become qualified specialists and practice is also guided by individual state practice acts. Training of specialists can occur either within the individual institution or at another institution that offers ECMO courses to outside individuals. The training program usually consists of didactic lectures and time in a lab setting learning and perfecting the skills needed to be adept at managing these complicated patients.

At the beginning of each shift, the ECMO Specialist should conduct a full check of the circuit. Patients who are on ECMO have separate data collection requirements from other required patient care activities to be documented. Bypass flow, sweep gas flow, and blended FiO$_2$ to the membrane oxygenator are documented hourly. Patient arterial blood gases are done every 2 - 4 hours or hourly (depending on institutional policy) if changes are made that will affect the patient's blood gas. Parameters for management are written by the physician every day. Changes in bypass flow, sweep gas, or blended FiO$_2$ are made based on arterial blood gas results, in-line saturation monitors, and the physician parameters. These changes are documented by the specialist. Each institution must determine the method to use for monitoring and regulating anticoagulation. Regardless of the method used, monitoring of the patients' anticoagulation status is done hourly and PRN. These results are also recorded and monitored by the specialist.

It is the responsibility of the ECMO Specialist to keep the ECMO physician up to date on any issues related to ECMO and the patient. The ECMO Specialist should contact the ECMO physician for abnormal laboratory findings or altered ECMO flow/oxygenation.

Management of Bypass by the ECMO Specialist

ECMO bypass must be maintained at a sufficient rate to adequately perfuse the patient and allow for "lung rest" to occur. In most cases this will be achieved at 60 - 80% of the patient's cardiac output. The cardiac output in infants is difficult to measure due to the presence of left to right shunts, but has been estimated from 120 - 300 cc/kg/min. Cardiac output in children is referenced by using

their cardiac index which is more accurate given the many weight ranges. It is 3 to 4.5LPM/ m^2/BSA (cardiac output divided by m^2 body surface area). Adult cardiac output range is 4 to 8 LPM. Average ECMO flows for children: 90 to 120ml/kg/min. Adults: 3 to 8LPM

There are several factors which will influence the ECMO specialists' ability to achieve and maintain extracorporeal bypass. These factors are:

- Size and length of the venous catheter
- The patient's hemodynamic status
- Hydrostatic column
- Size of circuit tubing
- Catheter position

Drainage of blood from the patient to the venous side of the ECMO circuit is accomplished by gravity. Frequently ECMO patients experience difficulty in maintaining adequate venous return to the circuit. The height of the patient's right atrium above the venous reservoir (bladder) determines the hydrostatic column. Volume status, specifically hypovolemia, can also be a problem for ECMO patients especially at the initiation of bypass. Centrifugal circuits are particularly sensitive to preload and afterload to maintain pump flows at desired rates. Many ECMO patients experience "capillary leaking" due to large amounts of volume given in the pre-ECMO period. Once on bypass, the capillary leaking continues and volume expansion may be necessary in order to maintain venous return to the ECMO circuit. An adequate daily protein intake will help restore a good osmotic pressure gradient.

ECMO catheters can be very positional (and can kink) depending upon the type of catheter used. If the catheter is two high or two low, venous return to the circuit may be diminished and cause "chatter" and venous return monitor (VRM) alarms. Catheter position can be verified by chest x-ray or ultrasonography. Good catheter position can occasionally be achieved through manipulation of the patient's head position, and through the use of various sized neck rolls. Surgical repositioning of the catheters by the surgeons can be done if the problem is severe. Venous catheter sutures which are too tight can also cause "chatter" by partially obstructing flow to the circuit. Efforts should be directed towards maintaining bypass at all times. When the patient on bypass is experiencing difficulties with venous return, the specialist should try to discover the etiology of the problem. First attempts should include repositioning the patient's head and verifying catheter position on the most recent chest x-ray. Auscultation of the chest should be performed to ascertain if a change in breath and heart sounds has occurred, which could indicate the presence of a pneumothorax or pneumopericardium. If venous return continues to be a problem small boluses of volume could be given. Whenever venous return becomes a problem, the ECMO physician should be notified. Venous return can also be compromised when a patient is extremely agitated. The use of comfort measures and sedation should be utilized.

The ECMO specialist should perform a visual inspection of the entire circuit at the beginning of each shift, this includes ascertaining that all connections are tight and that Ty-bands are in place. The system should be thoroughly checked for air bubbles, especially in the bridge, bladder, top of the oxygenator, and in any line filters. The circuit should be examined for any clot formation and the approximate size and location documented according to institutional policy. Clot and fibrin formation can usually be seen in the bladder and oxygenator where "low flow" areas exist. The venous and arterial pressure limits should be checked at least once a shift, as well as an actual test of the VRM alarm to determine its functioning status. Back up units of blood should be available from either the blood bank or from a blood bank refrigerator on the unit (as per individual hospital policy). At the beginning of each shift, the ECMO specialist should familiarize themselves with any emergency protocols particular to their institution (i.e. emergency ventilator settings, etc.). ECMO patient care areas should be stocked adequately enough to perform most emergency procedures (i.e. extra raceways, pigtails, connectors, etc) with a minimum of delay. An example of a daily checklist for the bedside specialist is shown in figure 1.

Figure 1.

ROTAFLOW PUMP ECMO SHIFT CHECKLIST

QC document only---not part of permanent record

	0700-1900	1900-0700
Date		
Time	0700-1900	1900-0700
Check system tybands, check circuit for air, verify pump mode		
Check the VRM, observe for decrease in flows, VRM# to become more neg, audible alarm		
Clots Y/N (chart size & location in cerner under ECMO comments)		
Check water bath: a) note water temperature b) note blood temperature c) check water level (sterile water only)		
Examine Patient: a) check breath sounds b) cardiac murmur Y/N c) check incision site/surgical site/open chest window		
Check and verify alarm limits for channel I/Art and III/VRM		
Check, set and verify low flow alarm limit (20% < desired flow rate)		
Check vent settings		
Check for emergency unit of blood		
Verify that thrombin, surgifoam, heparin 1000u/cc and vecuronium are in the cart		
Check CO_2 tank level (>200 PSI) Tank changed Y/N		
Verify 8 clamps present/pump plugged into battery		
Pump ABG q 8hrs and PRN		
Send CBC @1600, AM labs: CBC, Fibrinogen, Measured O_2 sat, plasma free hgb, PT/PTT,(non-hep absorbed), mag and phos		
Change sticky stopcock		
Re-stock cart/clean cart Qshift		
Check for hand crank		
Check for ultrasonic paste		
Perform hemochron QC ("sticks") Q8(0700,1500,2300)		
Verify bladder functionality Qshift and PRN		
ECMO specialists initials		

References

1. Sheehan, A, Bedside nursing care and ECMO specialists responsibilities. Chapter 14, ELSO Specialists Training Manual, 2nd Edition, Editor, Van Meurs, K, pp 199-211, 2000.
2. Remenapp RT, WinklerPrins A, Nursing care of the patient on ECMO, Chapter 41, ECMO, Extracorporeal Cardiopulmonary Support in Critical Care, 3rd Edition, Editors, Van Meurs, K, Lally KP, Peek G, Zwischenberger JB, pp 595-606, 2005
3. Responsibilities of the ECMO specialists and nursing staff, IN: CNMC ECMO Training Manual, 13th Edition, Authors: Short, B, Mikesell, G, Rivera, O, pp. 109-116, 2008.

Chapter 20 Questions

1. Nursing assignments for bedside care of the ECMO patient should be made based on :
   a) institutional policy
   b) experience of the ECMO specialist
   c) acuity of the patient
   d) all of the above

2. Who is responsible for recording the hourly readings and manipulations of gas flow to the circuit?
   a) The ECMO physician
   b) The bedside RN
   c) The ECMO specialist
   d) The parent

3. A primary responsibility of the ECMO specialist or other member of the ECMO team during patient transport is:
   a) Clearing the hallways of equipment
   b) Securing the elevator
   c) Guarding of catheters and control of speed of transport
   d) Clean up of area after procedure

Chapter 20 Answers

1. d
2. c
3. c

21

ECMO Intra-Hospital Transport: Minimizing Risk
Logistics, Strategy, and Safety

Christine Small RN, Daniel H. Conway MD, Matthew Moront MD and Dominick M. Carella RN

Objectives

After completion of this chapter, the participant should be able to:

- Describe the risk and emergencies that can occur with transport of the intra-hospital ECMO patient and the application and implementation of crew resource management and situational awareness methodology to resolve potential issues.
- Describe the necessary equipment needed for safe intra-hospital transport of the ECMO patient.
- Describe the personnel needed and their role for safe intra-hospital transport of the ECMO patient.

Introduction

The transport of critically-ill patients is complex and carries inherent risks. The intra-hospital transport of the ECMO patient can result in catheter dislodgement, bleeding, and potentially adverse events. Transport risk can be reduced by the implementation of a set of guidelines that describe the personnel, equipment, and the transport process. These guidelines promote measures to ensure safe patient transport and formalize a line of communication among members of the team and a reporting structure that coordinates communication and decision making. We believe that intra-hospital transport of an ECMO patient can be safely performed using Crew Resource Management (CRM) and Situation Awareness (SA) methodologies.

A formalized set of guidelines should accompany the decision to transport the ECMO patient within the hospital with risk versus benefit assessed, i.e. need for additional diagnostic examinations or interventions. Risk management and the decision making of a risk assessment for diagnostic examinations such as cardiac catheterization with and without interventional therapy and computed axial tomography scans are weighed against potential risks and the evaluation of hazards such as a power failure of the ECMO circuit. Judgment of whether the need for additional care can be brought to the location of the patient should be assessed rather than the patient transported to an alternate location to obtain additional diagnostic or therapeutic care.

Successful intra-hospital transport of the patient is rational if the diagnostic examination or procedural intervention under consideration is likely to alter the management or outcome of the patient. The need for transport must be questioned if the transport significantly increases patient mortality and morbidity. The use of standard operating procedures (SOP's) in an efficient manner with appropriate equipment and qualified personnel and selecting the best decision using available up-to-date patient information can eliminate what was previously felt to be a far too complex maneuver; intra-hospital transport of the ECMO patient.

Background

The concept of Crew Resource Management (CRM) has been widely used to improve the operation of flight crews by facilitating team member communication, mandatory briefing and debriefings, and the extensive use of standard operating procedures. The intra-hospital transport of an ECMO patient is an interdependent process carried out by a team of individuals with advanced technical training. Their group dynamics are similar to other technically complex high-stress endeavors with a high potential for error. We think that the ECMO community can benefit from the application of CRM theory with regard to the intra-hospital transport of an ECMO patient.

Introduced and developed by the aviation industry, CRM composes a set of cognitive skills needed to manage the flight operations within commercial and military aviation systems. CRM training develops aircrew skills in recognizing and responding to the conditions that lead to aircrew error. Core principles of adaptability, flexibility, assertiveness, communication, decision making, leadership, situational awareness and mission analysis (briefings and debriefings) establish a systematic and efficient process when un-briefed situations arise, thus assuring flight safety.

The application of CRM to medicine and healthcare suggests that the behaviors that have been applied in the aviation industry are relevant to human performance and the reduction of human error and mishaps in other domains. While it is certain that patients can be safely transported within the hospital on ECMO, the success of CRM can be evaluated using a number of performance outcome measures including group process dynamics, safety, adverse events, and efficiency variables. Along with integrating the core principles of CRM, several principles can be highlighted as primary factors that lead to an adverse condition on transport attributing to human error and especially important during the intra-hospital transport where information flow can be quite high and poor decision-making can lead to serious consequences.

A lack of communication and understanding of the individual team member responsibilities and the responsibilities of other team members will result in a failure to detect cues on transport that may result in adverse events. Proper interpretation of the meaning of those cues establishes a priority through a prescribed process and promotes problem solving, evaluation of potential hazards, and application of appropriate control measures.

Methodology

The success of CRM in the intra-hospital transport of the ECMO patient establishes an open and professional atmosphere and ensures that the team understands the goals and mission of the transport. The ability to direct and coordinate the activities of the members of the transport team to work together as a team requires that each hospital have a formalized plan for intra-hospital transport. Intra-hospital transport processes can be divided into three phases: (1) pre-transport assessment and coordination of transport personnel and transport equipment (briefing of the transport objectives), (2) transport and monitoring en route and recovery of transfer (following the prescribed transport plan), and (3) stabilization and documentation of patient in the home unit following the transport (debriefing and analysis of the transport).

Preparation and Equipment

The first phase of pre-transport assessment and coordination involves designating a Team Leader (TL) who assigns the team member's their roles and responsibilities and reiterates the team's goals. The TL is also responsible for reviewing and walking the intended route and considering any other space considerations; including contingency planning in case of known or unknown hazards for example; the power failure of the pre-designated elevator for transport. The TL is responsible for communicating the timing of the intra-hospital transport to other departments involved in the transport, parents and/ or family caregiver, and supervision of the actual transport.

All team members are briefed on their role and charged with a collective understanding of the responsibility of the other team members. The briefing should be interactive and questions encouraged and information conveyed to the team should be pertinent. While the conduct of the transport is the responsibility of the TL, any member of the team can stop or curtail the transport if any aspect of the transport becomes unsafe. Unbriefed situations may arise; and an organized transport may turn into an emergent situation in which adaptability and flexibility will reestablish priorities.

Coordination of transport personnel and transport equipment is necessary in the conduct of the transport. Preparation includes notification of appropriate attending physicians, ECMO coordinators, ECMO specialists, respiratory therapists, nursing team members and the receiving hospital department. Coordination and establishment of a total time span is established after discussion between these disciplines and attention to a start time, length of time required for the transport and end time to develop contingency plans if needed for allocation and monitoring of additional personnel and equipment resources.

The intra-hospital ECMO team transport configuration begins with the TL; but will involve direct ECMO team members. We prefer that the TL is designated to be a separate individual with no direct responsibilities for the operation of the bypass pump. The ECMO team coordinator is responsible for bypass pump supervision and operation and may assist with movement of the bypass pump. The ECMO team specialist is also responsible for the bypass pump operation and may assist with movement of bypass pump. A novel idea of using additional ECMO team support is to designate an ECMO team "joiner." This team member is responsible for maintaining a "bridge" between the bed/stretcher, bypass pump and cannulae. Additional personnel maybe needed for assistance as ECMO team movers for the remaining equipment such as intravenous fluids, intravenous poles, intravenous pumps and battery supply systems.

Allocation of appropriate equipment includes a full oxygen cylinder set to the patient's sweep flow rate, and secured to the ECMO cart as an oxygen source for transport. An uninterrupted power supply (battery) needs to be fully charged, checked, and obtained if not incorporated already into your system. The ECMO specialist needs to scale down the ECMO circuit; remove all extra pumps, power cords, and lines not needed for transport and check the cannula sites to make sure they are secure for transport. An emergency grab-and-go transport pack should be available. This transport pack should include appropriate sized supplies matched for the circuit to include: straight connectors, sterile tubing, sterile scissors, sterile clamps (at least four), sterile gloves, intravenous fluids such as normal saline, dispensing

pins for intravenous fluids, varied-sized syringes, caps, needles, and spare circuit components.

Additional personnel may be needed to help on transport and the TL should ensure that all the disciplines are ready with their equipment, supplies, and monitors. An oxygen source, an electrical source and hand ventilation resuscitation bags will have to replace the central sources for these items. Emergency medications, sedatives, and paralytics should be available, along with the patient's record. The heat source from the ECMO circuit will be turned off during transport to minimize electrical amperage; so an alternative heat source such as portable heat packs or warm or thermal blankets will offer some support to maintain the patient's temperature.

Transport

Transport and monitoring en route is initiated when all members are ready; the ECMO specialist will unplug the ECMO pump and the pump will go onto battery power. The heater will be turned off then unplugged. Alternative heat sources will be applied to the circuit and/or patient. The sweep flow will be adjusted on the oxygen cylinder. In-line and non-invasive oxygenation saturation monitoring devices are turned off and unplugged. The ECMO specialist will monitor all ECMO circuit pressures, monitor the color of the circulating venous and arterial blood, and maintain pump flow. Once the ECMO circuit is stable on battery power, the ECMO coordinator and ECMO specialist will be in charge of the bypass pump operation and may assist with movement of bypass pump. The TL will ensure the intra-hospital ECMO team transport configuration and initiate the transport move. Again, any member of the team can stop or curtail the transport if any aspect of the transport becomes unsafe.

Once at the transport destination, the ECMO specialist will restore power to pump and heater (water bath) by plugging into the hospital designated emergency electrical outlets. The oxygenator will be attached to the main oxygen supply and the oxygen cylinder is turned off for the recovery phase. The heater (water bath) will be plugged in and turned on to maintain the patient's temperature. Plug in the oxygen saturation monitors. The ECMO specialist will monitor circuit pressures, monitor the color of the circulating venous and arterial blood, and maintain pump flow. Once the team and patient is at the receiving destination, the transfer of the patient to the procedure table is initiated and supervised by the TL. Extra care is taken to maintain the security of the cannulae during the transfer of the patient from the patient bed to the procedure table.

After the completion of the procedure(s) or diagnostic intervention(s), the intra-hospital transport process is done in reverse; all staff will monitor the patient's clinical condition throughout the transport and again; any member of the team can stop or curtail the transport if any aspect of the transport becomes unsafe. All portable sources of oxygen and battery supply are retuned to mainframe sources. After unloading of the patient when the patient arrives back in the home unit, the ECMO specialist will continue to monitor the ECMO circuit as was done prior to the transport. Documentation of the intra-hospital transport, monitoring and return to the unit includes a complete total time span of the transport and any interventions performed. The intra-hospital transport should provide the same quality of care during transport as the patient would receive in an appropriate intensive care unit at the hospital while on ECMO.

Conclusions and Recomendations

We believe that a strict adherence to established guidelines utilizing CRM and team situation awareness has led to our success. The application of these processes is essential to the safe intra-hospital transport of the ECMO patient and will minimize adverse outcomes (no ECMO circuit or patient complications). Transporting a patient while on extracorporeal life support is a complex challenging endeavor and data suggests that intra-hospital transport is not infrequent and that a defined strategy for this maneuver is needed. The implementation of CRM and situational awareness methodology improves team member confidence and satisfaction, as well as improving efficiency and safety. These principles apply in a broad range of applications in critical care medicine and resuscitation.

Centers with limited experience in intra-hospital transport of the ECMO patient should participate in "dry run" exercises and perform briefing and debriefing analysis with a focus on the safety and transportation responsibilities. To meet the requirements to complete such intra-hospital transports, teams must train and configure their staff properly to conduct these types of operations and orient their staff in a secure team-focused manner. With proper attention to logistics, strategy, and safety, intra-hospital transport of patients on ECMO can be performed by most institutions with relatively low risk to the patient and ECMO circuit for adverse events.

Editorial

Billie Short, M.D.

Transport of the ECMO patient requires organization and team work as outlined in this chapter. Each center should develop a well defined Policy/Procedure for this. An example is included at the end of this chapter.

References

1. Andrew, J. Resuscitation, stabilization, and transport in Perinatology. Current Opinion in Pediatrics. 1993; 5:150-155.
2. Coppola, C., Tyree, M., Larry, K., DiGeronimo, R. 22-year experience in global transport extracorporeal membrane oxygenation. Journal of Pediatric Surgery. 2008; 43: 46-52.
3. Duncan, B., Pediatric Mechanical Circulatory Support. ASAIO Journal. 2005; 51: 9-14.
4. Foley, D., Pranikoff, T., Younger, J., et al. A Review of 100 Patients Transported on Extracorporeal Life Support. ASAIO Journal. 2002; 48: 612-619.
5. Haneya, A., Philipp, A., Foltan, M., et al. Extracorporeal circulatory systems in the interhospital transfer of critically ill patients: experience of a single institution. Ann Saudi Med. 2009; 29(2): 110-114.
6. Henderson, C. Cockpit/Crew Resource Management Training Program. Available at: http://www.e-publishing.af.mil/shared/media/epubs/AFI11-290.pdf. Accessed March 9, 2010.
7. Heulitt, J., Taylor, B., Faulkner, S., et al. Inter-Hospital Transport of Neonatal Patients on Extracorporeal Membrane: Mobile-ECMO. Pediatrics. 1995; 95:562-566.
8. Kaber, B., Endsley, M. Team Situation Awareness for process Control Safety and Performance. Process Safety Progress. 1998; 17: 43-48.
9. Mainali E., Greene, C., Rozycki, H., Gutcher, G. Safety and efficacy of high-frequency jet ventilation in neonatal transport. Journal of Perinatology. 2007; 27:609-613.
10. Mills, L., Redpath, S., Liddell, M., et al. Predictors of clinical outcome for infants transferred for extracorporeal life support consideration. Arch Dis Child Fetal Neonatal Ed. 2007; 92: F-233 Letters.
11. Naval Aviation Schools Command. Crew Resource Management. Available at: https://www.netc.navy.mil/nascweb/crm/crm.htm. Accessed February 28, 2010.
12. Pizzi, L., Goldfarb, N., Nash, D. Crew Resource Management and its Applications in Medicine. Available at: http://www.ahrq.gov/clinic/pt-safety/chap44.htm. Accessed March 10, 2010.
13. Prodhan, P., Fiser, R., Richard, T., et al. Intra-hospital transport of children on extracorporeal membrane oxygenation: Indications, process, interventions, and effectiveness. Pediatric Critical Care Medicine. 2010; 11(2):227-233.
14. Warren, J., Fromm, R., Orr, R., et al. Guidelines for the inter- and intrahospital transport of critically ill patients. Critical Care Medicine. 2004; 32: 256-262.
15. Woodward, G., Insoft, R., Pearson-Shaver, A. et al. The state of pediatric interfacility transport: Consensus of the Second National Pediatric and Neonatal Interfacility Transport Medicine Leadership Conference. Pediatric Emergency Care. 2002; 18:1.

Chapter 21 Questions

1. Which set of established methodology is considered an application template to ensure the safe patient transport of the intra-hospital ECMO patient that describes personnel, equipment and the processes involved?
   a) Hospital guidelines
   b) ELSO guidelines
   c) Crew Resource Management
   d) ECMO guidelines

2. Lack of communication and understanding of the individual team member responsibilities and the responsibilities of the other team members will result in a failure to detect cues on transport that may result in adverse events.
   a) True
   b) False

3. What are the three phases of intra-hospital process?
   a) Pre-transport assessment, transport, and stabilization
   b) Transport, plan, and documentation
   c) Debrief, transport, and plan
   d) Stabilization, debriefing, and documentation

4. Only the Team Leader (TL) can stop or curtail the transport if any aspect of the transport becomes unsafe.
   a) True
   b) False

5. Who needs to be notified when the decision to transport an ECMO patient is made?
   a) Attending physician
   b) ECMO coordinator
   c) ECMO specialist
   d) Respiratory therapist
   e) Nursing team
   g) Receiving department
   h) All of the above

6. What are the two most important supplies needed for transport of an ECMO patient to run the ECMO circuit?
   a) Emergency medications and blood products
   b) Intravenous fluids and oxygen cylinder
   c) Full oxygen cylinder and fully charged battery
   d) Charged battery and emergency medications

7. The heat source from the ECMO circuit will be plugged into the battery during transport.
   a) True
   b) False

8. What are the responsibilities of the ECMO specialist during transport of the ECMO patient?
   a) Once the circuit is on battery power the ECMO specialist's job is complete
   b) Once the circuit is on battery power the ECMO specialist is to maintain the function of the circuit while helping move the circuit
   c) Once the circuit is on battery power the ECMO specialist is to take over for the Team Leader (TL)

9. Once you arrive at your destination the ECMO specialist will stay on battery power until you return to base unit.
   a) True
   b) False

10. The implementation of Crew Resource Management (CRM) and situation awareness methodology improves team confidence and satisfaction as well as improving efficiency and safety.
    a) True
    b) False

Chapter 21 Answers

1. C
2. A
3. A
4. B
5. H
6. C
7. B
8. B
9. B
10. A

EXAMPLE: POLICY/PROCEDURE FOR INHOUSE TRANSPORT OF THE ECMO PATIENT

SUBJECT: Transport of the ECMO patient	**DATE ISSUED:**
SERVICE: ECMO	**DATE EFFECTIVE:**
	POLICY NUMBER:

I. **Purpose** – To outline the equipment and personnel needed, and the procedure for conducting the transport of the ECMO patient to other area of the hospital as needed for patient care or diagnostic testing.

II. **Implementation**
   A. *The Process - Responsibilities*
   - The ECMO physician will notify the ECMO Manager, Core Team, or Perfusionist of the need for transport. If no Core Team member is available, a designated (approved by ECMO Manager) RD specialist will take the place of the Core Team member.

   - The ECMO specialist will notify the charge nurse, bedside nurse, and the respiratory therapist of the impending transport.

   - The ECMO specialist is responsible for assembling supplies and equipment that will be utilized during transport and in the receiving department.

   - The ECMO specialist is responsible for assuring that all daily safety checks are completed prior to transport.

   - The unit charge nurse will be responsible for recruiting additional personnel to assist with the transport.

   - The receiving department will notify the ECMO specialist of the time of the appointment.

   - The ECMO physician will confirm that the receiving department is ready to receive patient before the move begins.

   - Personnel planning to remain with the ECMO patient during the procedure must wear appropriate attire, (O.R. scrubs, O.R. caps and masks etc.) before leaving the critical care area.

   - The charge nurse/designee is responsible for obtaining access to the keyed elevator, and carrying the blood product cooler (if necessary).

   - The assigned bedside nurse or respiratory therapist will be responsible for disconnecting the infant from the ventilator, and hand ventilating at minimal settings as specified by the ECMO physician.

234

- The ECMO physician will be responsible for assuring the overall stability of the patient, ECMO circuit and cannula during transport.

- The respiratory therapist is responsible for assuring that the ventilator arrives in the receiving department and is set up and functioning.

- The Core Team member, perfusionist, or RD specialist will be the Team Leader and will:
    o Assign roles to staff assisting with the transport.
    o Maintain stability of the ECMO cannulas during transport
    o Control the speed of the transport and redirect other team members as needed to ensure patient safety during transport
    o Notify the attending physician if there are any significant concerns regarding the safety of the transport; if concerns still exist, the Team Leader will notify the pediatric or neonatal ECMO director as appropriate.

- The second ECMO specialist will be responsible for:
    o Pushing the ECMO pump during transport
    o Maintaining bypass before, during and after transport

- Once the ECMO patient arrives in the receiving department the ECMO Core Team member, perfusionist, or RD specialist and physician will be responsible for the transfer and stabilization of the ECMO patient, catheters, and pump.

B. *Equipment*

1	Battery pack
1	Transport monitor
2	Oxygen tanks E cylinders: 1 with a flow meter, 1 with a 50 PSI
1	Air tank E cylinder
1	Air/Oxygen extension hoses
1	Laerdal bag and mask
1	Ventilator/ Intubation equipment (RT responsibility)
1	Hand crank for centrifugal pump

Transport bag

C. *Supplies: the following items will be maintained in a transport bag in a ready- to-go state by the Core Team.*

10	Hemochron tubes
1	Hemochron machine
1	250cc bottle of 5% albumin
1	Bag NS for fluid resuscitation
2	3 way stopcocks
2	2 way stopcocks
20	1cc syringes
20	3cc syringes
4	60cc syringes
2	pigtails

1	sterile raceway
20	Betadine swabs
30	0.7cc flushes (NS or 1/2 NS)
20	2cc flushes (NS or 1/2 NS)
1	Blood infusion set
1	Platelet infusion set
1	Sterile Trauma scissors
1	I-STAT blood gas analyzer
4	#3 I-STAT cartridges
4	#7 I-STAT cartridges
	patient ID stickers
	ECMO flow sheets for backup if Cerner is down

D. Meds to be drawn up by clinical staff prior to transport:

      iv. Per ECMO physician

E. *Personnel* For the smooth, efficient, and safe transport of the ECMO patient, the following personnel have been designated as essential to the success of an ECMO transport.

- ECMO physician
- ECMO Core Team Member or Perfusionist or approved RD specialist
- ECMO specialist
- Bedside RN
- Charge nurse
- Additional RN (as necessary)
- Respiratory Therapy
- PCT/PSA for moving in equipment

F. *Procedure:*

- RT will secure 2 Oxygen and 1 Air E cylinders, to bottom of the patient bed

- Air cylinder and 1 oxygen tank must have 50psi adapters attached so the ECMO pump has temporary gas source during transport. Other oxygen tank is used for ambu bag.

- Place transport monitor on the patient bed

- Cover the patient with blankets.

- Disconnect all unessential IVs and put them to heparin locks, ie., intralipids, PA pressure line, etc.

- Secure the remaining IMED pumps.

- Place any chest tubes to water seal.

- Attach and secure chest tube pleurovacs to the patient bedside

- Connect the patient to the portable monitor.

- Disconnect the patient from the ventilator, hand ventilate the patient from this point on, using minimal settings.

- Take the battery on its moveable platform.
  - This is the electrical source for transport
  - Be sure hand crank is attached to ECMO pump in the event of an emergency
  - The pump should be unplugged just before the whole team is ready to move

- Transfer ECMO pump gas sources from the wall to the E cylinders

  - **CHECK YOUR GAS GAUGES ON THE FLOW METER TO BE CERTAIN YOU HAVE GAS FLOW TO THE MEMBRANE OXYGENATOR.**

- You are now ready for transport.
  - Check to make sure that the patient and pump are completely portable.
  - The ECMO Core Team member/designee will dictate the direction of movement for transport. Upon arrival in the receiving department, transfer ECMO pump gas sources from E cylinders to the wall sources. The E cylinders must be turned off as soon as wall source gas has been established, as the tanks will run dry

- Plug battery pack into wall source

- Check the patient's temperature and reset water bath to previous set point

- Move the IV pumps from the patient bed and secure them on an IV pole and plug them into wall electricity.

- Move any chest tube pleurovac from the patient bedside and secure to the procedure table in relation to the patient's head
  - Attach chest tubes to suction and be certain the correct amount of suction is being applied

- Transfer the patient to the procedure table.
  - Once on the procedure table, the eggcrate mattress, code board and warming mattress can be removed from under the patient if necessary

- Place the patient on the ventilator that the respiratory therapist has set up
  - Check the ventilator settings

- Secure the ECMO catheters to the procedure table, the same as if the patient is in the critical care area.

22

Outcome After Neonatal ECMO

Penny Glass, PhD

Objectives

After completion of this chapter, the participant should be able to:

- Describe the typical medical problems seen in an ECMO patient prior to discharge from the hospital.
- Describe the recommended follow-up for an ECMO patient.
- List some neurodevelopmental problems seen in the ECMO survivor at school age.

Introduction

ECMO has been shown to reduce mortality in critically ill neonates with severe cardiorespiratory failure which has been refractory to conventional ventilator management.[1,2,3] Given the severity of illness prior to ECMO treatment and the risks inherent with the procedure, it is important to recognize the expected short term and long term problems identified among the survivors and identify care practices that may improve outcome.

Mortality

Mortality risk factors for ECMO-treated neonates have included: primary diagnosis prior to cannulation, necessity for cardiopulmonary resuscitation, severe bleeding complications during bypass and birthweight. Less than 60% survival is reported for neonates with CDH, compared to 90% or better for neonates with severe MAS. In a recent review of the ELSO registry, Doski et al., reported poorer survival for ECMO treated neonates who required CPR prior to cannulation.[4] Approximately one-half of the ECMO deaths are associated with significant bleeding complications, although bleeding itself is not necessarily the cause of death. Lower birthweight, even among near-term neonates treated with ECMO, is also associated with poorer survival.[5]

Morbidity

Morbidity following neonatal ECMO is most frequently recognized during three time periods: the post-ECMO/pre-discharge period, around 1-2 years of age, and again at preschool or school age.

Post Cannulation and Discharge Status

For some ECMO-treated neonates, neurological status after decannulation and extubation is consistent with moderate to severe hypoxic-ischemic encephalopathy. By appearance, the infant may be lethargic, hypotonic, and hyporeflexic. Patients often require weaning from narcotic or other sedative medications given for pain management. A significant rate of clinical and encephalographic seizure activity is reported in the neonatal period, and some infants at discharge are still on anticonvulsant medication. Hearing screening (e.g. BAER) may identify elevated thresholds in 25%, but this is usually transient.

The most significant neurologic finding in the neonatal period is the extent and severity of hemorrhagic and non-hemorrhagic abnormalities identified by routine cranial ultrasounds during bypass and head CT or MRI scans prior to hospital discharge. Moderate to severe abnormalities occur in approximately 10-15%, with an additional 25% having smaller or more focal lesions. The majority of the lesions are bilateral, with the unilateral lesions distributed fairly equivalently to left or right hemisphere.[6] Major factors contributing to CNS injury include underlying hypoxic/ischemic injury and reperfusion following cannulation, systemic anticoagulation, alteration of cerebral blood flow, and loss of cerebral autoregulation.

A major developmental issue for post-ECMO patients centers around establishment of oral feeding. The majority of ECMO neonates have difficulty initiating a coordinated suck/swallow pattern even in the presence of a fairly good non-nutritive suck on a pacifier. The difficulty has been variously attributed to their respiratory status, generalized CNS depression, poor hunger drive, soreness in the neck from the surgical procedure or in the throat from intubation, and manipulation of the vagus nerve during cannulation and decannulation. Oral feeds are often facilitated by small amounts fed slowly but more frequently, and by oxygen via nasal cannula to support respiratory effort. The presence of a nasogastric tube may itself cause obstruction of airway sufficient to interfere with successful oral feeding. The majority of ECMO infants respond sufficiently within 1-2 weeks to transition to all oral feeds.

Infants who fail to transition to all oral feeds when other discharge parameters are sufficiently stable, may be successfully sent home on nasogastric feeds. A common finding has been that parents generally do not replace the nasogastric tube once it comes out (usually within a week) and most infants adapt well to the consistent caregiver and more ad lib feeding. Even so, closer tracking of intake and weight gain in the first weeks and, in some cases, months after discharge by key medical personnel is essential.

A small but significant proportion of ECMO infants, usually those with chronic lung disease, may develop food refusal which can stem from overly stressful oral feeding practices that begin in the hospital and may be carried over by the parent after discharge home. ECMO neonates with a diagnosis of CDH have complex feeding issues such as gastroesophageal reflux, in addition to difficulty establishing oral feeds as described above and may require placement of a gastrostomy tube to support adequate growth.

Post-ECMO Outcome at 1-2 Years

In spite of all the early feeding difficulty, normal growth should be expected for almost all ECMO-treated neonates after discharge home with the exception of the CDH infant. Linear growth is often affected in the first couple of years in the CDH group even with good caloric intake. In ECMO survivors, head circumference below the 5th percentile occurs at a higher than expected rate (10%) and, if it occurs in conjunction with significant brain lesion, is frequently associated with a major handicapping condition at five years of age.[7,8] Macrocephaly has also been reported, which follows a pattern consistent with venous obstruction observed on neonatal neuroimaging. It may resolve without surgical intervention, but needs close monitoring. Macrocephaly may also signify late hydrocephalus following earlier intraventricular hemorrhage.

Significant respiratory sequelae are reported for ECMO survivors during the first two years of life. According to parental report, as many as 25% of ECMO children are likely to have at least one episode of pneumonia before age two. Even so, reactive airway disease, as defined by recurrent episodes of wheezing requiring treatment with bronchodilators and/or corticosteroids, occurs at a lower rate for ECMO-treated neonates when compared to similar infants treated with conventional therapy.[8,9]

There is a typical pattern of neurodevelopmental sequelae following hospital discharge. As a general rule, by 4 months of age the typical ECMO-treated neonate is developing in the normal range on formal testing (e.g. Bayley Scales of Infant Development), with both the mental scale and motor scale scores being 85 or above (mean = 100 ± 15). Residual hypotonia or mild asymmetry persists in about 25% of the infants. Mild motor delay typically accompanies the hypotonia. The prognosis is generally good for these patients. Infants who exhibit more significant problems at this time are usually referred for community early intervention programs. In a manner similar to preterm children with chronic lung disease, resolution of the lung disease is generally followed by improvement in motor milestones, unless the problem is accompanied by significant brain lesion. By 1-2 years of age, significant neurologic abnormality and/or Bayley scores < 70 are reported in

10-15% of the children. A larger proportion (25%) exhibit a more specific delay in either language or visual/perceptual abilities.

Long-term Outcome Following Neonatal ECMO

Among our 5-year ECMO cohort, 15% were taking some form of asthma medication at the time of our study and 10% of the cohort had been hospitalized at least once for asthma. The prevalence of asthma in our urban population of 5-11 year old children is estimated around 5%.

Major disability or handicap is reported in approximately 15% of ECMO-treated neonates by age five.[7] The most common disability is mild to moderate mental retardation. Severe or profound impairment is uncommon (< 5%). Motor handicap is unlikely to occur alone, but rather as an accompaniment to more severe degrees of mental retardation, reflecting more diffuse brain injury. Surprisingly, epilepsy is rare (2%) by age five, even among the ECMO children who had sustained significant neonatal brain injury.

Sensorineural hearing loss is reported in the range of 4-21% of ECMO-treated neonates by preschool age. Factors associated with hearing loss in non-ECMO patients include: asphyxia, hyperventilation, hypocapnia, and prolonged diuretic usage. There is no evidence that the ECMO procedure itself increases the risk for hearing loss. For many infants this hearing loss is progressive, following normal BAERs in the newborn period.

Isolated cases of visual disability have been reported, primarily cortical visual impairment as would accompany severe brain damage. In spite of the relatively hyperoxic condition sustained during bypass, retinopathy of prematurity is rarely a concern, since the lower birthweight limit of standard ECMO treatment has been 2 kg or 34 weeks gestation.

The majority of ECMO neonates at school entry are functioning in the normal range on measures of general intelligence, although the mean IQ scores and standard scores on measures of specific neuropsychological functioning are lower than in the normal population.[7] In a manner similar to other neonatal high risk populations, such as very low birthweight infants, non-handicapped five year old

ECMO-treated children are at increased risk for learning problems at school age.

Predictors

As in other populations of at-risk neonates, neurodevelopmental outcome is affected by the severity of chronic medical conditions such as bronchopulmonary dysplasia and failure to thrive. As expected, the strongest neonatal predictor of handicap in childhood is the extent and severity of abnormality on post-ECMO neuroimaging.[10] Even so, a significant proportion of children who had moderate to severe abnormality on neonatal neuroimaging have normal IQ scores in childhood.

Family Stress

The often unexpected and acute crisis surrounding ECMO therapy is traumatic for the parents and family of the neonate and the effect can be long lasting. It is helpful to remember that the parent has had to face the fact that ECMO is a treatment of last resort, that there is a time frame for their baby to recover or treatment will be stopped, and there may be significant brain injury. What may appear to be routine to the ECMO team is often overwhelming to the parents. Often, their emotional release is delayed until after the baby is discharged home.

Neurodevelopmental Follow-up

Long-term follow-up of ECMO patients is essential. The ECMO team can offer ongoing support to the family after discharge to ease the transition. Families should be guided to appropriate community resources as needed, especially if they are unable to return for follow-up at the ECMO site. Direct communication with the child's pediatrician is also important.

The current ELSO recommendation for follow-up after discharge are for evaluations at the ages of 4-6 months, 1 year, 2 years, 3 years, and 5 years. An age appropriate neurodevelopmental evaluation should occur at each of these visits. Behavioral hearing testing and language screening are also recommended.

For the majority of ECMO-treated neonates, the critical issues are developmental needs and psychosocial support. However, comprehensive multidisciplinary follow-up is essential for CDH children or other ECMO children who have significant medical and developmental issues. A team approach and case management is essential to prioritize the needs of the child and to relate directly to the parent and community pediatrician. In this manner, avoiding contradictory patient care plans and insufficient staff communication across multiple disciplines (e.g. Surgery, Neonatology, Pulmonary, Gastroenterology/Nutrition, Neurology, and Developmental Specialists) can be avoided. The long-term management and follow-up of the ECMO patient represents the final challenge to the ECMO team.

References

1. Bartlett R, Dietrich R, Cornell R, Andrews A, Dillon P, Zwischenberger J. Extracorporeal circulation in neonatal respiratory failure: a prospective randomized study. Pediatrics 1985;76:479-87.
2. O'Rourke P, Crone R, Vacanti J, Ware J, Lillehei C, Parad R, Epstein M. Extracorporeal membrane oxygenation and conventional medical therapy in neonates with persistent pulmonary hypertension of the newborn: a prospective randomized study. Pediatrics 1989;84:957-63.
3. UK Collaborative ECMO Trial Group. UK collaborative randomised trial of neonatal extracorporeal membrane oxygenation. Lancet 1996;348:75-82.
4. Doski J, Butler J, Louder D, Dickey L, Cheu H. Outcome of infants requiring cardiopulmonary resuscitation before extracorporeal membrane oxygenation. J Pediatr Surg 1997;32:1318-21.
5. Revenis M, Glass P, Short B. Mortality and morbidity rates among lower birth weight infants (2000 to 2500 grams) treated with extracorporeal membrane oxygenation. J Pediatr 1992;121:452-8.
6. Bulas D, Glass P. Neonatal ECMO: Neuroimaging and neurodevelopmental outcome. Seminars in Perinatology, 2005;29(1):58-65
7. Glass P, Wagner A, Papero P, Rajasingham S, Civitello L, Kjaer M, Coffman C, Getson P, Short B. Neurodevelopmental status at age five years of neonates treated with extracorporeal membrane oxygenation. J Pediatr 1995;127:447-57.
8. Walsh-Sukys M, Bauer R, Cornell D, Friedman H, Stork E, Hack M. Severe respiratory failure in neonates: mortality and morbidity rates and neurodevelopmental outcomes. J Pediatr 1994;125:104-10.
9. Vaucher Y, Dudell G, Bejar R, Gist K. Predictors of early childhood outcome in candidates for extracorporeal membrane oxygenation. J Pediatr 1996;128:109-17.
10. Glass P, Bulas D, Wagner A, Rajasingham S, Civitello L, Papero P, Coffman C, Short B. Severity of brain injury following neonatal extracorporeal membrane oxygenation and outcome at age 5 years. Dev Med Child Neurol 1997;39:441-8.

Chapter 22 Questions

1. Increased mortality for ECMO treated infants is associated with:
    a) CPR prior to cannulation
    b) Lower gestational age
    c) Bleeding complications
    d) Diagnosis of CDH
    e) All of the above

2. A normal hearing screening (BAER) in the neonatal period indicates the absence of hearing loss. Therefore, hearing need not be tested at later follow-up visits.
    a) True
    b) False

3. At the 4 month old visit, the most common neurodevelopmental abnormality noted is:
    a) Hypotonia
    b) Areflexia
    c) Hypertonia
    d) Hyperreflexia

4. At 1 year of age, the typical ECMO-treated patient will have neurodevelopmental scores in the normal range (100 ± 15).
    a) True
    b) False

5. At school age, specific delays in language or visual/perceptual abilities will occur in _____% of ECMO-treated children.
    a) 5%
    b) 15%
    c) 25%
    d) 40%

6. The ELSO recommendations for ECMO follow-up include what 3 elements:
    a) EEG
    b) Formal age-appropriate neurodevelopmental testing
    c) Behavioral hearing testing
    d) Language screening

7. Children who perform well on neurodevelopmental testing a age 4 months need not **b** re-evaluated at later ages.
    a) True
    b) False

8. Major disability is reported in 15% of ECMO-treated patients by age 5. The most common disability is mild to moderate mental retardation.
    a) True
    b) False

9. Non-handicapped 5 years old ECMO-treated children with normal IQ scores continue to be at risk for specific learning problems.
    a) True
    b) False

10. While normal growth is expected in the first 2 year of life for the majority of ECMO-treated patients, infants with a diagnosis of _____ often experience failure to thrive and gastroesophageal reflux.
    a) Meconium aspiration syndrome
    b) Sepsis
    c) Respiratory distress syndrome
    d) Congenital diaphragmatic hernia
    e) Persistent pulmonary hypertension of the newborn

Chapter 22 Answers

1. e
2. b
3. a
4. a
5. c
6. b, c, d
7. b
8. a
9. a
10. d

23

Outcome Following Pediatric ECMO

Heidi J. Dalton, MD

Objectives

After completion of this chapter, the participant should be able to:

- Better understand the available techniques and tests that can assist with neurologic outcome following extracorporeal support
- Understand the neurologic outcome observed in the pediatric ECMO follow-up literature and contained within the ELSO registry.
- Have improved understanding of the changing demographics of ECMO support and how they impact further needs for neurologic outcome research

Introduction

With the increasing use of extracorporeal life support in patient groups outside the neonate with respiratory failure, the need for more intricate and longitudinal neurological follow-up is becoming more and more important. While there is still little information available for older patients, we will examine here what we know, what we surmise and what we need to focus on in the future.

While in the past, ECMO was applied primarily to neonates with respiratory failure, improvements in prenatal and perinatal care, coupled with improved patient support techniques, have seen a drastic reduction in the need for ECMO in these critically ill neonates.[1-3] Over the past few years, ECMO support has become more common in patients with underlying cardiac disease, sepsis, or as a resuscitative tool in refractory cardiac arrest.[3-16] In addition, ECMO support is now being applied to adults, a group in which skepticism has delayed any acceptance into common practice.[17-18] The recently published CESAR trial, which found improved survival in patients considered for ECMO as compared to those treated with only conventional ventilation, may increase the acceptance of ECMO in adults in the future.[19] The need to develop standardized neurological evaluation procedures, collect uniform data and collaboratively share obtained results is the most pressing issue in the extracorporeal life support field today.

Patients undergoing ECMO are at risk of neurologic damage from hypoxia, acidosis, hypotension, induced alkalosis prior to ECMO, and from hemorrhage or ischemia related to systemic heparinization and alterations in cerebral blood flow from ligation of the carotid artery and internal jugular vein.[20-24] Nevertheless, two-thirds of the neonatal respiratory failure survivors appear to have a normal neurodevelopmental outcome. The remaining third suffer from mild to severe deficits in motor or cognitive function. Sensorineural hearing loss has been noted in 23% of patients, an incidence comparable to that in infants with persistent pulmonary hypertension treated conventionally. Another study of neonatal ECMO found sensorineural hearing loss in 26% of patients Of those affected neonates, 72% had progressive sensorineural hearing loss, with 48% having a delayed onset of hearing loss identified. Factors identified with increased risk for sensorineural hearing loss were a primary diagnosis of congenital diaphragmatic hernia, duration of ECMO therapy >7 days and the total number of days children received aminoglycoside antibiotics.[25] Long-term effects of carotid artery and jugular vein ligation are unknown.

While neonatal ECMO patients have been followed up to 15 years now from their initial event, with between 10-30% having some neurologic dysfunction, there are few reports on long term neurologic outcome in children. [26-28] One study from Italy detailing outcome in 12 neonates and 9 children found that a negative neurologic outcome (Glasgow Outcome Score different from "good recovery" or a neurodevelopmental score <70) at 12 months following ECMO was present in 8.3% of neonates and 30% of children who survived. [29] When followed over an additional 24 months, no further deterioration was noted. In this single center report, the most abnormal EEG (p=0.017), the first EEG obtained after ECMO (p=0.028), the neuroimaging score obtained from CT or ultrasound (p=0.016), and somatosensory evoked potentials performed after ECMO (p=0.014) were all associated with a negative neurologic outcome. Other variables assessed in the pre-ECMO period (oxygenation index, pH, paO_2) and during the ECMO run (pH, paO_2, duration of ECMO, activated clotting time and EEG) were not predictive of risk for a negative neurologic outcome.

Severe chronic respiratory disease in patients treated with ECMO is uncommon.[30] Most reports relate an incidence of bronchopulmonary dysplasia (defined as the need for oxygen beyond the first month of life) from 4% to 27%. Most cases occurred in patients who had required extreme ventilator settings for more than 7 days before ECMO rescue. A follow-up report of neonates treated with ECMO and evaluated at 10-15 years post-ECMO found that although the ECMO patients had some diminished lung function by pulmonary function testing, they had similar aerobic capacity and were able to reach anaerobic exercise goals similar to those of age-matched healthy controls.[31]

Of 4,000 pediatric respiratory ECMO patients listed in the Registry through July 2009, nine percent of patients had intracranial infarct or hemorrhage found on CT examination. Brain death occurred in 6% of the patients and 6% of patients had reported seizures. Long term neurologic outcome data is sorely missing in the pediatric population. Few centers maintain regular follow-up clinics and patients are often referred for ECMO from distant sites, which makes follow-up difficult as well. In one report of 15 pediatric and 4 adult patients, 58%

survived to discharge. Patients were evaluated by use of the Pediatric Cerebral Performance Category (PCPC, which measures cognitive impairment) and the Pediatric Overall Performance Category (POPC, which measures functional morbidity).[32] Overall, 64% of survivors had normal PCPC scores, 27% had mild disabilities and 9% had moderate cognitive disability. Functional morbidity was normal in 27% while 45% had mild disability, 18% moderate disability and 9% were severely disabled.[32] 5(45%) had mild disability, 2 (18%) moderate disability and 1 (9%) was severely disabled.

Of interest, when 161 patients with ARDS, entered in the ELSO-sponsored randomized pediatric ECMO trial from the 1990's, were evaluated for PCPC and POPC scores following hospital discharge, findings were similar. Overall survival was 65%. Of survivors, 53% were normal, 19% had mild disability, 18% moderate disability and 10% had severe disability as per their POPC prior to the admission.[33] At the time of discharge, 87% had no change in their PCPC, 7% had a one category change and 6% had a more than one category change. Of the patients with a more than one category change in POPC/PCPC, 4 had a trauma related disability (e.g. spinal cord injury). When these patients were removed from the analysis, only 2% of ARDS survivors had a more than one category change in their PCPC and 10% demonstrated a change in the POPC. None of the patients in this study were randomized to receive ECMO. However, this information does provide some glimpse into outcome from severe respiratory failure in patients not receiving ECMO that might be used as a comparison.

In the UK collaborative ECMO trial, which focused only on neonatal respiratory failure, moderate to severe disability was noted in 13% of the children supported with ECMO at 4 years follow-up.[34]

Neurologic complications in cardiac patients who receive ECMO parallels that of respiratory failure patients. Four percent of patients developed brain death, 3% had intracranial infarct and 6% had intracranial hemorrhage. Since many cardiac patients are in a state of prolonged low cardiac output or sudden cardiac arrest prior to ECMO, the ability to assess neurologic function once ECMO is instituted is vitally important. Paralysis and sedation should be minimized until a neurologic examination can occur. This information is especially important in patients who are being listed for transplantation to avoid transplanting a viable organ into an inappropriate recipient.

A recent study which sought to identify risk factors for acute neurological injury in children undergoing ECPR, found 22% patients had acute neurological injury, which they defined as occurrence of brain death, brain infarction or intracranial hemorrhage identified by ultrasound or computerized tomography imaging.[35] Brain death occurred in 11% , cerebral infarction 7% and intracranial hemorrhage in 7%. The in-hospital mortality rate in patients with acute neurological injury was 89%. During ECMO, neurologic injury was associated with ECMO complications including pulmonary hemorrhage, dialysis use and CPR during ECMO. Pre ECMO factors including cardiac disease and pH > 6.8 were associated with decreased odds of neurological injuries.

The long-term follow-up of children with cardiac disease who required mechanical circulatory support during a decade of experience at Children's Hospital, Boston was recently analyzed.[36] Thirty-seven children (26 ECMO and 11 ventricular assist device (VAD) survivors) were followed for an average of more than four years. Only a single patient died in either group for an overall long-term survival of 95%. Eighty percent of the patients in both groups were described as exhibiting good to excellent general health. Both low patient weight at the time support was originally instituted and long duration of hypothermic circulatory arrest in operative patients were associated with poor neurologic outcome. The majority of patients with these characteristics were supported with ECMO. Neurologic impairment of moderate to severe degree was noted in more than 60% of the ECMO patients and in 20% of VAD survivors. Adverse neurologic outcomes were not associated with pre-support cardiac arrest, carotid cannulation or carotid reconstruction. Other series have noted neurologic complications in 20-30% of cardiac ECMO patients.[37, 38] Survivors are generally described as "normal" neurologically, although the extent of examination or radiologic assessment of the brain is unknown.

A new report from California, not yet published, is the first to provide a large review of ECMO patients over time and perhaps heralds a new era of focus on longitudinal outcome well past the hospital discharge period.[39] This study reviews outcome of non-neonatal patients treated with ECMO in California over a period from 1999-2006, including subsequent hospital readmissions, development of long-term morbidities and long term survival. Patients were identified and assessed using the California Patient Discharge Database. This is a hospital discharge database of all nonfederal hospitals in the state of California. A discharge abstract for each inpatient hospitalization is recorded which includes patient demographics, admission and discharge details, patient disposition and up to 24 diagnoses and 20 procedure codes. The accuracy of the data is validated internally through nine levels of checkpoints with an error tolerance level of <2%. Prior reports of health outcomes in both adult and pediatric patients using this database have been published.

In the current study, all children between the ages of 1 month and 18 years who had undergone ECMO at 13 of the 516 licensed California hospitals were extracted from the database. Patients with congenital heart disease were excluded. While 1,313 children were identified who had undergone ECMO in the 8 year study period, 896 were neonates and 229 had congenital heart disease, leaving 188 children from 13 California hospitals who received ECMO for non-neonatal disease. The median age was 3 years and 46% survived to discharge. Late deaths (after discharge) occurred in 5% of children. Indications for ECMO included acquired heart disease in 81, pneumonia in 56, other forms of respiratory failure in 22, sepsis in 8, trauma in 8 and other indications in 12. Fifty six of 87 survivors were followed over a period of 3.7 years. Hospital readmission rate was 62% with a mean time to first readmission of 1.2 years. Readmissions were most frequent for respiratory infections (34%) while 7% of patients had reactive airway disease. Neurologically debilitating conditions occurred in 16% of patients, 7% with epilepsy and 9% with development delay. Of readmitted survivors, the cumulative length of stay during rehospitalization was 8 days with an average hospital charge of $43,000. Regarding the initial ECMO hospitalization, patients had an average length of stay of 23 days with median hospital charge of $423,000. Dialysis was common, occurring in 17% of patients. Survival to discharge among the California cohort was not different from that recorded in the ELSO registry (46% to 49%, p=0.29). Survival based on indication for ECMO was not statistically different between groups. In the 5% of patients who suffered late death, all were related to acquired heart disease requiring cardiac transplantation during the ECMO hospitalization. Thus, the overall long term survival rate was 42%. By multivariate regression analysis, a positive volume-outcome relationship was identified after controlling for ECMO indication, age, and whether the patient was transferred from another facility (HR 0.98/case,p<0.01). Thus, comparing hospitals with a mean volume of 14 cases to those one standard deviation above the mean (26 cases), there was a 1.34 times higher likelihood of survival with increased hospital volume. This finding has not been described previously. Further evaluation will be required to ascertain if this is a consistent finding or just among this one-state cohort.

This complex evaluation of patients from California will hopefully provide a springboard for future efforts to perform similar analysis of ECMO patients in the future. Issues of maintaining patient confidentiality and HIPAA restrictions are still controversial in many arenas and this study may provide a framework to allow other states or database registries to develop similar patient tracking systems which ensure confidentiality. Resolution of some of these issues will likely make future evaluations either easier to perform or so difficult that only a prospective, controlled study will allow appropriate data collection to follow patients longitudinally outside a single center

Other series of pediatric respiratory failure treated with ECMO have been small and are quite old compared to the current era. In one series, 26 patients were evaluated 1-3 years after ECMO. [40] In pre-school age children, 5/13 (38%) were normal, 4/13 (31%) patients had abnormalities prior to ECMO (cortical atrophy, Goldenhar's syndrome, Trisomy 21 and child abuse) and remained at their pre-ECMO baseline and 4/13 (31%) were abnormal. None of these patients had evidence of cerebral hemorrhage or infarct on CT examination, although cortical atrophy with mild hydrocephalus was present in several patients. Whether observed abnormalities following ECMO were related to pre-ECMO hypoxemia or ischemia is not known. In school age children assessed by parental report, 10/13 (77%) were normal, 2/13 (15%) were below average and 1/13 (8%) was above average. For patients over 5 years of age at the time of ECMO, 4/5 were normal. No CT abnormalities in the normal children were found. The single child with development delay had evidence of hypoxic/ischemic encephalopathy on CT examination.

In a review of patients treated with ECMO at the University of Michigan following cardiac surgery between 1995-2001, 74 patients were analyzed. In this period, 69% were placed on ECMO following 2 ventricle repairs while 28% had single ventricle physiology. [41] Final outcomes found that 32% died when separated from ECMO and an additional 18% died within 48 hours after removal from ECMO. In all, 50% of patients survived to hospital discharge. Survival was not affected by age, mode of ECMO, site of cannulation (35% cervical) or cardiac arrest prior to ECMO. Patients placed on ECMO during CPR had significantly less survival (20% vs 80% survival in those not receiving CPR). Patients with 2 ventricle repairs trended to improved survival (58% vs 34% single ventricle). Need for renal replacement therapy and elevated lactate 48 hours after cannulation for ECMO were both associated with poor outcome. Neurologic dysfunction in the form of seizures was found in 14% of patients (n=10) although presence of seizures was not correlated with death. Intracranial hemorrhage or stroke noted on radiologic examination was found in 7% (n=5) of patients, again without relation to death. This review gives little information on the cause of death or reason for removal from ECMO in non-survivors so the extent of neurologic injury among these patients cannot be ascertained. No long term neurologic function results are described among survivors.

In perhaps one of the first most detailed descriptions of neurodevelopmental outcome following ECMO outside the neonatal respiratory failure population, Hamrick reported on 53 infants treated following cardiac surgery. [42] Average age at followup was 55 months, or about 2.5 years following ECMO in most patients. Overall, only 13% were described as "completely intact" based on overall testing and clinical examination. Among the 17 survivors, 16 were available for follow-up and 50% had normal cognitive outcome. In 3 (21% of survivors), cognitive outcome was 1-2 SD below the mean while 4 patients (29%) were abnormal (>2 SD below the mean). Neuromotor outcome was normal in 72% of survivors, 7% were "suspect" and 21% had abnormal neuromotor performance. This report also found that no patient with an aortic cross-clamp times >40 minutes had normal cognitive outcome. This factor has not been found to be predictive of outcome in other studies. As with other reports, the need for renal replacement therapy was associated with poor outcome. Cardiac arrest was also found to be predictive of death in this study, although this center did have a rapid-resuscitation circuit or protocol in place over the study period and this likely contributed to this factor as a risk for death. Neurologic hemorrhage noted by ultrasound was cited as an indication to withdraw support in 25% of patients, with specific details of extent and location of damage not described. Among survivors, abnormalities in neuro imaging by ultrasound or MRI correlated with observed neurologic deficits.

More recently, an excellent review of mental and motor outcomes in 39 children supported with cardiac ECMO in Edmonton, Alberta (Canada) for a 5 year follow-up period was presented.[43] All patients treated with venoarterial ECMO for cardiac disease who were less than 5 years of age were eligible between 2000-2004. Consent for long-term follow up was obtained from parents/caregivers once survival off ECMO was likely. Information was obtained through specific chart review and from existing neonatal follow-up clinics throughout the provinces where patients resided. All assessments were done at least 6 months following ECMO. A family socioeconomic status tool used in previous reports that incorporates income, education, "prestige" factor of employment among a population using the Blishen index was recorded. Pediatricians trained in neurodevelopmental follow up assessed evidence for cerebral palsy or visual impairment. Hearing was tested. Patients were given the Bayley Scare of Infant Development II if <42 months of age at testing and the Wechsler Preschool and Primary Scale of Intelligence if assessed after 48 months of age. A developmental quotient score of less than 70 indicates mental delay. Parents completed the Adaptive Behavior Assessment System and Multiattribute Health Status Classification System questionnaires to assess perceived motor, development, behavior and self-care function. Factors relating to the pre-ECLS period, indication for ECLS, and ECLS variables for up to 120 hours following initiation were recorded. Patients were divided into 3 groups: single ventricle anatomy, biventricular anatomy and myocarditis. Of the 39 patients placed on ECLS during the study period, no demographic, pre-ECLS or ECLS related variables were different between the 3 descriptive groups. Overall survival was 46% to discharge and 41% at 2 years. No difference in mortality was noted between groups.

Among the entire cohort, only 18% had no adverse outcomes reported (n=39). Disability was found in 23% of survivors and 59% of the entire cohort had died by 2 years. Overall, 50% of survivors had mental delay, all 3 survivors with chromosomal abnormality (1 Turners, 2 chromosome 22) being abnormal and 38% of survivors without chromosomal abnormality having abnormalities. Predictive models for death and delay found that death at 2 years was associated with days of hospitalization, lactate on admission to the ICU, platelets infused over the first 120 hours of ECMO, single ventricle anatomy, ventilator days, pre-ECLS highest lactate, admission weight and seizures. Logistic regression found that lactate on admission to the ICU and single ventricle anatomy was associated with death at 10 days. Comparison of survivors with and without mental delay found only presence of chromosomal abnormality to be predictive (p=0.06) Continuous variables were examined to obtain correlation with mental score in 16 survivors. Of note, CPR before ECLS, during initiation of ECLS and duration of CPR were not associated with either increased risk of death or mental delay.

In another recent review of neurologic morbidity in children receiving ECMO for cardiac disease, Chow et al examined the outcomes of 90 children treated at the Hospital for Sick Children in Toronto between 1990-2000.[44] Short term outcomes assessed included: seizures, paresis, dystonia or chorea, coma, gaze palsies or visual field defects or other findings such as brachial plexus injury.

Long term outcome was determined by contacting families with a standardized questionnaire by phone (19 pts), in cardiac outpatient clinic (5 patients), neurodevelopmental clinic (1 pt) and during rehospitalization (1 pt). Deficits were divided into motor impairment, cognitive/behavioral impairment, seizures and other. Results from neuroimaging and autopsy studies were also reported. All neuroimaging results were evaluated by a radiologist blinded to the clinical details and outcomes. The median age of patients was 0.77 years. Sixty-one patients were neonates and 42 were male. Patients had underlying diagnoses of: myocarditis (n=10), cardiomyopathy (n=9) or structural heart disease (n=78, 58 with biventricular repair, 7 single ventricle repair and 6 without surgical intervention). Of patients with repair of congenital defects, 40 children were placed on ECLS directly from cardiopulmonary bypass. Three patients were bridged to heart transplant and 8 patients had multiple ECMO runs (7 patients had 2 runs and 1 patient 3 ECMO runs). Thirty-seven [34] percent of children required CPR for cardiac arrest prior to ECMO. Thirteen children were bridged to heart transplant from ECMO (2 expired) and 13 had an intracardiac repair performed while on ECLS (11 died).

In eight children who had neuroimaging prior to ECLS, 1 had a subdural hematoma noted while one had an infarct. Overall survival in these 8 patients was 25%. Thirty-eight children underwent neuroimaging either during or after ECMO, distributed as 35 head ultrasounds, 17 CT and 2 MRI. Abnormalities were noted in 24 patients, with 9 hemorrhages, 4 infarcts, 7 ventriculomegaly and 4 with cortical atrophy. No scans demonstrated hydrocephalus. In 11 non-survivors who had autopsy findings available, 7 brain hemorrhages were noted, 3 had infarcts and 1 had cerebellar tonsillar herniation. Long-term outcome assessment in survivors was performed at an average of 4.5 years following ECMO (range 4 months-9 years). Evidence of seizures was noted in 22% of children during their initial hospital course. Of these, 10/20 (50%) of patients died, 5 had long-term neurologic sequelae and 5 were "normal" at follow up. Overall, only 15/90 (17%) of the total study population were neurologically normal, while 11 had long term neurologic abnormalities. Thus, 39% (11/28) survivors had long term neurologic

sequelae on follow up exam. Patients with congenital cardiac defects had worse outcome than patients with myocarditis or cardiomyopathy (68% vs 32%, p=0.03). There was no difference in outcome based on whether ECMO was used for resuscitation, for inability to separate from bypass, for myocardial dysfunction or for postoperative low cardiac output state. There was also no statistical difference in outcome based on whether patients were preoperative, postoperative, intraoperative or non-operative. Univariate analysis found that congenital heart disease and abnormal neuroimaging were predictive of short-term neurologic sequelae. Both the presence of congenital heart defects and the presence of short-term neurological events were associated with death. Logistic regression, however, only noted that abnormal neuroimaging was associated with short-term neurological events (p=0.03, OR 10.5, 95% CI 2.2-50). Age, sex, previous ECMO, CPR, type of repair, congenital heart disease versus myocarditis, were not found to be significant factors. To assess for long term neurologic outcome and long term mortality, factors of age, sex, previous ECMO, previous CPR, short-term neurological event, type of repair, abnormal neuroimaging during admission, and presence of congenital heart disease versus myocarditis were entered into regression analysis. Previous CPR predicted lack of long-term survival (p<0.001, OR 2.6, 95% CI 1.47-4.47). No significant predictors of long term neurologic outcome were identified.

Overall outcome from this report noted a 66% short term mortality, with another 3% of patients expiring following hospital discharge for an overall survival rate of 28%. Short-term neurologic events occurred in 22% (20/90) of patients and long term sequelae were noted in 12% (11/90), which accounted for 39% (11/28) of survivors. The report highlights the need for prospective studies which will further assess the impact of risk factors on survival, short-term and long-term outcome and neurodevelopmental function. From these investigations, potential strategies to prevent adverse outcomes may be developed to improve outcomes.

In one evaluation of outcomes following extracorporeal life support applied during cardiac arrest at the Children's Hospital of Philadelphia, 50% of 66 patients with CPR events were decannulated and survived for at least 24 hours.[45] Overall 33%

of children undergoing ECPR survived to hospital discharge. Neurologic outcome was evaluated by review of medical records and discharge summaries. A meaningful neurologic impairment was prospectively defined as a new seizure disorder, loss of developmental milestones, loss of muscle tone, or focal weakness. Admission and discharge PCPC and POPC were calculated for survived children >2 months of age. Of 21 survivors, 24% were noted to have significant neurologic impairment at discharge, 3 with stroke and three with seizure disorder. Admission and discharge PCPC and POPC were available in 10/13 survivors who were >2 months of age. Of 3 patients >2 months of age who survived after >60 minutes of CPR, 2 had no change in these scores while 1 patient had a change of 1 in the PCPC and POPC scores. In 3 infants <2 months who had CPR for >60 minutes, 2 developed a new seizure disorder and 1 had no apparent sequelae. Thus, 3/6 patients with >60 minutes of CPR prior to ECMO had no gross neurologic injury at discharge. Of 10 patients who died within 24 hours of ECMO decannulation, 3 had support withdrawn due to neurologic devastation, 2 from ongoing multiorgan failure, 3 suffered an additional cardiac arrest from which resuscitation was not successful and the cause of death was unclear in 2 patients. Another finding from this review was that patients with underlying cardiac disease (19/43, 44% survival) had improved outcome as compared to those with other medical conditions (2/21, 9.5%). Whether this reflects intrinsic differences in patient physiology, patient selection or access to ECPR itself is unclear. When compared to 79 cardiac arrest events in the same institution between 2000-2002 who did not receive ECMO for resuscitation, 36% survived to discharge. However, 0/10 conventional CPR patients survived after >30 minutes while 14/43 ECPR patients survived.

In a review of the ELSO registry focused on ECPR outcomes between 1992-2005, 682 patients were evaluated. [46] The median age was 3 months and median weight 4.6 kgs. Among diagnostic groups: cardiac disease (n=499, 73%), congenital heart disease (n=398), myocarditis and cardiomyopathy (n=101), sepsis (n=54, 8%), pediatric respiratory failure (n=43, 6%), miscellaneous (n=35, 5%), neonatal respiratory failure (n=34, 5%) and accidental injury (n=17, 2%). Although ECPR use increased over time, survival did not improve over the study period. Mortality was lower in children with neonatal respiratory disease and cardiac disease than with other diagnostic categories. Children who survived had higher median paO_2 and arterial pH before ECMO than children who died. Of 421 ECPR nonsurvivors, 221 patients (52%) died within 72 hours of ECMO initiation and brain-death criteria were met in 85%. Predictors of death in ECPR patients included need for CPR during ECMO (OR 3.06, 95% CI 1.42-6.58), arterial blood pH <7.2 on ECMO (OR 2.23, 95% CI 1.23-4.06), radiologic evidence of CNS injury during ECMO (OR 2.79, 95% CI, 1.55-5.02), pulmonary hemorrhage (OR 2.23, 95% CI 1.11-4.5) or renal injury (OR 1.89, 95% CI 1.17-3.03). The major limitation of the ELSO registry is that there is no long-term neurologic information provided in the database, no quality of life information and no data on CPR techniques or other adjunct therapies such as hypothermia. As with other reports, this review highlights the need for specific, prospective evaluation of these factors as well as neurologic outcome in patients undergoing ECPR.

In addition to pediatric patients, use of ECMO as a resuscitative tool in adults with refractory cardiac arrest is also increasing. Survival to discharge is often quoted as between 30-40%. [47] As with other studies, many reports outlining outcome in adults refer only to neurologic function at time of discharge and no specific long term testing and evaluation are available. Survival obtained with ECMO from these pilot reports have triggered a renewed interest in expanding the use of ECPR techniques to patients in adult emergency departments. The recent flurry of adult ECMO for H1N1 influenza has also increased awareness of ECMO in the adult community. These events may well significantly increase the use of ECMO internationally.

New equipment, which is smaller, easier to use and portable, combined with better understanding of patient management techniques may herald a new frontier for ECMO use. Close attention to functional outcome and quality of life among survivors of ECMO, as well as analysis of cost-benefit ratios, are mandated to avoid excessive use of ECMO techniques or to help more firmly establish their beneficial role in the medical treatment armentarium.

References

1. ECLS Registry Report of the Extracorporeal Life Support Organization (ELSO), Ann Arbor, University of Michigan, July 2009.

2. Dalton HJ, Weise K, Davis K et al. Survival in Pediatric Respiratory Failure: Is It Really Improving? Pediatric Critical Care Colloquium, Chicago, IL, 1998;14.

3. Wilson JM, Bower LK, Thompson JE. ECMO in evolution: the impact of changing patient demographics and alternative therapies on ECMO. J Pediatr Surg 1996;31:1116-1123.

4. O'Toole G, Peek G, Jaffe W. Extracorporeal membrane oxygenation in the treatment of inhalation injuries. Burns 1998;24:562-5.

5. Goldman AP, Kerr SJ, Butt W, et al. Extracorporeal support for intractable respiratory failure due to meningococcal disease. Lancet 1997;349:466-469.

6. Michaels AJ, Schreiner RJ, Kolla S, et al. Extracorporeal life support in pulmonary failure after trauma. J Trauma 1999;46:638-645.

7. Linden V, Karelen, J, Olsson M et al. Successful extracorporeal membrane oxygenation in four children with malignant disease and severe pneumocystis carinii pneumonia. Medical and Pediatric Oncology 1999;32:25-31.

8. Dalton HJ, Thompson AE. Extracorporeal membrane oxygenation. In. Pediatric Critical Care, Second Edition, Eds: Fuhrman BP and Zimmerman JJ, Mosby, St. Louis, MO, 1998:562-575.

9. Kanter KR, Pennington DG, Weber TG, et al. Extracorporeal membrane oxygenation for postoperative cardiac failure in children. J Thorac Cardiovasc Surg 1987;93:27-35.

10. Del Nido P. Extracorporeal membrane oxygenation for cardiac support in children. Ann Thorac Surg 1996;41:365-384.

11. Kulik T, Moler F, Palmisano J. Outcome-associated factors in pediatric patients treated with extracorporeal membrane oxygenation after cardiac surgery. Circulation 1996;94:1163-68.

12. Klein MD, Shaheen KW, Whittlesey GC, et al. Extracorporeal membrane oxygenation for the circulatory support of children after repair of congenital heart disease. J Thorac Cardiovasc Surg 1990;100:498-505.

13. del Nido P, Armitage J, Fricker J. Extracorporeal Membrane Oxygenation Support as a Bridge to Pediatric Heart Transplantation. Circulation 1994;90:1167-69.

14. Dalton H, Siewers R, Fuhrman B. Extracorporeal membrane oxygenation for cardiac rescue in children with severe myocardial dysfunction. Crit Care Med 1993;21:1020-28.

15. Duncan BW, Ibrahim AE, Hraska V, et al. Use of rapid-deployment extracorporeal membrane oxygenation for the resuscitation of pediatric patients with heart disease after cardiac arrest. J Thorac Cardiovasc Surg 1998;116:305-311.

16. Duncan B, Hraska V, Jonas R. Mechanical Circulatory support in children with cardiac disease. J Thorac Cardiovasc Surg 1999;117:529-542.

17. Kolla S, Awad SS, Rich PB, Schreiner RJ, Hirschl RB, Bartlett RH. Extracorporeal life support in 100 adult patient with severe respiratory failure. Annals of Surg 1997;226-544-566.

18. Zapol WM, Snider MT, Hill JD, Fallat RJ, Bartlett RH, Edmunds LH, Morris AH, Peirce EC 2nd, Thomas AN, Proctor HJ, Drinker PA, Pratt PC, Bagniewski A, Miller RG Jr.Extracorporeal membrane oxygenation in severe acute respiratory failure. A randomized prospective study. JAMA. 1979 Nov 16;242(20):2193-6.

19. Peek, GJ, Mugford M, Tiruvoipati R, Wilson A, Allen E, Thalanany MM, Hibbert CL, Truesdale A, Clemens F, Cooper N, Firmin RK, Elbourne D. Efficacy and economic assessment of conventional ventilatory support versus extracorporeal membrane oxygenation for severe adult respiratory failure (CESAR): a multicentr randomized controlled trial. Lancet; 373:1351-63.

20. Matamoros A, Anderson JC, McConnell J, et al: Neurosonographic findings in infants treated by extracorporeal membrane oxygenation (ECMO). J Child Neurol 4(suppl):S52, 1989.

21. Krummel TM, Greenfield LJ, Kirkpatrick BV, et al: The early evaluation of survivors after extracorporeal membrane oxygenation for neonatal pulmonary failure. J Pediatr Surg 19:585, 1984.

22. Schumacher RE, Barks JD, Johnston MV, et al: Right-sided brain lesions in infants following

extracorporeal membrane oxygenation. Pediatrics 82:155, 1988.

23. Adolph V, Bonis S, Falterman K, Arensman R: Carotid artery repair after pediatric extracorporeal membrane oxygenation. J Pediatr Surg 25(8):867, 1990

24. Towne BH, Lott IT, Hicks DA, et al: Long-term follow-up of infants and children treated with extracorporeal membrane oxygenation (ECMO): A preliminary report. J Pediatr Surg 20:410, 1985.

25. Fligor BJ, Neault MW, Mullen CH, Feldman HA, Jones DT Factors associated with sensorineural hearing loss among survivors of extracorporeal membrane oxygenation therapy. Pediatrics 2005; 115:1519-1528.

26. Lott IT, McPherson D, Towne B, et al: Long-term neurophysiologic outcome after neonatal extracorporeal membrane oxygenation. J Pediatr 116:343, 1990.

27. Hofkosh D, Clouse H, Smith-Jones J, et al: Ten years of ECMO: neurodevelopmental outcome among survivors. Pediatr Res 27:246A, 1990.

28. Adolph V, Ekelund C, Smith C. Developmental outcome of neonates treated with extracorporeal membrane oxygenation. J Pediatr Surg 1990;25:43-46.

29. Amigoni A, Pettenazzo A, Zacchello F et al. Neurologic outcome in children after ECMO: prognostic value of diagnostic tests. Ped Neurology 2005; 32:173-179

30. Koumbourlis AC, Motoyama EK, Mutich RL. Lung mechanics during and after extracorporeal membrane oxygenation for meconium aspiration syndrome. Crit Care Med 1992; 20:751-756.

31. Boykin AR, Quivers ES, Wagenhoffer KL, Sable CA, Chaney HR, Glass P, Bahrami KR, Short BL. Cardiopulmonary outcome of neonatal extracorporeal membrane oxygenation at ages 10-15 years. Crit Care Med. 2003 Sep;31(9):2380-4.

32. Heulitt MJ, Moss MM, Walker WM. Morbidity and mortality in pediatric patients with respiratory failure. Extracorporeal Life Support Meeting, 1993;41.

33. Heulitt M, personal communication, 1998

34. UK Collaborative ECMO Group The Collaborative UK ECMO Trial: Follow-up to 1 Year of Age. Pediatrics 1998;101(4).

35. Barrett CS, Bratton SL, Salvin JW, Laussen PC, Rycus PT, Thiagrajan RR Neurological injury after extracorporeal membrane oxygenation use to aid pediatric cardiopulmonary resuscitation Pediatr Crit Care Med 2009;10:445-451.

36. Ibrahim AE, Duncan BW, Blume ED, Jonas RA Long-term follow-up of pediatric cardiac patients requiring mechanical circulatory support. Ann Thorac Surg. 2000 Jan;69(1):186-92.

37. Raymond TT, Cunnyngham CB, Thompson MT, Thomas JA, Dalton HJ, Nadkarni VM; for the American Heart Association National Registry of CPR Investigators. Outcomes among neonates, infants, and children after extracorporeal cardiopulmonary resuscitation for refractory in-hospital pediatric cardiac arrest: A report from the National Registry of CardioPulmonary Resuscitation. Pediatr Crit Care Med. 2009 Nov 17. [Epub ahead of print]

38. Kulik T, Moler F, Palmisano J. Outcome-Associated Factors in Pediatric Patients Treated With Extracorporeal Membrane Oxygenator After Cardiac Surgery. Circulation 1996; 94:II63-68.

39. Jen HC, Shew SB. Pediatrics (in submission, with permission) 2010.

40. Fajardo EM. Outcome and follow-up of children following extracorporeal life support in ECMO: Extracorporeal cardiopulmonary support in critical care. (Zwischenberger JB, Barlett RH eds, Extracorporeal Life Support Organization pub., Ann Arbor, MI) 1975;373-381.

41. Kolovos NS, Bratton SL, Moler FW, Bove EL, Ohye RG, Bartlett RH, Kulik TJ. Outcome of pediatric patients treated with extracorporeal life support after cardiac surgery. Ann Thorac Surg. 2003 Nov;76(5):1435-41.

42. Hamrick SE, Gremmels DB, Keet CA, Leonard CH, Connell JK, Hawgood S, Piecuch RE. Neurodevelopmental outcome of infants supported with extracorporeal membrane oxygenation after cardiac surgery. Pediatrics. 2003 Jun;111(6 Pt 1):e671-5.

43. Lequier L, Joffe AR, Robertson CMT, Dinu IA, Wongswadiwat Y, Anton NR, Ross DB, Rebeyka IM Two-year survival, mental, and

motor outcomes after cardiac extracorporeal life support at less than five years of age, J Thorac Cardiovasc Surg. 2008; 136:976-83

44. Chow G, Koirala B, Bohn D, de Veber G et al Predictors of mortality and neurological morbidity in children undergoing extracorporeal life support for cardiac disease. Eur J Cardiothorac Surg 2004;26:38-43

45. Morris MC, Wernovsky G, Nadkarni VM Survival outcomes after extracorporeal cardiopulmonary resuscitation instituted during active chest compressions following refractory in-hospital pediatric cardiac arrest. Pediatr Crit Care Med. 2004 Sep;5(5):440-6Kulik T, Moler F, Palmisano J. Outcome-Associated Factors in Pediatric Patients Treated With Extracorporeal Membrane Oxygenator After Cardiac Surgery. Circulation 1996; 94:II63-68.

46. Barrett CS, Bratton SL, Salvin JW, Laussen PC, Rycus PT, Thiagrajan RR Neurological injury after extracorporeal membrane oxygenation use to aid pediatric cardiopulmonary resuscitation Pediatr Crit Care Med 2009;10:445-451.

47. Hemmila MR, Rowe SA, Boules TN, Miskulin J, McGillicuddy JW, Schuerer DJ, Haft JW, Swaniker F, Arbabi S, Hirschl RB, Bartlett RH Extracorporeal life support for severe acute respiratory distress syndrome in adults. Ann Surg. 2004 Oct;240(4):595-605

Chapter 23 Questions

1. The majority of patients who received cardiac ECMO were placed on bypass with the following diagnosis:
    a) Bridge to transplant
    b) Myocarditis
    c) Cardiac arrest
    d) Following repair of congenital heart disease

2. Neuroimaging abnormalities have no relationship to observed outcome in ECMO patients
    a) True
    b) False

3. The following abnormalities have been noted in > 5% of pediatric ECMO survivors treated for respiratory failure EXCEPT:
    a) Stroke
    b) Hydrocephalus
    c) Mild to moderate mental retardation
    d) Chronic renal failure

4. The neurologic complications seen in survivors of cardiac ECMO differ greatly than those seen in ECMO survivors treated for respiratory failure.
    a) True
    b) False

5. The following statement correctly describes the changing ECMO demographics noted in the medical literature or ELSO Registry:
    a) Most patients in cardiac failure receive venovenous ECMO
    b) Neonatal ECMO for respiratory failure has increased
    c) ECMO has never been successfully used during resuscitation from cardiac arrest
    d) Adults with respiratory failure are currently the largest group of patients who are placed on ECMO support
    e) None of the above

Chapter 23 Answers

1. d
2. b
3. b
4. b
5. e

24

Case Scenarios - Neonatal, Cardiac, ECPR, Adult, Pediatric

Patricia English, MS, RRT-NPS and Jeanne Braby, MSN, RN, CCRN

Objectives

After completion of this chapter, the participant should be able to:

- List the questions that need to be answered when considering whether a patient is a candidate for ECMO support
- List several parameters that indicate adequate oxygen delivery during venovenous ECMO support
- List several complications associated with providing ECMO support
- Describe common technical causes of acute desaturation during ECMO

Introduction

The scenarios presented in this chapter are designed to highlight physiological and technical issues associated with managing patients on both venoarterial and venovenous ECMO support. It is hoped that after reviewing the situations presented, the specialist will be better prepared to respond to ECMO complications.

The five scenarios presented are based on actual patient situations. Some events have been changed to de-identify the patient. Some situations have been expanded or exaggerated to allow the reader greater learning opportunities. Further explanations associated with the discussion points raised with each scenario can be found in various chapters in this manual as well as chapters in the ECMO Extracorporeal Cardiopulmonary Support in Critical Care, 3rd edition.

As the scenarios play out, responses to situations are suggested. It is important for the reader

to know that the suggested responses will be the philosophy of some centers but may not be the standard approach for other centers. Throughout each scenario discussion points are highlighted. These discussion points are written to help ECMO Specialists reflect on how a similar situation might be handled in their center.

Neonatal Case Scenario

Baby J is a 41 week gestational age, 3.5 kg infant born by normal spontaneous vaginal delivery. Meconium stained fluid was noted and the baby was limp and without spontaneous respiration. The infant was intubated twice, each time suctioned for large amounts of meconium. The baby remained apneic with a heart rate of 60. Positive pressure via bag mask ventilation with 100% oxygen was given. After 30 seconds the infant had a heart rate of 120 and began to breathe spontaneously. The infant was taken to the special care nursery breathing spontaneously on nasal cannula oxygen. Over the next hour the baby developed increasing respiratory distress. He was transferred to the NICU, intubated and placed on a mechanical ventilator. Surfactant was administered before a chest x-ray (CXR) confirmed the endotracheal tube (ETT) was in the right mainstem bronchus. The ETT was repositioned. A right–sided pneumothorax was also noted. A pigtail catheter was placed and the pneumothorax resolved.

Two hours later the infant had an acute desaturation. Decreased breath sounds were noted bilaterally and a repeat CXR showed bilateral pneumothoraces. A pigtail catheter was placed on the left and a second pigtail placed on the right. The baby continued to decompensate and an ECMO center transport team was called. The baby arrived at the ECMO center hypercarbic, hypoxic, hypotensive, on vasopressors and nitric oxide. Attempts to improve hemodynamics, oxygenation, and ventilation were made over the next four hours. Air leak continued from two pigtail catheters. The infant's best PO_2 was 42 mmHg and the lactic acid level continued to rise. A cardiac ECHO showed suprasystemic pulmonary artery pressures, right to left shunting at the ductal level and at the foramen ovale, with poor biventricular function. A head ultrasound was negative for hemorrhage. A coagulation panel was sent and no coagulation issues were identified. The decision was made to place the infant on VV ECMO.

An ECMO circuit was primed with PRBC, heparin, tham, albumin, and calcium gluconate. The infant received a bolus of heparin prior to cannulation. A 12 Fr double lumen cannula was placed in the mid right atrium and the infant was started on VV support. ECMO flow was increased to 400 mL/min (114/kg/min) over twenty minutes using a roller pump and a silicone membrane oxygenator. The sweep flow was started at 1 lpm, at 70% oxygen. Oxygen saturation improved from 68% to 78%.

Discussion points:

- With pump flows set at nearly 115 mL/kg/min why didn't the patient's arterial saturations increase further?
- What is the normal cardiac output of a 3.5 kg infant?
- What are concerns with VV ECMO that may limit the potential to support this patient?
- Should the patient have been cannulated for VA support instead of VV support?
- Is twenty minutes an appropriate amount of time to ramp up the pump flow to 400ml/min?
- What are specific concerns associated with the use of a double lumen cannula?
- What are signs of significant recirculation?
- What can be done to minimize recirculation?
- Could the pump occlusion be set inappropriately?
- How can the pump occlusion be verified after support has been started?

Arterial, pre-membrane and post-membrane blood gases were obtained and the results are listed in Table 1.

The color of the blood in the drainage line resembled the color in the return line, both appearing well saturated. The cannulating surgeon was made aware of the concern and repositioned the cannula. Decreased recirculation resulted as evidenced by desaturated blood in the drainage line. The infant's arterial saturations improving to 92%. The mean arterial blood pressure (MAP) improved and the vasopressors were weaned slightly maintaining a MAP between 45 and 60 mmHg. The ventilator settings were weaned and the infant's saturations remained stable in the low 90's. An ACT was obtained soon after support was started. The results were higher than desired so an ACT was obtained every 30 minutes until the ACT decreased to 250 seconds. A continuous heparin infusion was started at 20 units/kg/hour and ACTs were followed hourly with a goal of maintaining ACTs at 200 seconds.

On ECMO day two the infant's sedation had been weaned and he was moving all extremities and opening his eyes. His blood pressure was stable and his oxygen saturations were in the high 80's to low 90's. An audible alarm sounded on the console of the SS III and the flow rate was noted to be ramping down and then stopped. The baby's color quickly became dusky and his oxygen saturations fell from 89% to 75%. A drop in MAP to 32 mmHg was noted.

Table1. Blood Gas Results

	pH	PCO_2 mmHg	PO_2 mmHg
Pre-membrane	7.42	40	68
Post-membrane	7.44	38	240
Arterial	7.36	48	52

Discussion points:

- When the pump stops should hand cranking be immediately initiated?
- Which alarm(s) could have sounded and activated the flow ramping, then stopping the pump?
- If the bladder (negative) pressure alarm sounded what are the most likely causes?
- What causes acute changes in right atrial volume?
- What are indications that the pump flow is too high?
- What could acutely restrict flow out of the drainage lumen?
- If a clot occurred where would it most likely have lodged?
- If the cannula is kinked what is a likely cause in an awake moving patient?
- If a high pressure alarm (post-pump) sounded what are the most likely causes?
- What effect does the patient's blood pressure have on the circuit pressures during VV support?
- What is the most likely reason the blood pressure fell?
- Where is the most appropriate place to begin to determine the cause of a high pressure alarm?
- How should the patient be managed while the cause of the problem is being identified?
- Should the alarm limits be changed in order to get some support to the patient?

After identifying that the negative pressure alarm caused the pump to stop, the specialist observed that the baby had turned his head toward the cannula and created a kink in the cannula. The baby's head was repositioned, the kink resolved and the pump support was restored to baseline.

At ECMO hour 54 the SPO$_2$ suddenly decreased to from 90 to 72%. The infant appeared dusky, became tachypneic and tachycardiac.

Discussion points:

- What is a likely reason for a sudden increase in respiratory rate during ECMO support?

- Why would a patient being supported with ECMO suddenly become dusky?
- Could the pump flow have been inadvertently changed?
- Does the blood coming out of the oxygenator appear well saturated?
- Is the sweep flow connected to the oxygenator?
- Is the sweep flow connected at the gas source and is the flow rate still the same?
- If the gas source is an oxygen blender, could the blender have failed?

Knowing that acute changes in saturation and ventilation are most likely signs of technical issues, the ECMO specialist started a rapid visual inspection of the ECMO system. The pump flow remained at 400 mL/minute. The system pressures were unchanged and the sweep flow meter was running at 1 lpm. The team was called to the bedside. The ventilator FIO$_2$ was turned up to 1.0 with minor improvement in SPO$_2$. The specialist then noted that blood coming out of the oxygenator was quite dark and quickly inspected the oxygen supply tubing. The tubing had become disconnected at the oxygenator. The tubing was re-attached to the oxygenator. The infant's SPO$_2$ improved, heart rate (HR) and respiratory rate (RR) returned to baseline.

Later the same night the patient's vasopressor requirement was increased in order to maintain a MAP > 45 mmHg. The pump speed began slowing down and a pump flow of only 75 mL/kg was obtainable. A recent CBC revealed a drop in platelets from 105K to 88K and a decrease in hematocrit from 35 to 30%. The last ACT was high at 250 seconds on 35 units/kg/hr.

Discussion points:

- Could a 5% decrease in hematocrit indicate the patient is actively bleeding?
- Where are likely sources for bleeding?
- Should the patient immediately receive a transfusion?
- What are other possibilities for a 5% decrease in hematocrit?
- Should the hematocrit be repeated if there are no obvious clinical signs of bleeding?

- The patient's ACT was 50 seconds above the prescribed range. Is that likely causing the patient to bleed?

During the period when the hematocrit decreased, the chest tube output which had been 1-2 mL/hour for several hours had increased to 25 mL from the right side and 15 mL from the left side. In response to the increased bleeding from the chest tubes the target ACT was lowered to 160-180 seconds. The heparin infusion was reduced from 35 units /kg/hr to 20 units/ kg/hr. The patient received a platelet transfusion and 10 ml/kg transfusion of PRBC. Over the next few hours the chest tube output lessened and the patient's blood pressure stabilized.

On ECMO day five the infant was stable hemodynamically, off all vasopressors, and on low ventilator support with a SPO_2 in the low 90's. There had been no clinical evidence of ductal shunting for >48 hours and a repeat ECHO confirmed decreased pulmonary artery pressures with improved biventricular function. The CXR showed good lung expansion bilaterally. The tidal volume increased from 2 mL/kg to 5 ml/kg. The sweep flow was weaned from 1 lpm to off over 6 hours. The ventilator support was adjusted to provide adequate CO_2 removal. The patient's SPO_2 remained stable on 40% oxygen. The patient was trialed off ECMO support with the membrane capped. The pump flow continued at 400 mL/min.

Discussion points:

- What is the purpose of "capping" the membrane?
- What needs to be monitored closely during the trial off period?
- Are the venous saturations useful during a trial off of VV support?
- What are indications of a failed trail off ECMO support
- When weaning VV support does the pump flow need to be weaned?

After four hours the patient remained hemodynamically stable with SPO_2's in the low 90's on 40% oxygen. The arterial blood gas showed adequate

CO_2 and pH. The patient was decannulated and discharged to home on day of life 21.

Cardiac Case Scenario

A 2 ½ month old male with a history of truncus repair was placed on ECMO for cardiac support after an unsuccessful attempt at chest closure. He was born at 30 weeks gestation with a birth weight of 1266 grams. At the time of cannulation, his weight was 2.9 Kg. He had one mediastinal and two pleural chest tubes. A 16 Fr DLP cannula was placed directly into his right atrium and an 8 Fr DLP cannula was placed in his aorta. A roller pump with a Carmeda-coated circuit, a hollow fiber oxygenator, and a silicone bladder was used. The cardiovascular surgeon ordered that heparin not be used for 24 hours because the patient was at risk for bleeding. The initial pump flow was 500 mL/min (172 mL/kg/min.). The initial pre-oxygenator pressure was 218 with a post-oxygenator pressure of 202 and a gradient of 16. The initial ACT was 344 using an ACT+ cuvette with the Hemochron Signature Plus analyzer. The next hour's ACT was 171. Target range for a patient at risk of bleeding is 160-180 seconds using this instrument and the ACT+ cuvette. At hour 5 of ECMO, the ACT was 145, with a repeat of 134 seconds. The information was relayed to the new attending MD in the following way, using the SBAR tool for communication.

Situation: "The ACT is now 145 seconds."
Background: "Dr. CV did not want any heparin started for 24 hours."
Assessment: "The ACT has fallen below the range of an unheparinized patient. I am oncerned that clots will begin to form in the circuit if the ACTs remain this low."
Recommendation: "I would like to start the heparin and get the ACT back within range."

The MD agreed to start the heparin at 10 units/kg/hr, and increase the drip as needed to maintain ACT's 160-180 seconds. Table 2 shows the resulting ACT's along with the heparin dose.

Discussion points:

- What is the best way to communicate information?
- How do you deal with conflicting orders from different physicians?
- What are the risks/benefits of not running heparin in a circuit?
- What are the risks/benefits of using uncoated circuits?
- What is considered the normal range of heparin drips on ECMO?
- What could affect the increased need for heparin?
- What else should be considered?
- What affects the pre and post-oxygenator pressures?

At hour 9 an antithrombin III (AT III) activity level was sent. It came back @ 47% (normal laboratory reference range for this age patient is 48-108%). At hour 12, the ECMO specialist noted a clot in the arterial cannula. The patient was removed from ECMO and the surgeon was able to remove the clot from the cannula. The urine output ranged from 25-80 mL/hr (8-27 mL/kg/hr). AT III concentrate was given at hour 14, and the heparin rate was decreased to 50 units/kg/hr.

The patient's heparin requirements continued to increase on day 2 of ECMO. The heparin drip needed to be increased to100 units/kg/hr in order to maintain the ACT within the range of 180-200 seconds. The AT III activity level was 128%.

Discussion points:

- What else could affect the heparin requirements?
- What other test results would be important to know?
- When should FFP be given?
- When should Vitamin K be given?
- When should cryoprecipitate be given?
- When should you verify the concentration of the heparin syringe or bag?
- How does AT III effect heparin requirements?

Table 2. ACT and Heparin dose

ECMO hour	ACT	Heparin bolus (u/kg)	Heparin drip rate (u/kg/hr)
5	145/134	10	10
5 ½	123	20	20
6	150	10	25
6 ½	130	20	35
7	146	10	45
7 ½	135	30	50
8	148	20	55
8 ½	147	20	60
9	137	30	65
9 ½	153	30	65
10	165		65

Table 3 below shows the results of a DIC screen

The platelet count ranged from 80-120K, and the patient was requiring 1-2 units of platelets per day. A heparin level was drawn and it came back at 0.3 units/ml, which was considered adequate.

On day 3 of ECMO, the pump flow was gradually decreased from 400 mL/minute (138 mL/kg/min.) to 200 mL/ min (69 mL/kg/min.). The mean BP's had been >40 mmHg on a pump flow of 400 mL/min. When the pump flow was decreased to 200, his mean BP dropped to 30 mm Hg. His SPO_2 decreased from 95 to 80%.

Discussion points:

- On VA ECMO, what parameters would indicate that a pump wean is successful?
- What are other indicators of perfusion?

On day 4 of ECMO, the patient's PCO_2 was 71 mmHg on an ABG. The orders were to maintain the PCO_2 40-60. The ECMO pump flow was at 400 mL/min. and the gas (sweep) flow was at 0.3 L/min.

Discussion points:

- What adjustment should be made to the pump?
- How do you determine what is the low and high limit of sweep flow?
- When do you worry that the oxygenator is failing?
- What devices do you have to monitor the effect of pump flow or sweep changes?

The sweep flow was increased to 0.4 L/min and the resulting patient PCO_2 was 56 mmHg.

On day 5 of ECMO, the circuit was changed due to large amount of plasma leakage from the hollow fiber oxygenator, as well as for the appearance of multiple fibrin strands coating the tubing.

Discussion points:

- How does a circuit change affect medications the patient is receiving?
- Is it beneficial to pre-medicate with steroids prior to a planned circuit change?
- Will the patient need platelets after a circuit change?

The heparin was stopped for a planned chest exploration. The pump flow was increased to 900 mL/minute (310mL/kg/min.) during the surgery. When the ACT dropped to 170 seconds, the heparin was started at 10 units/kg/hr. Factor VIIA (Novoseven) was given for large amount of bleeding from the chest tubes.

After discussion with the parents, the patient was decannulated after 172 hours on ECMO due to futility.

Discussion points:

- What is the dose for Factor VIIA?
- What are the risks of factor VIIA administration during ECMO?
- How do you determine when to discontinue ECMO?
- How should the subject of discontinuing support discussed with the family?
- How do you debrief/support the staff after a long ECMO run?

Table 3. DIC Screen

		Normal ranges
PT	15.8 sec	(12.1-14.2) sec
INR	1.38	
PTT	>200 sec	(23.8-35.0) sec
TT	>100	(13.1-19.8) sec
Fib	200	(200-400mg/dl)
D-Dimer	1.70	(<0.46 ug/ml)

ECPR Patient Case Scenario

A 9 month old 7 Kg female with a diagnosis of hypoplastic left heart syndrome status post stage II palliation with a Glenn at 6 months of age, was admitted to an outside hospital emergency room for fever and increased irritability. She had a 2 day history of increased stools. Her vital signs were reported as HR 236, RR 38, SPO_2 of 70%, and temperature of 105.1 F. She was given acetaminophen and ibuprofen. An IV was started, and she was given a dose of an antibiotic. When the transport team arrived, they noted that the patient clinically appeared to have evidence of poor cardiac output.

Discussion points:

- What is the expected SPO_2 for a single ventricle patient who is status post a Glenn-Surgery?
- What are some clinical symptoms of decreased cardiac output?

She had grunting respirations, cool and clammy extremities, and poor pulses. An attempt to repeat a fluid bolus of 20 mL/kg of normal saline resulted in IV infiltration, so an intraosseous line was placed and she received another fluid bolus and was started on an epinephrine drip at 0.1 mcg/kg/min. Her hemodynamics remained unstable and she became increasingly tachypneic. During this time, her heart rates were in the 250s. The transport nurse was unable to obtain a blood pressure or a pulse oximeter reading and the child was intubated. The epinephrine was increased to 0.2 mcg/kg/min, and a milrinone drip was started at 0.5 mcg/kg/min. On the flight back, her HR decreased from 250's to 160's and 170's. A BP of 113/75 with a mean of 86 was obtained. Her epinephrine was turned down to 0.1 mcg/kg/min. Her pulse oximetry was intermittently obtained with SPO_2 readings of 63% with poor tracings. Her extremities remained mottled and her pulses, skin temperature, and capillary refill time were poor.

Upon arrival to the PICU, attempts were made to place arterial and central lines. Epinephrine was rapidly escalated to 1 mcg/kg/min and a norepinephrine infusion was started and escalated to 1 mcg/

kg/min. The HR dropped to 100, and the nurse was unable to obtain a blood pressure or palpate a pulse. Compressions were started, and the child's head was packed in ice. Venous blood gas showed pH 6.88, PCO_2 103, PO_2 38.6, venous sat 35.6% and base deficit of 22.2. The Hct was 58.8, glucose 31, and lactic acid 52 (normal 4.0-15.0 mg/dl).

Discussion points:

- At what point should the ECMO team be called?
- What tests, labs, etc. need to be done prior to ECMO?
- What factors determine if the patient is an ECMO candidate?
- Who should make the final decision?

The patient was placed on a Biomedicus (centrifugal) pump with a Carmeda-coated circuit and a Minimax Plus hollow fiber oxygenator. An 8 Fr Carmeda coated Biomedicus cannula was placed in the right common carotid artery. A 10 Fr Carmeda-coated Biomedicus cannula was placed in the right internal jugular vein and it was connected with to a10 Fr FemFlex cannula that was placed in the right Femoral Vein. The initial pump flow was 850 mL/min (120 mL/kg/min) with the pump RPMs at 2680.

Discussion points:

- What special cannulation techniques are necessary when a patient has had a Glenn procedure?
- What temperature do you want to "cool" the patient after a cardiac arrest?
- How long do you want to keep them cool?
- How high of an ECMO pump flow is necessary for a single ventricle patient?
- What determines how high you can adjust your RPMs?
- What is an adequate blood pressure?
- How does preload and afterload affect pump flow with a centrifugal pump?

The first ABG on ECMO was pH 7.11, PCO_2 52.6, PO_2 174, sat 98% with a base deficit of 12.3. On hour 6 of ECMO, her ABG was pH 7.22, PCO_2

56.1, PO_2 129, SPO_2 98% with a base deficit of 5.3. By ECMO hour 24, her pressors were able to be weaned off, and her mean BP's remained in the mid 50's. The water temperature was set in the blood warmer to maintain her core temperature between 32 and 34 degrees Celsius. Her HR was in the 140-150 range. Her pre- and post-oxygenator pressures were in the 320-340 range. Urine output was low at 1 ml/kg/hr, and was blood-tinged. Her BUN and creatinine are listed in Table 4 below. She was at a positive fluid balance of 1 liter.

Discussion points:

- When using a centrifugal pump when should you be concerned about high oxygenator pressures?
- What can you do to lower oxygenator pressures?
- How do you know if hemolysis is occurring?
- Under what conditions should hemofiltration be considered?
- Where should the hemofilter shunt be placed in the circuit?
- How do you assess actual pump flow with a hemofilter in place?

Hemofiltration was started on ECMO day 3 to remove 20 cc/hr. The RPMs were decreased to 2360 with a resulting pump flow of 720 mL/min (102 mL/kg/min). The pre- and post-oxygenator pressures

Table 4 BUN and Creatinine*

ECMO day	BUN	Creatinine
1	49	1.1
2	62	1.3
3	72	1.8
4	96	2.2
5	118	2.7

*Normals BUN 5-20 mg/dl, Creatinine 0-0.5 mg/dl

decreased to 250-260 range. At ECMO hour 50, the oxygenator had started to leak, and the urine continued to be bloody. The decision was made to switch to a roller pump circuit.

On ECMO day 4 the head ultrasound showed a left frontal and parietal area lobe hemorrhage with a questionable area representing a cerebrovascular event. The patient was transported for a CT scan. A head CT showed a right middle cerebral artery stroke with multiple petecchial hemorrhages. ECMO was discontinued after discussion with the family and the parents were assisted in holding their child. She expired 4 hours later.

Discussion points:

- Is a CT necessary?
- What do you need to consider prior to an in-house ECMO transport?
- What personnel should be present to assist with a transport?
- How can the cannulas be cut and clamped from the circuit to enable a family to hold the child easily?

Adult Respiratory Failure Patient Case Scenario

A 54 year old 60 Kg female was diagnosed with necrotizing pneumonia. On day two of hospitalization she began having increasing respiratory distress resulting in intubation and moderate ventilator support. On day 3, her CXR showed bilateral lower lobe and right middle lobe consolidation with a small right pleural effusion.

On day 5 of hospitalization, her CXR revealed new consolidations in both upper lobes and bilateral effusions, right side greater then left. On day 6 the patient became increasingly more hypoxemic, hypercarbic and acidotic. Arterial blood gas results were as follow: pH 7.15; pCO_2 82; PO_2 46; SPO_2 77%; SVO_2 47% on significant ventilator settings: RR 26; VT 360; PIP 50; PEEP 17; FIO_2 1.0. She was on multiple vasopressors and her vital signs were HR 156, BP 80/56 with a mean BP of 66 mmHg. The ECMO team was consulted.

Discussion points:

- When should ECMO be considered for adult respiratory failure?
- What level and length of time on ventilator support is considered a relative contraindication to ECMO?
- Is there an age and/or weight limit above which ECMO should not be considered?
- Is ECMO an appropriate option with more than one organ system failure?
- Would a patient with a coagulopathy be an ECMO candidate ?
- Is there a reasonable expectation for a good quality of life post-ECMO?

In this case, ECMO was considered when the patient did not improve on escalated ventilator settings. At the level of ventilator support being used, ventilator induced lung disease was a significant concern. Consideration was given for the duration of ventilator support, but except for the last 16 hours pre-ECMO, she had been on moderate levels of ventilator support. It was felt that her lung process was likely reversible and that she had no other organ system failure. She was not coagulopathic. The expectation of a good quality of life was reasonable.

Discussion points:

- What type of support is most appropriate for this patient -VA or VV support?
- What are the goals of support (adequate O_2 delivery/ CO_2 removal, cardiac support, minimize barotrauma)?
- Do existing central venous lines complicate cannulation?
- Are any potential cannulation sites infected?
- What is the center's experience with managing various types of ECLS?
- What type of equipment is needed?
- Are appropriate size and type cannulas available?

The primary goals for this patient were adequate oxygen delivery while minimizing the potential for barotrauma. Her degree of hemodynamic stability was considered and it was felt that with adequate oxygen delivery on ECMO, her cardiac function would improve and her vasopressor requirement would diminish. The decision was made to place her on VV support. A 23 French right internal jugular cannula was placed for drainage and a 17 French cannula was placed in the left femoral vein as a return cannula. Her right groin was not used for cannulation since a previously placed right groin central line had a positive blood culture. A roller pump was used with a Quadrox D oxygenator. The initial pump flow was 3.5 liters per minute (lpm) and the sweep gas flow was 6 lpm.

Discussion points:

- Would the patient be better supported if the drainage cannula was in the femoral vein and the return cannula in the RIJ?
- What are the advantages of one site over another?
- How much pump flow is needed to provide adequate oxygen delivery?
- How is oxygen delivery assessed during VV support?
- Is recirculation a concern?

In this case, the jugular vein was used as the drainage cannula as the RIJ was able to accommodate a significantly larger cannula than the left femoral vein. A higher pump flow was likely to be achieved draining from the larger cannula. The determination of adequate oxygen delivery was made as vasopressor requirement decreased, baseline heart rate decreased from 156 to 90, lactic acid levels decreased, urine output increased, and the capillary refill time decreased from 5 seconds to < 3 seconds. Recirculation was not a significant factor. Desaturated blood was observed in the drainage line. Additionally the pre-oxygenator saturation was 70% while her arterial saturations were in the mid 80's. The ventilator FiO_2 was able to be lowered to 0.6.

On ECMO days 1-2, her vasopressor requirements were decreased further and her HR remained 85-90, with a BP of 110/60 and a MAP of 84. Her SPO_2 was 88-90%, on a pump flow of 3.5 lpm and 60% oxygen from the ventilator. Her ventilator support included PEEP of 20, a pressure control of 10, and a rate of 10. Her pH and PCO_2 improved; however, her total body fluid balance was 8 Liters positive. She remained stable and by ECMO days 3-6, she was able to be weaned off all vasopressors, and her oxygenation improved on a FiO_2 of 0.5 on the ventilator. In addition a vigorous diuresis was ongoing.

Discussion points:

- What are "acceptable" ventilator settings on VV ECMO?
- Would prone positioning be useful?
- Are ventilator recruitment maneuvers indicated?
- What is the effect of a positive fluid balance?
- Would hemofiltration be helpful?

In this case, the ventilator was set so that pressure did not exceed 30 cmH_2O to decrease the potential for ventilator induced lung injury. CO_2 removal was achieved using a sweep flow of 12 lpm. The FiO_2 was weaned maintaining the SPO_2 $\geq 85\%$. Daily lactic acid levels were followed to help evaluate adequacy of tissue oxygenation. The patient continued to diurese well on her own, diuretics and hemofiltration were not needed.

On ECMO days 7-9, daily bronchoscopies were done, removing large amounts of purulent secretions. By ECMO day 10 her SPO_2 improved to the low 90's on a FiO_2 of 0.5. On ECMO days 10-13, the PEEP was weaned from 18 to 12 but resulted in significant lung volume loss on CXR and worsening compliance. In hope of regaining lung volume the PEEP was increased to 24 cmH_2O.

Discussion points:

- How is best PEEP level determined?
- Should daily bronchoscopies be standard practice for adult respiratory failure patients on ECMO?
- What is the effect of PEEP on venous return?
- Does PEEP interfere with achieving the desired pump flow?

In this case, the PEEP of 24 did not appear to impact venous return since the pump flows could be maintained. The increased PEEP resulted in increased lung volume by CXR and improved compliance.

On ECMO day 14, a small increase in pre-membrane pressure was noted with no change in the post-oxygenator pressure. A few hours later, the pre-oxygenator pressure increased by 100 mm Hg, again with no increase in post-oxygentor pressure. The pump flow was decreased to maintain system pressures within desired range and the patient's SPO_2 remained above 88%. The d-dimers were elevated significantly.

Discussion points:

- Is the change in pre-oxygenator pressure significant?
- What is the maximum pre-oxygenator pressure?
- What affects pre-oxygenator pressure?
- With rising oxygenator pressures should the oxygenator be replaced or is a complete circuit change indicated?
- Should steroids be given prior to a circuit change?
- Should a new circuit be crystalloid or blood primed?
- What effect will a new circuit and/or oxygenator have on drugs/platelets/heparin?
- How is the patient supported the during a circuit change?
- What are other indicators to help decide when a circuit needs to be changed?

The high pre-oxygenator pressure indicated that the resistance in the oxygenator had increased, likely from clot formation The decision was made to change out the entire circuit because the patient had already been on ECMO for 2 weeks, was not likely to be weaned off ECMO in the next day or two, clots were visible in other parts of the circuit, and d-dimers were rising. An adult circuit was crystalloid primed and 25% albumin was added to decrease blood surface interactions. The ventilator support was adjusted and medications were readily available. The circuit was changed with only a brief interruption in support to the patient. Post circuit change PRBCs were given to achieve a hematocrit within the desired parameters. Platelets were not needed after the circuit change, likely because the Quadrox D oxygenator has little effect on platelets.

On ECMO days 15-17, the PEEP was gradually weaned from 24 to 15, and the patient remained well ventilated with stable oxygenation on a FIO$_2$ of 0.4. The patient's lung compliance improved significantly and her CXR began to show improvement. The sweep flow was decreased from 8 to 5 to 3 lpm and then removed. She remained well saturated, hemodynamically stable over the next two hours and was decannulated from ECMO. Two days post-decannulation a percutaneous tracheostomy was placed for long term ventilation. She was eventually weaned from ventilatory support and her tracheostomy was removed. On hospital day 40 she was discharged, neurologically intact, breathing room air.

Pediatric Respiratory Failure Case Scenario

A fifteen month old 11 kg. previously healthy child was admitted to an outside hospital and diagnosed with RSV bronchiolitis and respiratory failure. On hospital day one he was intubated and placed on a conventional ventilator. Over the next twenty-four hours he became increasingly more difficult to ventilate and was transferred to an ECMO center. On arrival at the ECMO center his SPO$_2$ was 82% on 100% oxygen. His PCO$_2$ was 166 with a pH 7.05. Despite ventilator adjustments, muscle relaxants with adequate sedation, an inhaled nitric oxide trial, and intravenous and inhaled steroids, his respiratory distress worsened. His PCO$_2$ remained greater than 150 mmHg and his oxygenation was marginal. He remained hemodynamically stable with good urine output for about twenty-four hours. The following morning his blood pressure began to decrease requiring vasopressors. A sputum sample sent at the outside hospital was now reported to be positive for adenovirus. An infectious disease consult was obtained and the recommendations of the I.D. team were instituted. His CXR showed diffuse bilateral airspace opacities consistent with multifocal pneumonia along with small bilateral pleural effusions. A cardiac ECHO was obtained with no structural defects noted and by ECHO his cardiac function was quite good. His coagulation panel showed no gross

coagulopathy. His oxygenation remained marginal and on hospital day 4 any attempt to provide care to the child resulted in significant desaturation with long recovery periods to achieve a saturation in the 80's. The decision was made to initiate VV ECMO.

An 18 Fr double lumen cannula was placed in the child's right internal jugular vein. The cannula was connected to a circuit consisting of 3/8 inch tubing with a 1.5 m2 silicone membrane oxygenator. Pump flow of 800 mL/min (72 mL/kg/min.) was achieved and the SPO$_2$ increased from the 60's to the low 80's. Five hours post-cannulation a kink was noted in the cannula and the maximum achievable pump flow was 500 mL/min. SPO$_2$ fell to the 70's. Surgery was consulted and a single lumen 18 Fr cannula was inserted into the RIJ along with a 14 Fr cannula inserted into the right femoral vein. A pump flow of 1 lpm was achieved and the patient's SPO$_2$ improved to mid 80's. The heart rate remained elevated at 155 and the blood pressure was labile. A fluid bolus was given twice and multiple vasopressors were added. Urine output dropped to 1 mL/kg/hour. Capillary refill was > 3 seconds and the plasma lactic acid level increased overnight. The ventilator FIO$_2$ remained at 1.0, PEEP of 16, pressure control of 14 with a tidal volume of 20 mL and a respiratory rate of 10. The sweep flow was at 4.5 lpm to achieve a patient PCO$_2$ of 80mmHg with a pH of 7.18. The following morning a 14 Fr arterial cannula was inserted into the right carotid artery and VA ECMO was initiated. A 2.5 m2 membrane was inserted into the circuit replacing the 1.5 m2. The maximum achievable pump flow was 1 lpm.

Discussion points:

- Is a pump flow of 1 lpm on VV support the same as a pump flow of 1 lpm on VA support?
- Would the amount of CO$_2$ removal be the same at a sweep flow of 4.5 lpm through a 2.5 m^2 membrane as it is through a 1.5 m^2 membrane?
- What would limit the maximum attainable pump flow to only 1 lpm?

On VA support with a pump flow of 1 lpm and sweep flow of 6 lpm the patient's condition was much improved: blood pressure was stable off pressors, heart rate decreased to 90, capillary refill < 3 seconds with an SPO$_2$ >95. The PCO$_2$ decreased to the 50's with a pH 7.33. The patient's lung compliance remained poor at 1.4 cc/cmH2O. The ventilator support was decreased to ECMO "rest" settings at an FIO$_2$ of 0.3 and the pressure control was decreased to 10 with a set rate of 10.

On ECMO day 5 the specialist attempted to reposition the tubing in the roller pump (walk the raceway) to avoid tubing wear. During the procedure the tubing became pinched in the roller and a raceway rupture occurred.

Discussion points:

- Should the raceway be rotated or repositioned periodically?
- What precautions should be taken during the raceway repositioning?
- Should the pump flow be turned off, or slowed during the procedure?
- What equipment needs to be at the bedside in the event of a raceway rupture?
- What fluid should the replacement tubing/connectors be primed with?
- When a rupture is identified how should the patient be managed?
- During the time off support for a circuit repair should heparin continue to be administered to the patient?

The specialist immediately called for assistance managing the patient anticipating that the patient may become unstable. She clamped the circuit off separating the patient from the circuit and quickly identified the point where the rupture had occurred. She applied manual pressure at the rupture to minimize circuit blood loss and was able to quickly reposition the tubing in the pump with the point of rupture positioned before the pump. While manually applying pressure on the tubing without impeding flow, she was able to re-start ECMO support. The sterile raceway repair kit, which was kept at the bedside, was opened. Preparation for repairing the rupture included having the optimal number and type of care givers at the bedside, adjusting the ventilator settings and preparing medications to treat

the patient during the time off ECMO support. The specialist took the lead in outlining to others what needed to be done and individual responsibilities were identified. The patient was clamped off support, the pump stopped and the sweep flow removed from the oxygenator. The ruptured raceway section was cut out and a fluid filled connector was inserted in order to join the cut raceway segments. The pump and sweep flow were re-started, after assessing that the circuit was free of air and without any further leak ECMO support was returned to the patient. During the time off ECMO the patient's SPO$_2$ fell to 78%, his heart rate dropped to 65 and he was hypotensive. As the pump flow was re-started the SPO$_2$ increased to 97% and his heart rate and blood pressure stabilized. The ventilator support was reduced back to the pre-event settings. The patient continued to receive heparin during the repair. An ACT was obtained immediately after re-starting support.

On ECMO day 4 the child's platelet count, which had been slowly decreasing, dropped from 90 K to 40K over six hours. The level prescribed for transfusion was >60 K and the child received a platelet transfusion. Despite the transfusion, the platelet count did not rise. A second transfusion was ordered and a Platelet Factor (PF4) was sent to test for heparin induced thrombocytopenia (HIT). A hematology consult was obtained and the consulting physician confirmed the diagnosis of HIT.

Discussion points:

- How is anticoagulation maintained during ECMO once HIT is confirmed?
- If an alternative method of anticoagulation is used what is the best method of assessing the appropriate amount of anticoagulation?
- If the cannulas are heparin coated do they need to be replaced?
- Are ACT's a reliable indicator of anticoagulation when heparin is not being administered?

The decision was made to change the ECMO circuit and to use a direct thrombin inhibitor for anticoagulation. In this case Argatroban was ordered. The patient was given a bolus dose of Argatroban and heparin was discontinued. A continuous infusion of Argatroban was started. ACT's could no longer be considered reliable indicators of adequate anticoagulation. The Argatroban dose was titrated to maintain APTT between 60-90 seconds. A new circuit was also primed with Argatroban and the circuit was changed. The cannulas were not heparin coated and were left in place. The patient remained on ECMO support for nine additional days on the same circuit without any clotting or bleeding issues. He was eventually weaned from support and discharged to a rehabilitation hospital on a ventilator.

References

ECMO Specialist Training Manual 2nd edition

Van Meurs, K et al 2005 ECMO Extracorporeal Cardiopulmonary Support in Critical Care, 3rd Edition, Extracorporeal Life Support Organization, Ann Arbor , MI

Management of Mechanical Complications, University of Michigan Health Systems ECMO Program DVD

Chapter 24 Questions

1. When a patient receiving ECMO support has an acute desaturation the most likely cause is
    a) from a technical or mechanical malfunction
    b) cardiac failure
    c) respiratory failure
    d) bleeding

2. Increasing pre-oxygenator pressure with no change in post-oxygenator pressure indicates
    a) an increase in the patient's blood pressure
    b) an increase in resistance within the oxygenator
    c) the pump flow is too high
    d) the pump occlusion is set too tight

3. Indications that a patient is tolerating weaning from VA support include which of the following?
    a) the patient's blood pressure is stable
    b) the SVO_2 decreases
    c) the SVO_2 remains within the desired range
    d) a and c

4. During VV support a clear indication of severe recirculation is
    a) desaturated blood in the drainage line and desaturated blood in the return line
    b) well saturated blood in the drainage line and desaturated blood in the return line
    c) well saturated blood in the drainage and return line
    d) $SPO_2 > 95\%$

Chapter 24 Answers

1. a
2. b
3. d
4. c

25

Trouble Shooting: The What-If's of ECMO

Eugenia K. Pallotto, MD, MSCE, Barbara M. Haney, RNC-NIC, MSN, CPNP-AC, Jeanne Braby, RN, MSN, CCRN and Patricia English, MS, RRT-NPS

Objectives

After completion of this chapter, the participant should be able to:

- Provide a trouble-shooting algorithm for the ECMO Specialist
- Provide a quick guide for the approach of common ECMO clinical questions
- Give common solutions to common problems

Introduction:

The following tables provide a framework to guide the specialist in identifying and solving potential problems with the ECMO circuit and the ECMO patient. The specialist must be trained to troubleshoot the unique circuit issues at his/her institution. Understanding the appropriate time to remove the patient from bypass in order to safely correct a circuit problem is a critical part of specialist training.

There are multiple causes and solutions for each symptom listed. The table is not meant to imply that there is only one solution for each cause. It should not be viewed as a one to one relationship between cause and solution.

Trouble Shooting the ECMO Circuit

Problem	Symptoms	Causes	Solutions
Pump Failures	No lights on equipment	• Power cords dislodged to cart or pump • Power failure • Battery malfunction/ not charged • Individual pieces of equipment not turned on	• Hand crank until power available • Plug in properly • Use portable power supply

Problem	Symptoms	Causes	Solutions
	Pump without power	• Pump power switch off • ECMO cart power switch off • Pump not plugged in	• Hand crank until power available if circuit pressures are normal and without alarms • Turn switch on • Check for defective alarms • Plug in properly
Pump Failures – (cont.)	Pump shutting off or not turning	• System pressures alarming • Pump on/off knob turned off • Flow knob turned to zero • Bubble detector alarming and set to control pump • Error code flashing due to roller heads having been manually turned/hand-cranked • Cover lid open • Pump malfunction	• Correct reasons for pressure alarms • Check for air • Check flow knob for appropriate settings • Turn pump power switch off and back on to reset • Check lid cover • Hand crank only if circuit pressures are normal and without alarms (DO NOT hand crank if pump stopped for high [oxygenator] or low [bladder] pressure alarms) • Turn pump power button off and back on to reset
	Overheated pump	• Wet connections	• Check connections
	Pump rotating but no flow	• Inadequate occlusion • Pump malfunction	• Adjust occlusion • Replace pump as indicated
Negative Pressure Monitor Failure (*e.g.* bladder box, bladder/ compliance chamber, transducers)	Cavitation as pump continues to turn	• Bladder/Compliance Chamber **full**: outlet obstruction (kinks, twists, large dislodged clot blocking neck/tubing) • Bladder/Compliance Chamber **not full**: malfunction of bladder box toggle switch, connections, or plugs; malfunction of pressure transducer; clot in pressure transducer tubing or connections; pump or bladder box in override mode	• Correct obstruction • Correct toggle switch or connection problem • Change bladder and/or box • Flush, zero, replace pressure transducers • Verify integrity of pressure transducer lines or stopcocks and replace as needed • Verify pump and bladder box are not in override mode

Problem	Symptoms	Causes	Solutions
Negative Pressure Monitor Failure (*e.g.* bladder box, bladder/ compliance chamber, transducers) – (cont.)	Pump not stopping when venous line clamped	• Bladder/Compliance Chamber **full**: inadequate raceway occlusion; flow problem • Bladder/Compliance Chamber **not full**: malfunction of bladder box toggle switch, plug, or box charge; malfunction of pressure transducers; pressure transducer not connected or stopcock turned off; clot in pressure transducer tubing or connections	• Correct raceway occlusion or flow abnormality • Change bladder box • Flush, zero, replace pressure transducers • Verify integrity of pressure transducer lines or stopcocks and replace as needed
	No alarms	• Battery malfunction • Bladder box plug not connected • Power failure • Incorrect pressure alarm limit settings • Pressure transducer malfunction • Pressure transducer not connected, stopcock turned off, or clot in tubing or connections	• Change bladder box as indicated • Flush, zero, and replace pressure transducers as needed • Check and reset pressure limits • Verify integrity of pressure transducer lines or stopcocks and replace as needed
	Blood on floor	• Leak in bladder • Cracked connector	• Change or repair bladder / connector

273

Problem	Symptoms	Causes	Solutions
Low Flow/ "Cutting Out"	Negative pressure (bladder or venous line pressure) alarm	• Venous/cephalic catheter malpositioned • Cannula kinked • Cannula too small • Kink in tubing between the baby and the pump • Pressure alarm limit or thresholds set too low • Flow knob bumped too high • Pressure transducer malfunction • Clot in venous line, cannula, connectors, *etc.* • Intravascular volume depletion • Inadequate venous return due to patient condition (*e.g.* pericardial tamponade or increased abdominal pressure) • Bed/warmer height too low	• Reposition catheter, head, or neck • Check cannula position and manipulate as needed • Consider replacing or adding second catheter • Remove tubing kinks • Adjust pressure alarm and threshold settings • Check flow scale and lower blood flow • Flush, zero, and replace pressure transducers as needed • Check for clots • Consider fluid bolus • Evaluate for and treat patient condition causing inadequate venous return • Raise the height of the bed/warmer
	Positive pressure (oxygenator) alarm	• Kink in tubing between pump and the baby • Kink or malposition of arterial cannula • Oxygenator clotted • Arterial line filter clotted • Pressure alarm limit or thresholds set incorrectly • Pressure transducer malfunction	• Remove tubing kinks • Check cannula position • Replace oxygenator if indicated • Check for clots • Adjust pressure limits and thresholds • Flush, zero, and replace pressure transducers as needed • Verify integrity of pressure transducer lines or stopcocks and replace as needed • Replace arterial line filter
Raceway Rupture	Blood in roller pump	• Raceway tubing develops leak from wear and tear	• Replace or repair raceway segment

274

Problem	Symptoms	Causes	Solutions
Air in Circuit	Pre-oxygenator (venous line or bladder, compliance chamber, raceway)	• Cracked or open stopcocks, pigtails, or connectors in venous line • Air from IV infusions or volume pushes into circuit • Venous cannula connector loose or cracked • Venous cannula dislodged - side hole out of vessel • Air in right atrium - patient source (*e.g.* from central line infusion)	• Walk air to removal location - aspirate air from bladder, top of oxygenator, or bubble trap • Remove air - air blood interfaces will promote clot formation and risk air embolus to the patient • Check for leaks and secure connections • Replace pigtail and connector components • Correct cannula problems
	Oxygenator	• Air from IV infusion or volume pushes into the circuit • Air leak in oxygenator or gas outlet obstruction in oxygenator • Priming problem • Air leak from venous line, bladder, compliance chamber, raceway - as above	• Remove air - air blood interfaces will promote clot formation and risk air embolus to the patient • Replace oxygenator • Monitor closely for recurrence
	Post-oxygenator (some centers have an additional air trap prior to the arterial line)	• Air from IV, medication, or platelet infusions into circuit • Air leak from venous line passing through oxygenator • Air leak from oxygenator or gas outlet obstruction	• Remove air - air blood interfaces will promote clot formation: risk of air embolus to the patient • Stop air leak • Check air detector function, if present • Replace oxygenator • Clamp off ECMO if risk of air reaching arterial line

Problem	Symptoms	Causes	Solutions
Air in Circuit – (cont.)	Arterial line	• Massive air pumped from venous side • Air leak from oxygenator or gas outlet obstruction	• Emergency! - manually kink the arterial line to stop the flow and rise of air • Prevent patient transfusion with inadvertent air embolus • Find and stop leak • Replace oxygenator • Clear arterial line of air by re-circulation through the bridge and removing from an air trap
Exchanger Water Heater	Blood in water lines	• Crack in heat exchanger water/blood seal	• Emergency! - turn off the heater immediately, remove water hoses, and replace heat exchanger
	Water dripping	• Crack in outer plastic housing • Leak at water hose connections	• Try to seal with bone wax or replace • Turn water heater off, reseat the water hose connections
	Temperature alarm	• Temperature set improperly • Water heater pump malfunction • Large amount of cold water added to water reservoir • Unit just turned on • Temperature recently adjusted • Water level too low	• Check and reset temperature setting as needed • Replacement of water heater may be indicated • Add water to heater

Problem	Symptoms	Causes	Solutions
Exchanger Water Heater – (cont.)	Patient cold	• Heater unit malfunction - check water wheel - must be turning • Not turned on • Temperature set point too low • Temperature LED malfunction after power interruption - reading characters rather than temperature • Water shut off valves turned off • Water hoses kinked, occluding water flow • Radiant warmer malfunction • Heater unit set in FLUID mode without inline temperature probe • Large amount of cold water added to water heater reservoir	• Replacement of water heater may be indicated • Adjust set temperature on water bath or overhead heater • Check and reset temperature set point - turn heater off/on, then reset temperature set point • Verify water hoses are unobstructed and shut off valves are open • Check appropriate mode set on heater • Consider isolating patient from heater until water warms

	Patient hot	• Heater unit malfunction
		• Radiant warmer or patient temperature probe malfunction
		• Water temperature set too hot
			• Replacement of water heater may be indicated
			• Adjust set temperature on water bath or overhead heater
			• Consider patient may have fever
			• Radiant warmer overcompensating due to:
			  ○ water heater set point too low
			  ○ water heater turned off
			  ○ water shut off valves turned off or hoses kinked
			  ○ water heater malfunction

Problem	Symptoms	Causes	Solutions
Exchanger Water Heater – (cont.)	Water heating unit off	• Not plugged in • Not turned on • Overheated - exhaust fan occluded	• Turn on or plug in • Check exhaust fan
Oxygenator Failure	Low/decreasing pump arterial PO$_2$, decreased PCO$_2$ clearance, increased positive pressure, increased pressure gradient across membrane (if monitoring pre- and post-oxygenator pressures)	• Sweep gas line to oxygenator is loose, disconected or cracked • Oxygenator failure • Oxygenator clotting off • Increased condensation in gas phase • Oxygenator rated flow/efficiency exceeded • Sweep gas FiO$_2$ changed or source empty • Carbogen tank running out (some centers where carbogen mix is up to 95% oxygen) • Incorrect CO$_2$ / carbogen setting	• Reattach gas line to oxygenator • Troubleshoot gas line connections • Replace oxygenator • Increase sweep gas flow rate • Check rated oxygenator flow, decrease blood flow if indicated • Check arterial cannula/tubing for kinks causing increased pressure • Some centers will "sigh" oxygenator by increasing sweep gas flow to maximum manufacturer's recommendations at regular intervals • Troubleshoot pressure monitors/transducers • Replace correct CO$_2$ carbogen tank settings.
Oxygenator Gas Exhaust Blood Leak	Blood in gas exhaust	• Blood leak into gas portion of oxygenator	• Ensure gas exhaust remains patent; if gas outlet becomes obstructed, massive air leak can occur • Replace oxygenator • Some centers will conservatively observe and monitor small blood leaks

Trouble Shooting the ECMO Patient

Problem	Symptoms	Causes	Solutions
Decreasing Patient PO$_2$	Cyanosis, acidosis, poor perfusion, lethargy, worsening blood gases	• Inadequate ECMO flow • Pneumothorax, atelectasis, ventilator/ETT problem • Pericardial tamponade • Hemothorax/Effusion • Sweep gas line to oxygenator is loose, disconnected or cracked • Oxygenator failing • Seizures • Sepsis • Agitated patient • Hypervolemia, increased pulmonary perfusion prior to pulmonary recovery • Decreased cardiac output especially on VV ECMO • Significant recirculation on VV ECMO • Decreased patient hematocrit • Consider structural cardiac defect • Centrifugal pump: change in patient preload or afterload causing inadequate or altered blood flow • Carbogen tank running out (some centers where carbogen mix is up to 95% oxygen)	• Increase ECMO flow • Evacuate pneumothorax, hemothorax, effusion or tamponade • Aggressively strip chest tubes in the postoperative cardiac patient • Adjust ETT or ventilator as needed • Tighten sweep gas line connections or replace if needed • Increase blender FIO$_2$ to increase pump artery PO$_2$ • Replace oxygenator as indicated • Treat seizures • Treat sepsis • Calm or sedate patient • Evaluate blood volume and correct as needed • Administer diuretics • Transfuse if hematocrit low • Consider vasopressor support if VV ECMO • Minimize recirculation if VV ECMO • Consider conversion to VA if VV ECMO • Centrifugal pump: interventions to increase preload or decrease afterload as indicated clinically • Replace carbogen tank
	Patient looks well	• Improving cardiac output	• Consider ECMO weaning

Problem	Symptoms	Causes	Solutions
Increasing Patient PO_2	Cyanosis, acidosis, poor perfusion, worsening blood gases	• Decreased cardiac output • Hypovolemia • Pneumo/hemothorax/effusion • Pneumo/hemopericardium • Cardiac stun or inadequate VA flow • Cardiac tamponade • Central shunting • Sepsis with peripheral shunting • Tissue death with decreased O_2 consumption	• Increase ECMO flow • Administer volume • Evacuate pneumo/hemothorax/effusion • Drain pericardium • Aggressively strip chest tube in the postoperative cardiac patient • Treat sepsis
	Patient looks well	• Improving respiratory function • Altered ventilator FIO_2 • Cardiac stun on adequate VA flow	• Consider ECMO weaning • Adjust ventilator FIO_2 • Continue full ECMO flow
Decreasing Patient PCO_2	Apnea, alkalosis	• Sweep gas CO_2/Carbogen too low • Sweep gas flow too high • Overventilation • Improving respiratory function	• Increase or add CO_2/Carbogen to sweep gas • Decrease sweep gas flow • Wean ventilation • Consider ECMO weaning
	Tachypnea	• Sweep gas CO_2/Carbogen too high • Sweep gas flow too low • Underventilation • ETT problem	• Decrease or remove sweep gas CO_2/Carbogen • Increase sweep gas flow • Increase ventilation • Correct ETT problem
Increasing Patient PCO_2	Tachypnea, acidosis, agitation, hypertension	• Oxygenator failure • Sweep gas CO_2/Carbogen too high • Sweep gas flow too low • Patient agitated • Underventilation • ETT problem • Pneumo/hemothorax/effusion	• Replace oxygenator • Decrease or remove sweep gas CO_2/Carbogen • Increase sweep gas flow • Consider sedation • Adjust ventilation/ETT • Evacuate pneumo/hemothorax/effusion

Problem	Symptoms	Causes	Solutions
Inconsistent ACTs	High ACT	• Error/inconsistency in ACT technique, amount of blood used • New heparin lot • Error in calculation or mixture of heparin drip • Infusion pump malfunction or pump set incorrectly • Alterations/malfunction of ACT sampling site (*e.g.* clots, contamination) • ACT instrument or tubes/cartridges malfunction • Low or decreasing platelet counts • Sample drawn in a heparinized syringe • Heparin from another source (*e.g.* TPN/HAL, line flushed) • Vitamin K deficiency • Low AT III level • DIC due to circuit coagulopathy • DIC due to sepsis • Cartridge not warmed (device specific) • Alteration in device temperature (device specific) • Decreased urine output	• Review sampling technique, repeat test • Consider replacement of heparin drip • Consider commercially manufactured pre-mixed heparin drip bags • Check infusion pump, consider replacement • QC and replace ACT instrument as needed • Check coagulation parameters and correct as indicated • Evaluate for and treat sepsis • Change adaptors, stopcocks, and tubing as needed • Check platelet count, coagulation tests, and/or AT III level and correct as indicated • Correct cause of DIC (*e.g.* circuit change, sepsis) • Look for heparin administered in other sources (minimal amounts by continuous infusions usually will not cause ACT alterations) • Repeat in non-heparinized syringe • Assess for changing urine output and address as clinically indicated

Problem	Symptoms	Causes	Solutions
Inconsistent ACTs – (cont.)	Low ACT	• Error/inconsistency in ACT technique, amount of blood used • New heparin lot • Error in calculation or mixture of heparin drip • Infusion pump malfunction or pump set incorrectly • Alterations/malfunction of ACT sampling site (*e.g.* clots, contamination) • ACT instrument or tubes/cartridges malfunction • Recent platelet transfusion • Alterations/malfunction of heparin infusion site (*e.g.* tubing clamped, not connected, stopcock off, clots, obstructed flow) • Patient diuresing, large increase in urine output	• Review sampling technique, repeat test • Consider replacement of heparin drip • Consider commercially manufactured pre-mixed heparin drip bags • Check infusion pump, consider replacement • QC and replace ACT instrument as needed • Check coagulation parameters and correct as indicated • Evaluate and treat for sepsis • Change adaptors, stopcocks, and tubing as needed • Check infusion pump • Check heparin infusion site • Assess for changing urine output and address as clinically indicated
Decreased Urine Output	Oliguria	• Hypovolemia/hypotension • Capillary leak syndrome • Poor cardiac output • Ischemic renal disease	• Increase pump flow • Volume or pressor support • Stimulate cardiac output and renal blood flow • Hemofiltration • Diuretics

Problem	Symptoms	Causes	Solutions
Hemolysis	Plasma free hemoglobin > 50 mg/dl; tea colored urine; renal dysfunction	• Inaccurate sampling • Pump overoccluded • Water bath temperature too high • Clots in patient • Clots or kinks in system • Hemofiltration • Centrifugal pump, especially at low flows	• Repeat test - draw slowly, send specimen stat to lab • Turn down water bath temperature • Check for clots or kinks in circuit , hemofilter, or patient • Change circuit or circuit components if indicated • Consider pump cone replacement if centrifugal pump
Bleeding	Visible bleeding, decreased hematocrit, decreased blood pressure, increased heart rate, decreased urine output	• ACT too high • Platelets too low • DIC • Sepsis • Recent surgery • Agitation • Hypertension	• Decrease ACT parameter goal • Administer platelets • Other blood product replacement as indicated by laboratory values • Treat sepsis • Change circuit if suspect circuit DIC • Consider aminocaproic acid infusion or Novo7 • Sedation/paralysis • Treat hypertension • Local control if isolated site
Hypertension	Increased blood pressure	• Fluid overload • Pain • Agitation • Idiopathic • Improved cardiac output • High pump flow • Recent steroid administration	• Diuretics or hemofiltration • Treat pain and agitation • Anti-hypertensive medication • Decrease ECMO flow

Problem	Symptoms	Causes	Solutions
Seizures	Repetitive involuntary movement, increased blood pressure, increased heart rate, decreased heart rate, decreased SVO_2, hypoxia, cyanosis	• Ischemic brain injury • Cerebral edema • Infarction • Intracranial hemorrhage	• Anticonvulsants • Treat as indicated based on reason for ECMO, time course of ECMO, and underlying cause of seizure: • EEG, head ultrasound, CT scan as indicated for diagnosis
Hypotension	Decreased blood pressure	• Decreased cardiac output • Hypovolemia • Capillary leak syndrome • Massive hemorrhage • Sepsis • Low pump flow (VA)	• Support cardiac output as needed • Volume • Identify patient specific cause and treat as indicated • Increase pump flow if adequate right atrial volume
Arterial Line Tracing Flat	Patient well perfused, narrow pulse pressure	• High/full VA ECMO support • Pressure transducer malfunction • Decreased cardiac output	• May be appropriate with full VA nonpulsatile support - no intervention needed • Support cardiac output as needed • Flush, zero, replace pressure transducers as needed

Trouble Shooting the Biomedicus Centrifugal Pump

Regulating the revolutions per minute (RPM) of the electric motor controls forward flow; however, the Biomedicus pump is totally non-occlusive and is preload and afterload dependent. Flow will increase when preload increases or when afterload decreases. Conversely, a decreased preload or an increased afterload will decrease pump flow.

Similar to the roller pump, inlet and outlet oxygenator pressures can be measured continuously on the centrifugal pump. A pressure alarm may also be placed to measure the amount of negative pressure coming from the patient. This alarm can be helpful in alerting the ECMO specialist if there is any obstruction in venous return; however, there are not any alarms on the Biomedicus pump that can be set to **servoregulate** or stop the pump for any reason. For this reason, it is important that venous return is adequate or cavitation will occur.

Problem	Symptoms	Causes	Solutions
Flow Probe	No flow value is displayed on the pump console	• There is not a flow probe in line (probe may have fallen off tubing)	• Place flow probe in line
	A negative flow value is displayed on the pump console	• Probe is on backwards	• Place flow probe on correctly
	Will not "zero"	• Problem in pump console	• Replace pump console
	Flow probe indicates "0" flow	• Obstruction to flow somewhere in the circuit	• Locate and deal with the source of obstruction
	Flow probe # is flashing (indicates flow is suddenly changing)	• Patient blood pressure may be changing • Pump flow may be occluded	• Identify source and fix
RPM Display	RPM indicates "0" and dial is turned on	• Pump console may be broken	• Change out pump console
RPM Display – (cont.)	Unable to turn RPM dial below 2000	• Safety button engaged on dial	• Press down to release button
Pump Cone	No flow through pump cone	• Incorrect switch (external versus internal)	• Change to correct switch

Problem	Symptoms	Causes	Solutions
	Flow suddenly stops	• Pump cone is broken • Magnets in cone have decoupled • Strut is broken	• Replace pump cone
	Pump vibrates when RPMs are increased	• Pump cone is broken	• Decrease RPMs and replace pump cone ASAP
	Loud noise coming from pump cone	• Pump cone is broken	• Replace pump cone
	Air is entering circuit	• Stopcock is open • Kink or clamp on negative side causing cavitation	• Clamp patient off ECMO to replace pump cone to remove air (always clamp arterial side first) • De-air entire circuit before going back on ECMO
Biomedicus Battery	After transferring to battery, the RPMs decrease	• Problem with the battery	• Plug into AC power or change out pump console
	When using battery, the RPMs are insufficient	• Battery is not completely charged	• Plug into AC power or change out pump console
	Fan sounds quieter when switched to battery	• Normal - pump goes into energy saving mode	• No response necessary
Biomedicus Battery – (cont.)	Internal battery does not function	• Battery is not charged	• Plug into AC power
	Battery alarm indicator is flashing on the pump console	• Battery is not charged	• Plug into AC power
	Battery status indicator bars are not lit	• Battery is not charged	• Plug into AC power

References

1. Van Meurs K, et al. ECMO Extracorporeal Cardiopulmonary Support in Critical Care. 3rd ed. Ann Arbor, MI: Extracorporeal Life Support Organization; 2005.
2. Management of Mechanical Complications [DVD]. University of Michigan Health Systems' ECMO Program; 2006.
3. Pedersen TH, Videm V, Svennevig JL, Karlsen H, Ostbakk RW, Jensen O, Mollnes TE. Extracorporeal Membrane Oxygenation Using a Centrifugal Pump and a Servo Regulator to Prevent Negative Inlet Pressure. Ann Thorac Surg. 1997;63:1333-9.
4. Chapman RA, Schumacker RE, Bartlett RH. xtracorporeal Life Support Manual for Neonatal Patients. 10th ed. 1994.
5. Chapman RA, Bartlett RH. Extracorporeal Life Support Manual for Adult and Pediatric Patients. 1st ed. University of Michigan Medical Center; 1991.

Chapter 25 Questions

1. Signs of oxygenator failure may include all of the following except:
   a. Low/decreasing pump arterial pO_2
   b. Increasing patient pCO_2 despite decreased or no CO_2 titration and increased sweep flow rate
   c. Increased P_2 pressure
   d. Sweep gas line tightly connected to oxygenator

2. Possible explanations for decreasing ACTs despite increasing heparin drip infusion include:
   a. Heparin drip not connected to the circuit stopcock
   b. Crack in heparin drip infusion connection
   c. Incorrect heparin bag preparation
   d. ACT tube/Hemochron Response malfunction
   e. Patient diuresis
   f. All of the above

3. Indications for hand-cranking include:
   a. Loss of entire system & battery power
   b. Pump failure
   c. negative pressure alarms
   d. positive pressure alarms
   e. A & B
   f. All of the above

4. Possible causes of cyanosis, acidosis and poor perfusion in a patient on ECMO include:
   a. Pneumothorax
   b. Pericardial tamponade
   c. Sweep gas line loose or disconnected from oxygenator
   d. Recirculation
   e. All of the above

5. Blood in the water heater water lines is an emergency; immediately turn off the water flow and replace the heat exchanger
   a. True
   b. False

Chapter 25 Answers

1. d
2. f
3. e
4. e
5. True